Online Resources

Included with your purchase are multiple online resources. This includes the practice tests in an interactive format and a convenient study timer to help you manage your time.

Instructions for accessing these resources can be found on the last page of this book.

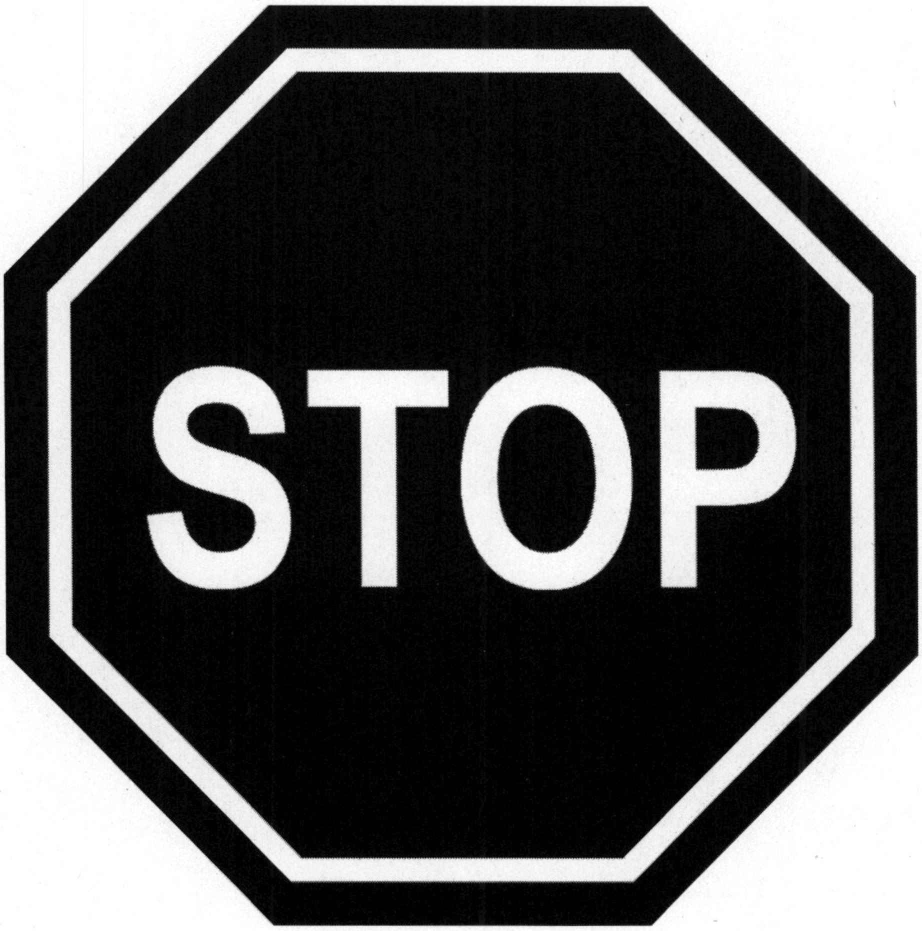

OCN® Study Guide 2026-2027

25 Full-Length Practice Tests and OCN Exam Prep [Updated for the New Outline]

Lydia Morrison

Written and edited by TPB Publishing.

ISBN 13: 9781637753170

Table of Contents

Welcome

Dear Reader,

Welcome to your new Test Prep Books study guide! We are pleased that you chose us to help you prepare for your exam. There are many study options to choose from, and we appreciate you choosing us. Studying can be a daunting task, but we have designed a smart, effective study guide to help prepare you for what lies ahead.

Whether you're a parent helping your child learn and grow, a high school student working hard to get into your dream college, or a nursing student studying for a complex exam, we want to help give you the tools you need to succeed. We hope this study guide gives you the skills and the confidence to thrive, and we can't thank you enough for allowing us to be part of your journey.

In an effort to continue to improve our products, we welcome feedback from our customers. We look forward to hearing from you. Suggestions, success stories, and criticisms can all be communicated by emailing us at support@testprepbooks.com.

Sincerely,

Test Prep Books Team

Quick Overview

As you draw closer to taking your exam, effective preparation becomes more and more important. Thankfully, you have this study guide to help you get ready. Use this guide to help keep your studying on track and refer to it often.

This study guide contains several key sections that will help you be successful on your exam. The guide contains tips for what you should do the night before and the day of the test. Also included are test-taking tips. Knowing the right information is not always enough. Many well-prepared test takers struggle with exams. These tips will help equip you to accurately read, assess, and answer test questions.

A large part of the guide is devoted to showing you what content to expect on the exam and to helping you better understand that content. In this guide are practice test questions so that you can see how well you have grasped the content. Then, answer explanations are provided so that you can understand why you missed certain questions.

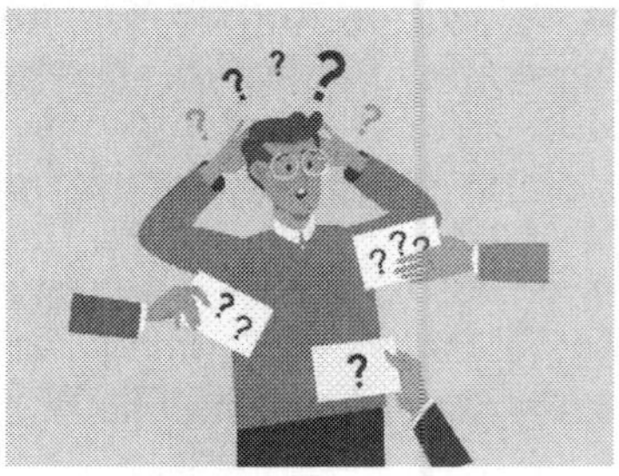

Don't try to cram the night before you take your exam. This is not a wise strategy for a few reasons. First, your retention of the information will be low. Your time would be better used by reviewing information you already know rather than trying to learn a lot of new information. Second, you will likely become stressed as you try to gain a large amount of knowledge in a short amount of time. Third, you will be depriving yourself of sleep. So be sure to go to bed at a reasonable time the night before. Being well-rested helps you focus and remain calm.

Be sure to eat a substantial breakfast the morning of the exam. If you are taking the exam in the afternoon, be sure to have a good lunch as well. Being hungry is distracting and can make it difficult to focus. You have hopefully spent lots of time preparing for the exam. Don't let an empty stomach get in the way of success!

When travelling to the testing center, leave earlier than needed. That way, you have a buffer in case you experience any delays. This will help you remain calm and will keep you from missing your appointment time at the testing center.

Be sure to pace yourself during the exam. Don't try to rush through the exam. There is no need to risk performing poorly on the exam just so you can leave the testing center early. Allow yourself to use all of the allotted time if needed.

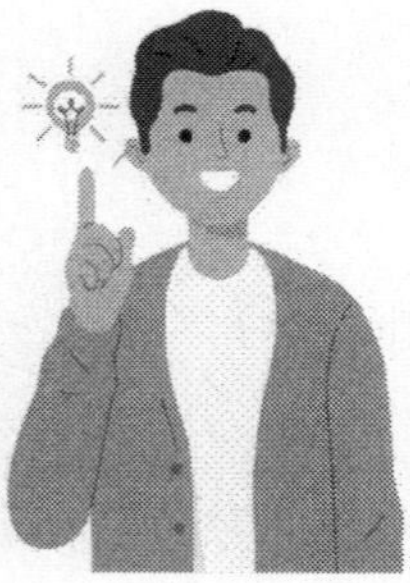

Remain positive while taking the exam even if you feel like you are performing poorly. Thinking about the content you should have mastered will not help you perform better on the exam.

Once the exam is complete, take some time to relax. Even if you feel that you need to take the exam again, you will be well served by some down time before you begin studying again. It's often easier to convince yourself to study if you know that it will come with a reward!

Test-Taking Strategies

1. Predicting the Answer

When you feel confident in your preparation for a multiple-choice test, try predicting the answer before reading the answer choices. This is especially useful on questions that test objective factual knowledge. By predicting the answer before reading the available choices, you eliminate the possibility that you will be distracted or led astray by an incorrect answer choice. You will feel more confident in your selection if you read the question, predict the answer, and then find your prediction among the answer choices. After using this strategy, be sure to still read all of the answer choices carefully and completely. If you feel unprepared, you should not attempt to predict the answers. This would be a waste of time and an opportunity for your mind to wander in the wrong direction.

2. Reading the Whole Question

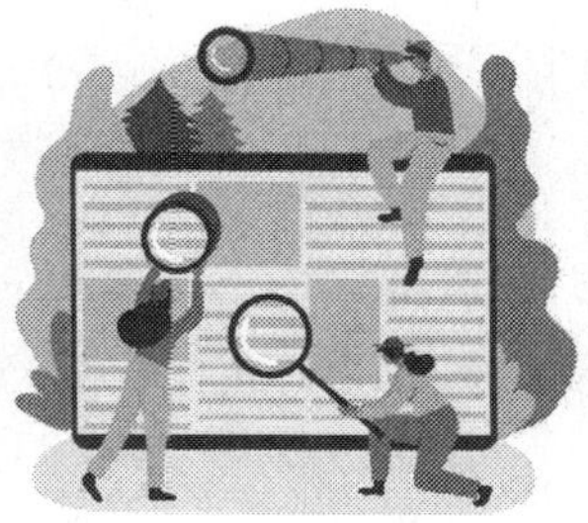

Too often, test takers scan a multiple-choice question, recognize a few familiar words, and immediately jump to the answer choices. Test authors are aware of this common impatience, and they will sometimes prey upon it. For instance, a test author might subtly turn the question into a negative, or he or she might redirect the focus of the question right at the end. The only way to avoid falling into these traps is to read the entirety of the question carefully before reading the answer choices.

3. Looking for Wrong Answers

Long and complicated multiple-choice questions can be intimidating. One way to simplify a difficult multiple-choice question is to eliminate all of the answer choices that are clearly wrong. In most sets of answers, there will be at least one selection that can be dismissed right away. If the test is administered on paper, the test taker could draw a line through it to indicate that it may be ignored; otherwise, the test taker will have to perform this operation mentally or on scratch paper. In either case, once the obviously incorrect answers have been eliminated, the remaining choices may be considered. Sometimes identifying the clearly wrong answers will give the test taker some information about the correct answer. For instance, if one of the remaining answer choices is a direct opposite of one of the eliminated answer choices, it may well be the correct answer. The opposite of obviously wrong is obviously right! Of course, this is not always the case. Some answers are obviously incorrect simply because they are irrelevant to the question being asked. Still, identifying and eliminating some incorrect answer choices is a good way to simplify a multiple-choice question.

4. Don't Overanalyze

Anxious test takers often overanalyze questions. When you are nervous, your brain will often run wild, causing you to make associations and discover clues that don't actually exist. If you feel that this may be a problem for you, do whatever you can to slow down during the test. Try taking a deep breath or counting to ten. As you read and consider the question, restrict yourself to the particular words used by the author. Avoid thought tangents about what the author *really* meant, or what he or she was *trying* to say. The only things that matter on a multiple-choice test are the words that are actually in the question. You must avoid reading too much into a multiple-choice question, or supposing that the writer meant something other than what he or she wrote.

5. No Need for Panic

It is wise to learn as many strategies as possible before taking a multiple-choice test, but it is likely that you will come across a few questions for which you simply don't know the answer. In this situation, avoid panicking. Because most multiple-choice tests include dozens of questions, the relative value of a single wrong answer is small. As much as possible, you should compartmentalize each question on a multiple-choice test. In other words, you should not allow your feelings about one question to affect your success on the others. When you find a question that you either don't understand or don't know how to answer, just take a deep breath and do your best. Read the entire question slowly and carefully. Try rephrasing the question a couple of different ways. Then, read all of the answer choices carefully. After eliminating obviously wrong answers, make a selection and move on to the next question.

6. Confusing Answer Choices

When working on a difficult multiple-choice question, there may be a tendency to focus on the answer choices that are the easiest to understand. Many people, whether consciously or not, gravitate to the answer choices that require the least concentration, knowledge, and memory. This is a mistake. When you come across an answer choice that is confusing, you should give it extra attention. A question might be confusing because you do not know the subject matter to which it refers. If this is the case, don't eliminate the answer before you have affirmatively settled on another. When you come across an answer choice of this type, set it aside as you look at the remaining choices. If you can confidently assert that one of the other choices is correct, you can leave the confusing answer aside. Otherwise, you will need to take a moment to try to better understand the confusing answer choice. Rephrasing is one way to tease out the sense of a confusing answer choice.

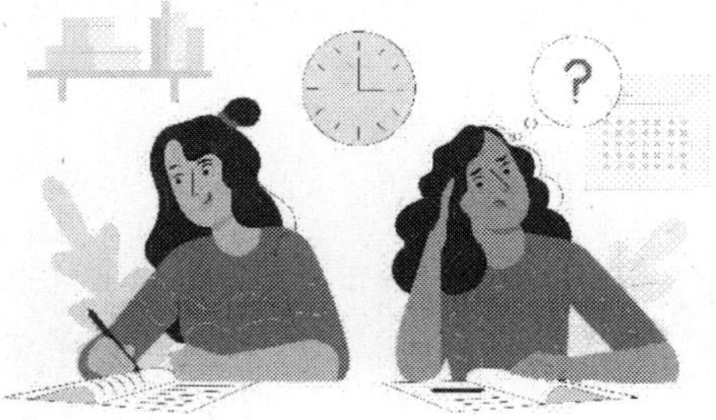

7. Your First Instinct

Many people struggle with multiple-choice tests because they overthink the questions. If you have studied sufficiently for the test, you should be prepared to trust your first instinct once you have carefully and completely read the question and all of the answer choices. There is a great deal of research suggesting that the mind can come to the correct conclusion very quickly once it has obtained all of the relevant information. At times, it may seem to you as if your intuition is working faster even than your reasoning mind. This may in fact be true. The knowledge you obtain while studying may be retrieved from your subconscious before you have a chance to work out the associations that support it. Verify your instinct by working out the reasons that it should be trusted.

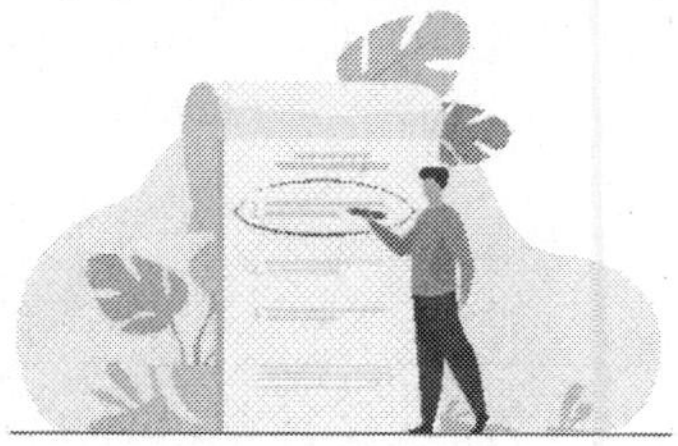

8. Key Words

Many test takers struggle with multiple-choice questions because they have poor reading comprehension skills. Quickly reading and understanding a multiple-choice question requires a mixture of skill and experience. To help with this, try jotting down a few key words and phrases on a piece of scrap paper. Doing this concentrates the process of reading and forces the mind to weigh the relative importance of the question's parts. In selecting words and phrases to write down, the test taker thinks about the question more deeply and carefully. This is especially true for multiple-choice questions that are preceded by a long prompt.

9. Subtle Negatives

One of the oldest tricks in the multiple-choice test writer's book is to subtly reverse the meaning of a question with a word like *not* or *except*. If you are not paying attention to each word in the question, you can easily be led astray by this trick. For instance, a common question format is, "Which of the following is…?" Obviously, if the question instead is, "Which of the following is not…?," then the answer will be quite different. Even worse, the test makers are aware of the potential for this mistake and will include one answer choice that would be correct if the question were not negated or reversed. A test taker who misses the reversal will find what he or she believes to be a correct answer and will be so confident that he or she will fail to reread the question and discover the original error. The only way to avoid this is to practice a wide variety of multiple-choice questions and to pay close attention to each and every word.

10. Reading Every Answer Choice

It may seem obvious, but you should always read every one of the answer choices! Too many test takers fall into the habit of scanning the question and assuming that they understand the question because they recognize a few key words. From there, they pick the first answer choice that answers the question they believe they have read. Test takers who read all of the answer choices might discover that one of the latter answer choices is actually *more* correct. Moreover, reading all of the answer choices can remind you of facts related to the question that can help you arrive at the correct answer. Sometimes, a misstatement or incorrect detail in one of the latter answer choices will trigger your memory of the subject and will enable you to find the right answer. Failing to read all of the answer choices is like not reading all of the items on a restaurant menu: you might miss out on the perfect choice.

11. Spot the Hedges

One of the keys to success on multiple-choice tests is paying close attention to every word. This is never truer than with words like *almost*, *most*, *some*, and *sometimes*. These words are called "hedges" because they indicate that a statement is not totally true or not true in every place and time. An absolute statement will contain no hedges, but in many subjects, the answers are not always straightforward or absolute. There are always exceptions to the rules in these subjects. For this reason,

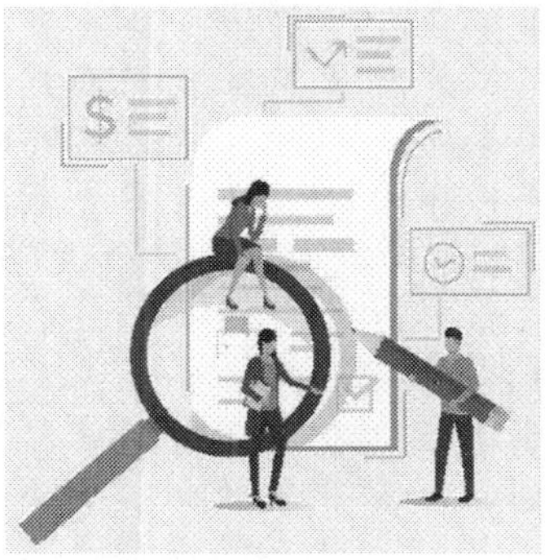

you should favor those multiple-choice questions that contain hedging language. The presence of qualifying words indicates that the author is taking special care with his or her words, which is certainly important when composing the right answer. After all, there are many ways to be wrong, but there is only one way to be right! For this reason, it is wise to avoid answers that are absolute when taking a multiple-choice test. An absolute answer is one that says things are either all one way or all another. They often include words like *every*, *always*, *best*, and *never*. If you are taking a multiple-choice test in a subject that doesn't lend itself to absolute answers, be on your guard if you see any of these words.

12. Long Answers

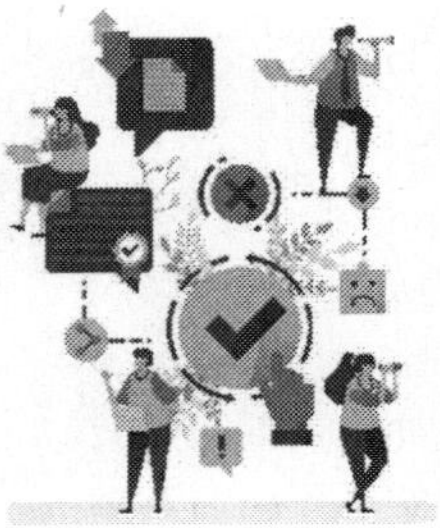

In many subject areas, the answers are not simple. As already mentioned, the right answer often requires hedges. Another common feature of the answers to a complex or subjective question are qualifying clauses, which are groups of words that subtly modify the meaning of the sentence. If the question or answer choice describes a rule to which there are exceptions or the subject matter is complicated, ambiguous, or confusing, the correct answer will require many words in order to be expressed clearly and accurately. In essence, you should not be deterred by answer choices that seem excessively long. Oftentimes, the author of the text will not be able to write the correct answer without offering some qualifications and modifications. Your job is to read the answer choices thoroughly and completely and to select the one that most accurately and precisely answers the question.

13. Restating to Understand

Sometimes, a question on a multiple-choice test is difficult not because of what it asks but because of how it is written. If this is the case, restate the question or answer choice in different words. This process serves a couple of important purposes. First, it forces you to concentrate on the core of the question. In order to rephrase the question accurately, you have to understand it well. Rephrasing the question will concentrate your mind on the key words and ideas. Second, it will present the information to your mind in a fresh way. This process may trigger your memory and render some useful scrap of information picked up while studying.

14. True Statements

Sometimes an answer choice will be true in itself, but it does not answer the question. This is one of the main reasons why it is essential to read the question carefully and completely before proceeding to the answer choices. Too often, test takers skip ahead to the answer choices and look for true statements. Having found one of these, they are content to select it without reference to the question above. The savvy test taker will always read the entire question before turning to the answer choices. Then, having settled on a correct answer choice, he or she will refer to the original question and ensure that the selected answer is relevant. The mistake of choosing a correct-but-irrelevant answer choice is especially common on questions related to specific pieces of objective knowledge.

15. No Patterns

One of the more dangerous ideas that circulates about multiple-choice tests is that the correct answers tend to fall into patterns. These erroneous ideas range from a belief that B and C are the most common right answers, to the idea that an unprepared test-taker should answer "A-B-A-C-A-D-A-B-A." It cannot be emphasized enough that pattern-seeking of this type is exactly the WRONG way to approach a multiple-choice test. To begin with, it is highly unlikely that the test maker will plot the correct answers according to some predetermined pattern. The questions are scrambled and delivered in a random order. Furthermore, even if the test maker was following a pattern in the assignation of correct answers, there is no reason why the test taker would know which pattern he or she was using. Any attempt to discern a pattern in the answer choices is a waste of time and a distraction from the real work of taking the test. A test taker would be much better served by extra preparation before the test than by reliance on a pattern in the answers.

Introduction to the OCN Exam

Function of the Test

The Oncology Certified Nurse (OCN®) exam is one of many exams offered by the ONCC (Oncology Nursing Certification Corporation) for registered nurses who have experience working with cancer patients, would like to expand their knowledge, and desire to gain specialty certification in oncology nursing. To be eligible to sit for the OCN exam, candidates must, when applying for and taking the examination, hold an unencumbered and valid RN license in the United States (or its territories) or in Canada, have experience as an RN for at least two years within the previous four years, and have at least 2,000 hours of practice in adult oncology nursing within the previous four years. Additionally, within the previous three years, candidates must have completed at least ten hours of approved continuing education related to oncology, with no more than five of those hours being devoted to continuing medical education (CME) or continuing pharmacy education (CPE). The continuing education hours must be shown to be awarded by NCC, ACCME, or ACPE if gained through Joint Accreditation/IPCE.

Test Administration

The OCN exam is computer based and offered year-round at PSI testing centers in the United States and its territories as well as Canada. The fee to take the exam is $300 for ONS/APHON members or $420 for nonmembers. International testing outside of these areas is offered for a short time each year and requires an additional fee of $75. There is a deadline to apply for international testing, so candidates should check ONCC's OCN test registration manual for current international testing dates and application deadlines.

The application to take the OCN exam must be filled out at www.oncc.org/get-certified. After applying, candidates can expect to receive the ATT (Authorization to Test) within fourteen to twenty-eight days. Candidates who are eligible to take the OCN exam will have ninety days to take the exam once they receive the ATT.

Candidates have the option of paying an additional non-refundable $100 fee when applying to take the exam that allows them to retake the exam if they do not pass with their first attempt. Test takers who need to retake the exam will have 180 days from the time of their first exam to apply to take the exam a second time. This option is only offered to test takers in the US, US territories, and Canada.

If accommodations for testing are needed due to disability, candidates have five business days after applying to take the exam to submit their requests. Requests for accommodations can be made by filling out the Testing Accommodations Request Form and sending it via fax, email, or mail. The form can be found on ONCC's website.

Test Format

Candidates have three hours to complete the exam, which consists of 165 multiple-choice questions that are based on content from six different domains. A certain percentage of the questions will be devoted to each domain as shown in the table below:

Domain	Percentage of Exam
Care Continuum	19%
Oncology Nursing Practice	17%
Treatment Modalities	19%
Symptom Management and Palliative Care	21%
Oncologic Emergencies	12%
Psychosocial Dimensions of Care	12%

Scoring

Of the 165 questions on the exam, only 145 are scored. The number of scoreable questions from each domain is based on the percentage of 145 questions. Possible scores range from 25–75, with passing scores being 55 and higher. When the exam is complete, a score will be shown on the screen, but results will also be sent via email within an hour of test completion. Test takers will need to wait 24 hours for results to become available on the PSI portal.

Study Prep Plan for the OCN Test

1 **Schedule** - Use one of our study schedules below or come up with one of your own.

2 **Relax** - Test anxiety can hurt even the best students. There are many ways to reduce stress. Find the one that works best for you.

3 **Execute** - Once you have a good plan in place, be sure to stick to it.

One Week Study Schedule

Day 1	Care Continuum
Day 2	Oncology Nursing Practice
Day 3	Treatment Modalities
Day 4	Oncologic Emergencies
Day 5	Practice Test #1
Day 6	Practice Test #2
Day 7	Take Your Exam!

Two Week Study Schedule

Day 1	Care Continuum	Day 8	Palliative Care Considerations
Day 2	Treatment-Related Considerations	Day 9	Oncologic Emergencies
Day 3	Oncology Nursing Practice	Day 10	Venous Thromboembolism
Day 4	Scope and Standards of Practice	Day 11	Psychosocial Distress
Day 5	Treatment Modalities	Day 12	Practice Test #1
Day 6	Chemotherapy	Day 13	Practice Test #2
Day 7	Targeted Therapies	Day 14	Take Your Exam!

One Month Study Schedule

Day 1	Care Continuum	Day 11	Chemotherapy	Day 21	Financial Concerns
Day 2	Advance Care Planning	Day 12	Immunotherapy	Day 22	Psychosocial Distress
Day 3	Survivorship	Day 13	Targeted Therapies	Day 23	Sexuality
Day 4	Treatment-Related Considerations	Day 14	Symptom Management and Palliative Care	Day 24	Take a Break!
Day 5	End-of-Life Care	Day 15	Palliative Care Considerations	Day 25	Practice Test #1
Day 6	Oncology Nursing Practice	Day 16	Pain Management	Day 26	Answer Explanations #1
Day 7	Site-Specific Cancer Considerations	Day 17	Take a Break!	Day 27	Practice Test #2
Day 8	Scope and Standards of Practice	Day 18	Oncologic Emergencies	Day 28	Answer Explanations #2
Day 9	Practice Quiz	Day 19	Cardiac Tamponade	Day 29	Take a Break!
Day 10	Treatment Modalities	Day 20	Venous Thromboembolism	Day 30	Take Your Exam!

Build your own prep plan by visiting the Online Resources page.

Instructions and a QR code can be found on the last page of this guide.

As you study for your test, we'd like to take the opportunity to remind you that you are capable of great things! With the right tools and dedication, you truly can do anything you set your mind to. The fact that you are holding this book right now shows how committed you are. In case no one has told you lately, you've got this! Our intention behind including this coloring page is to give you the chance to take some time to engage your creative side when you need a little brain-break from studying. As a company, we want to encourage people like you to achieve their dreams by providing good quality study materials for the tests and certifications that improve careers and change lives. As individuals, many of us have taken such tests in our careers, and we know how challenging this process can be. While we can't come alongside you and cheer you on personally, we can offer you the space to recall your purpose, reconnect with your passion, and refresh your brain through an artistic practice. We wish you every success, and happy studying!

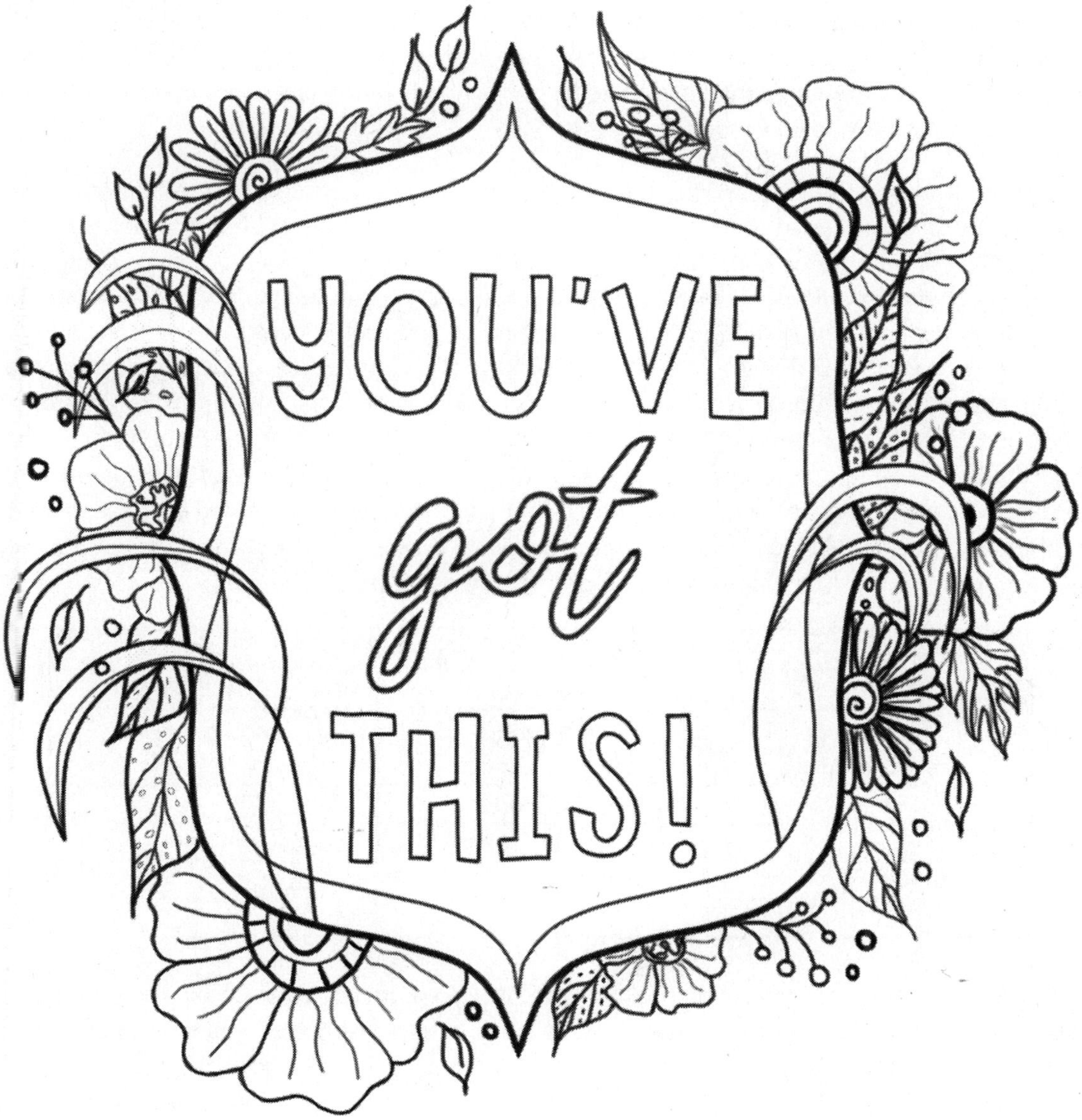

Care Continuum

Health Promotion and Disease Prevention

Health promotion refers to the process of encouraging patient attitudes and behaviors that contribute to disease prevention and health maintenance. The World Health Organization (WHO) broadens that focus to include environmental and social conditions that can affect at-risk populations. Practice guidelines that are consistent with the **Health Promotion Nursing Theory** have provided a framework for nursing practice. This theory is based on four general assumptions: individuals continually attempt to influence their own behavior; individuals interact with and exert effects on the environment; health professionals, including nurses, are part of the patients' environment and therefore have the ability to bring about changes in patient behavior; and changed behavior occurs when individuals initiate changes in their patterns of interaction with the environment. According to this model, nurses are uniquely qualified to provide patients with evidenced-based recommendations for beneficial healthcare practices, which may include regular exercise, weight management and nutritional plans, and smoking cessation. This teaching/learning process may occur in a "health fair" in the community, group sessions in the outpatient clinic, or one-to-one nurse-patient encounters in the acute care setting. Nurses also participate in health promotion activities that address the needs of the larger community by active involvement in the legislative process.

In addition to promoting disease prevention through screening studies and lifestyle changes, oncology nurses also focus on health promotion practices that improve the quality of life for patients with cancer. Improved survival times and the chronicity of many cancerous conditions means that patients being treated for cancer also frequently develop other chronic illnesses, due to aging or as the result of the treatments of their cancerous conditions. In this instance, in addition to health promotion activities related to chronic conditions, nursing behaviors associated with this form of health promotion may include pain management, alternative therapies to ease anxiety and fatigue, support of patients' social support resources, and individualized food plans to minimize the effects of therapy on the patient's nutritional status. While it is generally agreed that health promotion positively affects patient outcomes in this population, there is limited current research that supports the value of one of these elements over another element. The following table demonstrates an example of the three levels of prevention, primary, secondary, and tertiary, applied to the prevention of colorectal cancer.

Colorectal Cancer Prevention		
PRIMARY	**SECONDARY**	**TERTIARY**
Targeting Risk Factors	**Screening**	**Management**
Obesity	Fecal occult blood	Medical
Diet	Colonoscopy	Surgical
Physical Activity	Hct and Hgb	Rehabilitation
Smoking		

Primary prevention refers to preventing the incidence of cancer in a population by decreasing the exposure of group members to known causative agents or by increasing the population's resistance to the causative agents. **Secondary prevention** refers to the early detection and initiation of treatment of the cancerous condition, while **tertiary prevention** refers to the treatment and rehabilitation programs aimed at improving outcomes for individuals with cancer. In more general terms, prevention refers to eliminating personal behaviors that are associated with the development of a disease process while incorporating other behaviors that are believed to prevent the disease. Common cancer prevention strategies include dietary and lifestyle changes, detection and treatment of precancerous conditions with preventative medications, and surgical procedures. Although the strength of the supporting evidence may vary for these preventive measures, there is irrefutable evidence that smoking, including contact with second-hand smoke, and exposure to occupational and environmental carcinogens are associated with an increased risk for the development of cancer.

The other universally recommended lifestyle behaviors aimed at prevention include UV protection for the skin, weight management, and regular exercise. Although there is conflicting evidence of the benefits of specific foods for the prevention of specific cancers, there is general agreement that a calorie-controlled diet that includes generous amounts of fresh fruits and vegetables and avoids excess salt, red meats, processed meats, and alcohol provides the best possible level of prevention. Exercise guidelines are aimed at weight management and the reduction of the accumulation of abdominal fat, which is identified as a risk factor for several cancers, including endometrial, pancreatic, and colorectal cancers. **Chemopreventive medicines**, such as tamoxifen, raloxifene, and aspirin, may be used to reduce the risk of cancer in individuals with high-risk genetic profiles. Furthermore, surgical procedures, such as a bilateral mastectomy and ovarian ablation, may be considered to eliminate the risk of breast cancer in susceptible women.

Screening and Early Detection

Screening tests provide early detection of treatable diseases, which provides the opportunity for more timely interventions, such as lifestyle changes and medical treatments, that are often more effective in the early stages of the disease. The screening tests are most effective if individuals begin testing at the recommended age and continue with follow-up exams as necessary. **Colonoscopy** is recommended beginning at age 50, with repeat testing every 10 years if the results are normal. There is debate about the age at which women should have the first screening **mammogram**; however, many authorities agree that women should have an initial exam at 40 and repeat the exam yearly. Oncology nurses must be prepared to counsel women who receive an abnormal mammogram report. The **Breast Imaging-Reporting and Data System** (BI-RADS) identifies the results on the following scale: BI-RADS 0, meaning the screening exam is incomplete and more imaging or comparison views are needed; BI-RADS 1, which is normal; BI-RADS 2, when abnormalities are present but are considered benign; BI-RADS 3, when abnormalities are present that are most likely benign, but 6-month follow-up for two years is recommended; BI-RADS 4 and BI-RADS 5, which refer to probable and definite evidence of malignancy respectively and biopsy is recommended; and BI-RADS 6, which refers to findings that have already been previously identified as malignant on a biopsy. The timing for a **Pap smear** is also debated by some authorities. According to the current American College of Obstetricians and Gynecologists (ACOG) recommendations, women between 21 and 29 years of age should receive a Pap smear every three years, while women between 30 and 35 years of age have three options. These options include a Pap smear every three years, **HPV co-testing** every five years, or a Pap smear and HPV co-testing every five years. Annual full-body dermatology exams are also recommended as an important safeguard against skin cancer, which is the most common form of cancer in humans.

Early detection can also prevent the onset of the disease. For example, polyps of the large intestine can be identified and removed during a colonoscopy, which eliminates the progression of the polyps to colon cancer. There are rigorous criteria for screening tests that include measurements of sensitivity, specificity, positive predictive value, negative predictive value, and acceptability. **Sensitivity** is defined as the ability of the test to identify cancer in individuals who have the disease. **Specificity** refers to the validity of negative test results, which means that individuals who do not have cancer will have negative results. **Positive predictive value** is a measure of the probability that an individual who tests positive actually has cancer. In contrast, the **negative predictive value** measures the probability that an individual who tests negative does not have the disease. Oncology nurses understand that the interpretation of these two predictive values is dependent on the prevalence of the disease in the population. **Acceptability** refers to the willingness of people to agree to be tested. Additional criteria for screening tests include consideration of costs, availability of the necessary technology and trained personnel, and sufficient follow-up resources for patients with the disease.

Navigation and Coordination of Care

The **cancer continuum** spans the period from pre-diagnosis preventive cancer screenings to the end of life for patients who have been diagnosed with cancer. The continuum also includes the actual diagnosis period, treatment, survivorship, and relapse. Therefore, each stage brings its own set of needs. This can feel complex and overwhelming at a number of the different stages. **Oncology nurse navigators** (ONNs) are nurses who specialize not only in oncology nursing, but also in helping patients with their changing needs as they move across the cancer continuum. Lay navigators, volunteers, or allied health workers who have undertaken specific training can also play a useful role in working with patients to navigate the cancer continuum. They can also support ONNs when needed. In general, navigating the cancer continuum requires staff to be educated, experienced, culturally sensitive, and patient advocates.

The initial portion of the continuum deals with primary prevention, such as cancer screening and health counseling. All people fall in this section, whether they ever receive a cancer diagnosis or not. Under this section of the continuum, medical staff note a patient's risk for cancer, advise lifestyle choices that promote overall wellness, encourage screenings at certain ages (earlier for those who are predisposed to certain cancers), and provide general physical examinations that are conducive to early detection. This type of care is clinical in nature, but also encompasses health coaching and may include a focus on reimbursement mechanisms to ensure that patients can afford and access primary care.

Cancer detection is the next phase of the continuum. This may require further testing, taking a biopsy, or other investigative procedures to examine the cells and stage of cancer. Based on what is found as a result of this investigation, a proper diagnosis can be made. In addition to placing a focus on finances and ensuring that the patient knows reimbursement options, nurses may provide emotional support and advocacy during this time. Receiving a cancer diagnosis is acknowledged as an extremely stressful and challenging period for a person.

The next stage of the continuum focuses on treatment. Reimbursement and emotional support continue to be an important component of care; navigators may also help patients and their families with education about the disease and treatment, the prognosis, and providing other types of allied support that ease the patient and family burden. Even if treatment goes well, the transition into survivorship can be a major adjustment for patients and their families. Navigators can support patients in understanding the "new normal" of their life, linking them with resources and support groups to aid in understanding the complex feelings that come with survivorship and providing any other measures that may ease the burden of the transition.

Finally, navigators play an important role in palliative or end-of-life care, regardless of whether that period of the continuum arrives soon after diagnosis or much later in life. Navigators can help explain comfort measures that are available to both patients and their families (such as respite care); serve as a liaison to therapists, financial advisors, social workers, and other interdisciplinary professionals; share stress reduction and coping activities (especially for family members in bereavement); and research any other questions or needs shared by patients and their families.

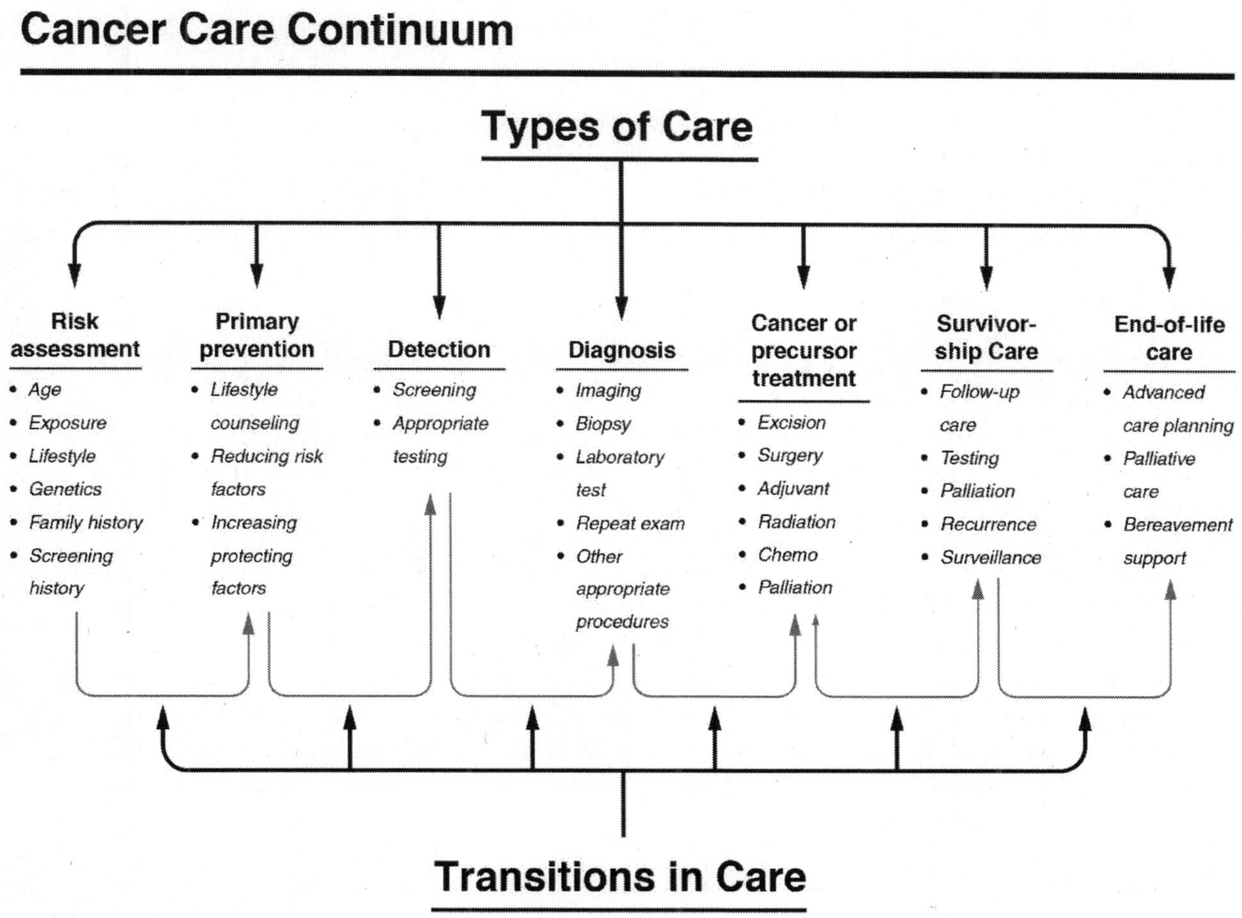

Palliative Care Considerations

Palliative care is a specialty that focuses on improving quality of life and enhancing comfort for individuals with serious chronic health diagnoses, such as cancer. It differs from hospice care in the following ways: patients may or may not have a terminal diagnosis; curative treatment may or may not be continued; care can be provided in any healthcare setting; Medicare is not required; and there is no life expectancy requirement to qualify for the service.

Palliative care practitioners address patients holistically and individually. For patients receiving cancer treatment, palliative care modalities supplement and support these standard treatments. Integrative approaches are used to blend standard medical care with complementary treatments. Points of focus are based on the unique needs of the individual, and multidisciplinary teams collaborate with other care providers to coordinate services. If patients are referred to palliative care from the point of diagnosis, baseline supportive treatment can occur as well as planning for potential changes or side effects throughout treatment. This can help patients avoid or limit side effects during cancer treatment.

Physical health is one major area of focus for palliative care. This includes management of common cancer-related symptoms such as pain or fatigue. Other physical issues that can be addressed by palliative care include treatment of side effects like nausea, vomiting, and insomnia. **Emotional health** is addressed through management of common issues experienced by oncology patients such as grief, depression, anxiety, and fear. On a spiritual level, palliative care providers can help patients explore their beliefs in order to process and accept their diagnosis.

Additional areas of assistance provided by palliative care providers include caregiver and resource support. Caregivers can also receive assistance to cope with the patient's diagnosis and manage caregiving responsibilities. Resources for various needs such as financial burdens, insurance concerns, advance directives, legal issues, and employment concerns can all be addressed with palliative care.

Advance Care Planning

Advance care planning consists of discussions to ensure that the values, preferences, and goals of patients are honored at the end of life. Despite the significance of this discussion, many patients and providers are resistant to having the conversation. This is due to fear of discussing death or the belief that their loved ones know their preferences. The oncology nurse is often in the position to initiate and navigate these conversations.

As cancer and its treatment are high risk and potentially life-threatening, it is important that advance directives are included in advance care planning for patients with treatable and terminal cancer. **Advance directives** are the patient's means of communicating what form of medical treatment they would like to receive at any point when they may be unable to express those decisions on their own. This includes whether the patient wants resuscitation measures if their heart stops or they stop breathing, what comfort measures may be acceptable, and who may be allowed to make medical decisions on their behalf. Whenever possible, advance directives should be discussed before the patient becomes too sick to make these decisions.

There are three distinct documents often used to communicate a person's wishes at the end of life. A **living will** is a legal document that communicates preferences about life-sustaining treatments in the event that a person is unable to communicate or make their own decisions. While it is legally recognized, it is not legally binding. However, it will guide a healthcare proxy or provider on interventions such as CPR, intubation, pacemakers, and artificial nutrition and hydration.

A **durable power of attorney** (DPOA) is another type of legal document that names a healthcare proxy or decision maker for a patient in the event that they become incapacitated. A DPOA can be appointed in addition to or independent of a living will. In the event that a DPOA has not been appointed, medical proxy will be determined by state law and is often passed to a spouse, parents, or adult children. Patients should be counseled that the next of kin indicated by the state may not be the person they would choose themselves. This is especially important in the case of unmarried partners.

A **Physician Orders for Life-Sustaining Treatment** (POLST) form is an order from a physician that communicates how to implement end-of-life care to align with a patient's wishes when they are unable to communicate those wishes themselves. A POLST is intended to be used by patients who are seriously ill, and it must be signed by the patient and the physician. A POLST will provide orders surrounding CPR, intubation, mechanical ventilation, IV antibiotics, IV fluids, and artificial nutrition. It is "portable" and thus valid across inpatient and outpatient care settings, including residential care facilities and patients' homes. Patients and caregivers should be counseled to provide the POLST form to emergency medical personnel if they are responding to a call at their residence.

Epidemiology

Epidemiology is defined as the identification and evaluation of patterns, etiologies, and effects of specific diseases in a target population. The analysis of this data serves as a guide for public health program planning decisions, development of population-based risk profiles, and evaluation of the effectiveness of treatment options for specific diseases such as cancer. Globally, cancer is the second leading cause of death, with 70 percent of those deaths occurring in low- and middle-income countries. The 2017 projections for the United States indicate that cancer will remain as the second most common cause of death after cardiovascular disease and stroke, while lung cancer is projected to continue as the leading cause of cancer deaths in both males and females. In addition, prostate cancer and breast cancer are projected to continue as the most commonly diagnosed conditions in males and females, respectively.

Modifiable Risk Factors

Oncology nurses understand that certain demographic characteristics such as the aging of the population and several modifiable lifestyle behaviors, including the use of reproductive technology, obesity, recreational drug usage, ETOH abuse, and smoking, put patients at risk for specific cancerous conditions. More than 50 percent of new cancers occur in individuals over 65, and while there is no single explanation for this finding, several contributing factors have been proposed. These include the cumulative effect of environmental exposure to sunlight, radiation, and food additives that may result in random DNA mutations, which initiate the development of the cancerous disorder. Other contributing factors that have been identified include the weakening of the immune system, the effects of oxygen free radicals on DNA structure, and the results of chronic inflammation.

There is also an increased risk of cancer in individuals with limited socioeconomic resources and individuals with occupational or environmental exposure to known carcinogens. Research indicates that depressed socioeconomic status in the United States is associated with an increased risk of lung, colorectal, cervical, stomach, and liver cancers. This disparity has also been linked to the incidence of smoking, obesity, sedentary lifestyle, alcohol use and abuse, and limited access to screening and treatment in this population. Sources of occupational or environmental exposure to carcinogens may include diesel exhaust; second-hand smoke; certain heavy metals such as cadmium, arsenic, and chromium; radiation; and air pollution. Oncology nurses are aware that there is also an increased risk for the development of cancer in individuals employed as roofing, paving, and painting contractors as well as chimney sweepers. In addition, there is also a possible link between the incidence of cancer and a history of tuberculosis.

Non-Modifiable Risk Factors

Inherited mutations in an individual's chromosomes, genes, or proteins may be harmful, beneficial, or have no effect on the individual's health. Harmful mutations increase the risk of diseases such as cancer, and research indicates that 5 to 10 percent of all cancers are genetically linked. Cancer-specific mutations have been identified, and the presence or absence of these defects in an individual can be confirmed with **genetic testing**. Oncology nurses understand that the existence of a cancer-related mutation is not always associated with the development of cancer, due in part to the inheritance pattern associated with cancer. The two main inheritance patterns include autosomal dominant and autosomal recessive. An **autosomal dominant** pattern means that the parent as well as the child will exhibit signs of the defective mutation. The **autosomal recessive** pattern means that the child will have an increased risk of cancer only if he/she receives a defective copy of the same gene from each parent. In this case, the parents do not generally have an increased risk of cancer. The genetic mutations also may not be expressed as predicted or the severity of the disease may vary from one individual to another.

Gene TP53, which produces a protein that suppresses tumor growth, is the most commonly mutated gene in all forms of cancer. Mutations of this gene cause **Li-Fraumeni**, a rare inherited disorder that is associated with an increased risk for several cancers. Hereditary breast and ovarian cancer syndromes, which result from mutations of the **BRCA1 and BRCA2 genes**, are associated with an increased lifetime risk for the development of breast and ovarian cancer. These two genes are thought to be responsible for 5 to 10 percent of all breast cancers in women and 100 percent of breast cancers in men. This inherited mutation is also associated with an increased risk for pancreatic cancer and prostate cancer. Mutations of **gene PTEN**, which also produces a protein that suppresses tumor growth, may result in an inherited disorder identified as **Cowden syndrome**, which is associated with an increased risk of breast, thyroid, and endometrial cancers. The most common inherited cancer is **Lynch syndrome**—or hereditary nonpolyposis colon cancer—, which occurs as the result of mutations in a group of five different genes.

Patient characteristics that are associated with inherited cancer syndromes include a history of cancer that was diagnosed at a very early age, simultaneous evidence of several different forms of cancer, cancer occurring in paired organs such as both kidneys or breasts, several first-degree relatives who have the same disease, evidence of certain birth defects that are associated with cancer, and being susceptible to cancer disorders due to gender, ethnicity, or race. Genetic researchers have identified inherited mutations for most, if not all, cancerous conditions, which means that individuals can identify their risks for the development of cancer with genetic testing. Health care providers are encouraged to strongly recommend **genetic counseling** when the following three criteria are met: the patient has a personal or family history that is consistent with an inherited cancer mutation, the test results will provide definitive information regarding the presence or absence of the disease, and the test results can be used to develop the plan of care.

Survivorship

Survivorship refers to the way people who have been diagnosed with cancer live after treatment has been completed. This is a broad term that encompasses all factors of living, including any lifestyle changes that patients make, follow-up care routines, career options, financial changes, spiritual choices, relationships with members of their support system, and so on. The impact of survivorship affects patients' psychosocial, cognitive, and physical quality of life. As patients move out of treatment and into survivorship, they may need to work through an adjustment period to acknowledge their cancer diagnosis and experience, any lifestyle transitions, and their expected prognosis. Patients may experience a wide range of emotions and desire to take specific actions based on their prognosis.

Psychosocial effects are those that relate to how patients interact with their environment, social and support systems, and other non-medical arenas of their life. Psychosocial effects also influence how patients perceive themselves and their relationships to others. Cancer survivors often must navigate new psychosocial parameters once treatment has ended. They may have new **internal stressors**, such as fear or anxiety about cancer returning and the effects the illness has on their families, especially on spouses and children. Survivors may feel uncomfortable having others continuously take care of them and may feel guilt or as though they are a burden. Survivors may also experience body image issues or self-esteem issues, especially if their physical appearance has radically changed (such as hair loss, major weight fluctuations, or removal of any body parts that were affected by or vulnerable to cancerous cells). This can heavily influence how they relate to people with whom they have romantic or sexual relationships or how comfortable they feel in group or social settings. If survivors experience low self-esteem or discomfort in public after treatment, it may cause them to distance themselves from others.

This can exacerbate feelings of depression and loneliness, as the isolation limits interactions with those people who potentially serve as the core of the survivor's social support system. Additionally, survivors may experience a number of external psychosocial stressors, such as financial problems. Cancer treatments can be long in duration, complex in nature, and costly overall, even with comprehensive medical insurance. This may deplete personal savings or cause families to go into medical debt. In addition, some survivors may need long term assisted care and regular follow-up appointments after treatment is over, which are additional expenses to maintain. Finally, a major psychosocial change includes the inherent quality of life that shifts after experiencing a disruptive, potentially life-threatening event such as cancer. Survivors may have some limitations to how their life used to be before their diagnosis; these can include physical limitations, financial limitations, or social limitations. They may also need to adopt new lifestyle habits, such as a new diet or exercise plan, in order to maintain their health while eliminating other habits that may have contributed to their diagnosis or would be harmful to their recovery. For example, smokers who have survived lung cancer will need to quit smoking, which is a highly addictive habit that is known to be stressful and difficult to quit. These sorts of lifestyle changes can be a major adjustment for both survivors and their families.

Rehabilitation

The rehabilitation process during the survivorship period should encompass the individual's holistic needs. Rehabilitation focuses on helping survivors acclimatize to life after their diagnosis and treatment, and they may need physical, emotional, mental, and psychosocial conditioning and support. Survivors' perceptions of a normal life may have drastically changed. Many medical facilities offer a transitional rehabilitation program to support survivors and their families as they adjust to a new way of living. Interdisciplinary health care professionals provide support in all aspects of healing.

Rehabilitation is a personal, subjective journey based on the individual's case, needs, and hopes. Almost all survivors will need some **physical rehabilitation** as they regain their strength after undergoing treatment. Most patients will not have engaged in much physical activity during their treatment, so their muscles and fitness ability may feel especially diminished. Additionally, most cancer treatments weaken the bones, so survivors should focus on weight-bearing exercising to try to rebuild bone density. Physical rehabilitation will likely begin gradually, with very gentle exercises such as mobility drills, stretching, or chair yoga, and increase in intensity as the survivor feels comfortable. In other cases, such as survivors who have lost limbs due to treatment, they may need to start in basic physical and/or occupational therapy settings (especially if they are learning how to use a prosthetic). The goal of these programs is to help the survivor learn to move efficiently and in a way that supports their daily living habits or work routines

Mental rehabilitation may focus on regaining cognitive clarity as the survivor recovers from the well-known cognitive "fog" or "haze" that tends to come with different chemotherapy medications. At first, cognitive functions such memory, decision making, and concentration may feel dulled. Different cognitive exercises such as matching games, puzzles, vision practices, fine motor control exercises that are linked to specific neural pathways (such as crossing an arm across the midline of the body, which requires both halves of the brain to communicate with one another), and reading comprehension practices may be employed. Speech practice may also be utilized in this setting. Often, cognitive disruption from cancers and their treatments affects patients' speech in terms of clarity and cohesiveness.

Psychosocial rehabilitation may include personal counseling, couples' therapy, and/or family therapy to allow the survivor to work through any fears, regrets, resentment, stressors, or other complex emotions that have resulted from their cancer experience. Couples' therapy can help partners who may have lost intimacy through one partner's diagnosis or help survivors who feels any sense of physical or emotional discomfort feel more comfortable with their partner. Couples' therapy can also be especially useful for parents of pediatric survivors if the relationship suffered during the emotional, intense experience of caring for a sick child. Family therapy can allow the family unit learn how to best support the survivors' "new normal", while also allowing an outlet for caregivers to receive support. Caregivers often feel complex emotions such as exhaustion, guilt, resentment, and fear, and family therapy can allow them to work through these emotions and utilize healthy coping mechanisms.

Recurrence Concerns

Cancer recurrence refers to cancer that returns after treatment is complete and after a definable period of remission where no cancerous cells could be found. Cancer recurrence can occur in the location it was initially found (local), in the same general area (regional), or in a completely different location (distant). If the cancer is the same type as the original cancer, it is considered recurrent regardless of the location. Recurrent cancer cells will have the same appearance and behavioral mannerisms as the initial cancer that was detected.

Secondary malignancies refer to cancers that occur as a result of treatment for the **primary malignancy**. Common cancer treatments, such as radiation and chemotherapy, are extremely offensive to the body. While they work to prevent cancerous cells from replicating, these treatments also add stress to healthy cells by inhibiting normal cell division and even causing some level of DNA damage. If enough healthy cells are affected, this can lead to secondary malignancies months or years later. Most commonly, secondary malignancies present as skin cancers. Generally, treatment protocols try to limit procedures that increase the risk of secondary malignancies. This may include practices such as administering radiation and chemotherapy treatments separately, spacing apart treatments of any kind, and keeping treatment dosing as minimal as possible for the patient's specific case. However, these prevention practices are not always feasible, especially in the advanced stages of cancer or if the patient is especially vulnerable (such as in pediatric patients). Pediatric patients experience secondary malignancy rates of up to 80 percent, with most secondary malignancies occurring in adulthood. These rates are higher in pediatric patients who were treated with radiation therapies. Additionally, some specific types of cancers have a higher correlation with developing secondary malignancies. Secondary malignancies are very common in patients diagnosed with **Hodgkin's lymphoma**, a cancer of the lymphatic system that has a relatively positive prognosis for the initial cancer; however, patients are told to expect a secondary malignancy and require more intensive follow-up care during survivorship. Common secondary malignancies with Hodgkin's lymphoma include breast, thyroid, and bone cancers. Additionally, breast cancer survivors experience increased vulnerability to secondary cancers as well. Secondary cancers are simply treated the same way they would be if they were found as a primary cancer; however, preventative screenings of all kinds are often performed at an earlier age and with more frequency in cancer survivors than they are in healthy individuals.

Family and Social Support Concerns

Family and social support is believed to be critical to the survivor's recovery experience. A number of studies indicate that if a survivor has a spouse, the spouse serves as the main pillar of support. Siblings, close friends, and colleagues also serve as important systems for the survivor. Survivors often lean on these relationships to make decisions, find comradery in new lifestyle changes (such as having exercise partners or sharing healthy meals), and ease the overall adjustment period. In addition, formal and informal support groups consisting of other survivors can also help survivors navigate their life after cancer. Studies also indicate that female survivors of breast cancer who report strong family and social support networks increase their chances of long-term survival without recurrence. Male survivors tend to have more difficulty building support systems, verbally expressing weaknesses or the need for emotional/physical support, and with sharing any personal vulnerabilities they may feel. Additionally, male survivors may feel pressure from societal and cultural norms to act strong for their families and place high expectations on themselves to provide resources and return to normalcy as soon as possible. All of these factors can be detrimental to the recovery and survivorship process. Families can work to create micro-cultures within their family unit to support the male survivor, encourage him to speak more about his perceived vulnerabilities and needs, and voice that their love and care for the male survivor is not contingent on any expectations he has placed on himself.

Sexuality Concerns

Both male and female survivors may experience concerns relating to their sexuality after treatment is over. First, survivors simply may feel exhausted, have a low libido, or experience temporary sexual dysfunction as they recover from their treatment period. It may take time for them to regain strength, for chemotherapy medications to fully leave their body, and to feel sexual desire again. Additionally, many types of cancers cause serious hormonal disruption that can cause women to experience early menopause and men to experience low testosterone or erectile dysfunction. If cancer affected the reproductive areas, survivors may feel pain upon sexual intercourse. Some studies indicate that older patients who are treated for reproductive cancers (such as cervical or prostate cancers) become voluntarily celibate for an indefinite period of time.

If treatment required the removal of certain parts that the survivor equated with sexuality (such as breasts or uterus in women, testes in men, or a large limb loss in either sex), survivors may experience body image issues and low self-esteem. This affects how the survivors view and value their physical appearance, perceived aesthetic appeal, and sexual capabilities. They may feel undesirable, depressed, sad about these changes, and angry. Other changes in appearance, such as grafts removed for skin cancers or physical facial alterations in head and neck cancers, can cause long lasting body disorder issues for survivors.

Post-cancer sexual dysfunction is reported as one of the main contributors to survivor depression and decreased quality of life during the survivorship period. Sexuality concerns are often not discussed or addressed during follow-up care, and survivors often feel ashamed or embarrassed to initiate the conversation themselves. Counseling sessions with a licensed sex therapist during the rehabilitation period is one way that survivors and their partners can get past these concerns and improve their quality of life. A sex therapist can help survivors understand and overcome their fears, shame, and limiting beliefs about themselves, as well as provide guidance for increased sexuality and sexual intimacy on a case-by-case basis.

Discrimination Concerns

Even though the federal ADA and state-regulated legislations exist to protect cancer survivors from organizational and **workplace discrimination**, they may not always work as intended since employers often do not want workers who may raise their health insurance costs or may be regularly absent from work. Employers may ask roundabout questions or make casual conversation that reveals a survivor's medical history if they are interviewing for a new job. If survivors are already employed, employers may cite a reason that cannot be otherwise disproven for terminating their position, such as a budget cut or restructuring. Often, the financial and time costs associated with a survivor taking an organization to court (especially if they are filing a lawsuit against a large organization that is well-funded and employs skilled attorneys) may be prohibitive and even destructive for the survivor. Additionally, even if survivors are able to maintain their employment status, they may experience intentional and unintentional stereotyping at work. Colleagues may display resentful attitudes if they have had to take on additional workloads while the survivor used FMLA leave. Supervisors may inadvertently act as though the survivor is less capable of completing tasks than they used to be and may not offer certain work challenges. Both colleagues and superiors may have difficulty knowing how to appropriately interact with the survivor after treatment has ended, and this may lead to unnecessary **workplace isolation** of the survivor. This would be a difficult experience for anyone, but many survivors are trying to regain a sense of normalcy and capability after treatment; therefore, awkward encounters in the workplace are especially detrimental to their re-adjustment. Organizations can prevent inadvertent forms of discrimination by having a well-versed human resources department that can support leadership in understanding discrimination laws, educated decision-making, and the genuine capabilities of survivors.

Delayed Treatment-Related Considerations

Delayed-Onset Side Effects

Delayed-onset side effects refer to those that do not appear until late in the treatment or after the treatment has concluded. These specific side effects may vary greatly depending on the patient's cancer and the patient's treatment for said cancer. For cancers that require surgical removal of organs or portions of organs, delayed-onset side effects vary depending on the organs removed. For example, removal of portions of the bowel in gastrointestinal cancer could later lead to bowel obstructions requiring further abdominal surgery. Removal of lymph nodes can later lead to lymphedema. Amputation of a limb due to cancer in the bone could later have the side effect of phantom limb pain. On the other hand, chemotherapy and radiation can have more systemic delayed-onset side effects. Patients may later find they suffer from infertility or early menopause due to hormone changes caused by certain types of chemotherapy. Additionally, depending on the course of chemotherapy or radiation used, some patients may be at greater risk of developing cardiovascular disease later in life. Coronary artery disease, heart failure, high blood pressure, and arrhythmias can occur in some patients taking medications such as Doxorubicin and Sorafenib. Chemotherapy and radiation can also cause damage to the lungs, which may later manifest in difficulties with breathing and oxygenation. Other delayed-onset side effects can include nerve damage causing neurological changes and decreases in bone density causing osteoporosis. It is important for oncology nurses to have a comprehensive understanding of disease and treatment-related side effects, including those with delayed onset. This knowledge prepares the nurse to provide patient-specific assessment, management, and education at any point in the patient's oncology journey.

Chronic Side Effects

While many common side effects associated with cancer treatment resolve quickly after treatment discontinuation (e.g., nausea/vomiting, diarrhea, sensitivity reactions, radiation burns, surgical wounds), it is important to recognize that this is not always the case. Some side effects can persist for weeks, months, or years after treatment is discontinued. Other treatment-related side effects can begin during treatment and remain indefinitely.

Chemotherapy medications are an example of a cancer treatment that can lead to **chronic side effects**. Chemotherapy drugs impact the body in vastly different ways. Some medications (e.g., anthracyclines) can cause damage to the heart (cardiotoxicity) and can result in chronic heart conditions like cardiomyopathy, arrhythmia, myocardial infarction, and coronary artery disease. Other medications (e.g., bleomycin) can cause pulmonary toxicity that can lead to chronic issues such as decreased lung function, fibrosis, and pneumonitis. The kidneys are another vulnerable organ that can be impacted by certain chemotherapy treatments, such as cisplatin. Kidney toxicity can result in varying degrees of chronic kidney disease. The liver is yet another susceptible site of organ toxicity, as certain medications (e.g., anthracyclines, taxanes, vinca alkaloids) heavily impact liver function. This can lead to cirrhosis and liver failure. Reproductive organs can be impacted by chemotherapy treatments. Infertility, impotence, and hormone changes are some examples of potentially chronic side effects of chemotherapy treatment. Lastly, chemotherapy medications have the potential to cause long-term neurological toxicities as well. Examples of this would include peripheral neuropathy, stroke, cognitive changes, hearing and vision changes, or development of seizures.

Radiation therapy is another example of a cancer treatment that carries a risk for the development of chronic side effects. Radiotherapy is performed by exposing cancer cells to very high levels of focused radioactive energy that results in damage to the DNA and cell death. The goal of treatment is to maximize radiation exposure of cancer cells while minimizing radiation exposure to healthy tissues and organs. However, tissue and organ injury can still occur. This damage to tissues and vasculature may result in varying degrees of decreased function, chronic inflammation, fibrosis, reduced blood flow, and/or tissue death to the affected areas.

Surgical cancer treatment is yet another treatment modality that can result in chronic side effects. One example of this is the development of chronic lymphedema following lymphadenectomy. Radical head and neck surgeries can result in many chronic issues ranging from nutrition deficits, airway challenges, dental issues, and osteonecrosis of the jaw. Other potentially chronic side effects from any surgery can include pain, stricture, complicated wound healing, and osteomyelitis.

Subsequent Malignancies

Chemotherapy and radiation therapy can be highly effective at treating and managing cancer. However, these treatments can increase a patient's risk for developing secondary malignancies. These treatment-related secondary cancers tend to develop within several years after initial exposure; therefore, adequate follow up and monitoring is critical to ensure the ongoing health of oncology patients.

Exposure to radiation from various sources, including radiation therapy, has been shown to be a risk factor for the development of blood and bone marrow cancers. This includes acute lymphoblastic leukemia (ALL), acute myelogenous leukemia (AML), and chronic myelogenous leukemia (CML). Additionally, patients exposed to radiation therapy are also at risk for developing myelodysplastic syndrome (MDS), which is a cancer of the bone marrow that leads to dysfunctional and deficient blood cells. About a third of patients with MDS will progress to AML. The risk of developing secondary leukemia or MDS after radiation therapy tends to be relative to the duration of treatment, the amount of total exposure, and how much bone marrow was exposed.

Patients who have undergone radiation therapy are also at risk for developing other types of cancer. **Solid tumors** (e.g., breast cancer, thyroid cancer, colorectal cancer, bone sarcoma) have been linked to exposure to radiation. Solid tumors tend to present ten or more years following initial exposure, and the younger the patient is at the time of treatment, the greater the chances of developing these tumors. Additional factors include the total dose and the specific location of treatment, as the amount of exposure and the site of exposure will impact the location and likelihood of developing secondary tumors.

Certain chemotherapy medications such as alkylating agents (e.g., cyclophosphamide), platinum drugs (e.g., cisplatin), and anthracycline topoisomerase II inhibitors (e.g., etoposide) have also been linked to the development of MDS and AML. As with radiation therapy, the dose and duration of treatment impacts the relative risk. More intensive treatment regimens (involving greater chemotherapy exposure over a shorter period) impact the patient's risk as well.

Lastly, it is important to understand that while newer immunotherapies are formulated with the intent to target cancer cells while minimizing harm to healthy cells, many of these medications do not have the longevity for researchers to know the long-term risks involved with their use. Therefore, ongoing education, research, and data collection will be required in the future to monitor for any potential links between specific targeted therapies and secondary cancers.

Follow-Up Care

Long-term follow-up is a crucial component of survivors' lives, since many cancers can and do return and developing secondary malignancies is a common effect of treatment. Long-term **follow-up care** is especially critical for pediatric survivors and young adult survivors, who have a much higher chance of developing secondary malignancies over the course of their lifespan. For these patients, routine care is much more intense than for an individual who simply goes for annual preventive well-visits. Based on the medical center, pediatric survivors will typically begin receiving cancer-focused follow-up care within one to two years of their cancer being in remission. In addition to a complete well-visit, survivors are regularly screened for cancer recurrence and secondary malignancies. Vital organs are also closely monitored for functioning. Since most pediatric patients' systems are not fully developed at the time of cancer diagnosis and treatment, medical professionals must check vital organs to determine whether treatment had any adverse effects on their functioning. Common delayed effects that occur in pediatric patients include endocrine system disruption during puberty as well as stunted growth of vital organs and bone length. Once pediatric patients become adults, they'll continue to receive similar screenings for the rest of their lives. However, care may change to include treatment focused on adult issues, such as infertility for survivors who are trying to conceive.

Older adults typically receive more health care, whether they have had a cancer diagnosis in their life or not. However, middle-aged to older cancer survivors who were diagnosed later in life often have a more intense component of psychosocial intervention in their follow-up care. This is because they spent many years of their lives as healthy individuals with routines, families they cared and provided for, careers, and so on; the disruption that a cancer diagnosis and treatment cause to these aspects of life can be a much more stressful adjustment for the older adult. Adult survivors will also receive follow-up appointments at quarterly intervals for the first few years after remission and then biannually after that.

In between follow-up visits, all survivors should remain vigilant about noticing and reporting any physical or cognitive changes they experience, especially changes in the skin (such as abnormal moles), as skin cancer is the most common secondary malignancy after treatment ends. Physical and cognitive changes should be reported and examined right away. This is an important discharge instruction to teach patients.

End-of-Life Care

End-of-life care is provided to individuals with a terminal condition. This is care that focuses on both the individual who is receiving it as well as his or her support systems. Planning for end-of-life care may begin upon receiving a terminal prognosis and should account for medical services the patient may need during the last few months of life, counseling options for family members, financial planning, estate planning, and so on. Direct end-of-life care activities are carried out in the final months of the recipient's life and directly related to preparing the individual and the individual's support system for the recipient's death.

Bereavement

Following the death of a patient, the oncology nurse often continues care and support for bereaved loved ones. This experience may be very different depending on the circumstances surrounding the patient's death. General nursing goals of care include providing emotional support and physical comfort, advocating for the patient's end-of-life wishes, and assisting with facilitation of spiritual, cultural, or personal post-mortem practices.

There are many factors that can impact how families experience the loss of their loved one. The care setting (e.g., at home alone, at home with family, emergency room, inpatient hospital, hospice unit), the surrounding circumstances (e.g., expected versus unexpected, calm versus chaotic), and the length of time from diagnosis to death all impact how families feel after the death of a loved one. Additional factors include individual beliefs and experiences of death, spiritual beliefs, and other cultural beliefs and practices surrounding end of life.

For oncology patients, research supports the idea that early **end-of-life planning** with the inclusion of family leads to more positive outcomes and perceptions. End-of-life planning with family is a way for the patient to feel empowered when they could otherwise feel helpless. There is an opportunity to discuss and plan which interventions and practices should ideally be included. Healthcare practitioners can provide comfort with counseling and education regarding death and dying. There is also less opportunity for family conflict or distress due to differences in expectations or wishes. Additionally, if the patient agrees to palliative care and/or hospice services, these specialties can provide additional support that can promote a more peaceful, meaningful end-of-life experience, which can have a profound positive impact on the surviving loved ones.

Oncology nurses often provide support prior to and following the death of a patient. Interventions include being respectful and mindful of the emotions and tone within the care area during interactions, ensuring the family is given privacy, limiting extraneous noise from outside the patient's care area, and maintaining a comfortable environment. Additionally, nurses advocate and facilitate the fulfillment of end-of-life, spiritual, or cultural practices.

Hospice Care

Hospice services are the most commonly utilized formal end-of-life and palliative services. They provide comfort measures and ensure that administrative and legal matters, such as estate planning, are complete. People typically elect hospice services when they do not want to receive any more treatment and/or have a terminal diagnosis. The goal for **hospice care** is to provide as much comfort and care as is needed on a daily basis to ensure the patient has high physical, emotional, mental, and spiritual support. Therefore, a hospice team usually consists of a physician, nursing staff, a social worker, a spiritual counselor of the patient's choosing, one or more therapists that focus on physical therapy and bereavement services, and other volunteers who may be specialized to the patient's specific situation. Hospice services can be as comprehensive as the patient wishes, ranging from providing occasional caregiver relief to providing continuous service around the clock. Through hospice services, patients can select which services they would like to receive and which pain measures they want to employ to maintain some level of control about their end of life. Most importantly, hospice service can be received in the comfort of the patient's own home. Even if they choose to go into a hospice facility, their family and friends can spend as much time as they wish with the patient. This can provide tremendous support and relief for the patient's family and caregivers.

Caregiver Support

Caregivers of oncology patients experience many challenges as they attempt to balance their own needs with the needs of the patient. This becomes especially challenging as a patient nears the end of life. Patients often require increasing levels of care, and the grieving process can create an emotionally taxing environment for the caregiver. Oncology nurses can assist caregivers in many ways. For instance, they act as an educator to the patient and caregiver by providing information on topics such as performing activities of daily living at home, providing medication management, assisting with side effect management, knowing when to contact the doctor, and knowing how to safely handle body fluids after chemotherapy treatment.

Nurses also act as patient and caregiver advocates by referring patients for appropriate services to support their at-home care. This can include home health nursing services, physical therapy, respiratory therapy, medical equipment, home health aide services, palliative care, and hospice care. By recognizing patients' needs and referring them to services, nurses can support caregivers who may have otherwise been responsible for managing the patient's medical needs at home.

In addition to patient resources and support, there is also caregiver support available. Caregiving education is one way to promote safe and effective caregiving. These services can range from individual sessions to group workshops that introduce basic information for caregiving and resiliency. Support groups are another effective outlet for caregivers to gain support and connection within a community of individuals going through similar circumstances. This provides an opportunity for expanded support systems, increased social interaction, better mental health outcomes, and ongoing caregiver education.

In situations where there is more than one available caregiver, nurses can assist in building a schedule of split care to reduce the strain on a single caregiver. Additionally, if applicable, **respite services** can provide periodic breaks for caregivers to maintain self-care and mental health needs. Lastly, caregivers may also seek mental health services for themselves to support healthy coping strategies when they are having difficulty managing caregiving responsibilities and the impending death of their loved one. Early access to these services and appropriate education and support for caregivers improves patient outcomes (e.g., fewer falls, fewer medication errors, reduced injury, increased at-home compliance with treatment plan), reduces risks for patient harm (i.e., neglect and abuse), and supports ongoing positive support systems for patients and families.

Interprofessional Team

Goals of care at the end of life shift from treating cancer to providing comfort measures and support to patients, families, and caregivers. To meet these goals and take advantage of the expertise of various disciplines, a multidisciplinary team is incorporated. The physician often plays the biggest role in helping patients and families decide whether to discontinue treatment. Along with mid-level providers (nurse practitioners and physician's assistants), physicians provide pharmacological measures to manage the symptoms of the death process, such as pain, confusion, dyspnea, and nausea.

Social work and spiritual care are incorporated to address the spiritual and emotional needs of patients and families at the end of life. Although social work and spiritual care roles seem similar, there are key differences. **Social workers** help patients and families navigate end-of-life planning, manage crisis, and connect to other support services that may be available. **Spiritual care** helps patients and families to process their beliefs surrounding death, understand what gives their lives meaning, and explore legacy. This may be in conjunction with a formal religion, but not always.

The nurse will play an important role in bridging the multiple disciplines and utilizing each one appropriately as the patient's and family's needs become apparent. In some settings, the nurse may have a direct role in caring for the patient as they near death, such as administering medications and comfort measures. In other settings, such as home hospice, one of the important roles the nurse will play is that of educator, making caregivers feel confident in providing care when healthcare workers are not present.

Comfort Measures

Comfort measures are the foundational component of palliative and end-of-life care, as the goal is to provide as much comfort and dignity as possible for patients. Depending on the patient's case, comfort measures may be pharmacologic or non-pharmacologic in nature. Often, comfort measures are an integrative approach of both.

Pharmacologic

In the context of palliative and hospice care, **pharmacologic interventions** are delivered with the intention of improving a symptom that is causing discomfort or embarrassment as soon as possible. The most common symptom that causes discomfort is pain. Pain is routinely managed with opioids that are delivered through titration in order to allow continuous pain relief without overwhelming patients' weakened systems. However, patients regularly experience side effects of nausea and constipation with opioids. Nausea may be treated through both prescription strength ondansetron and over-the-counter anti-nausea medications. Constipation may be treated with laxatives, including pure magnesium supplementation, polyethylene glycol solutions (including over-the-counter laxatives such as the brand name Miralax), or liquid lactulose. Other pain options may include prescription-strength oral or liquid ibuprofen, NSAIDs, or acetaminophen.

A number of cancers that are located in the gastrointestinal or reproductive regions may result in bowel obstruction. Additionally, as patients near the end of life, their appetite and liquid intake decreases, which can lead to bowel obstruction. Surgery in hospice patients should be avoided. Bowel obstruction can be prevented with regular laxative use; methylnaltrexone, which leads to increased bowel movements within four hours; and dexamethasone, which reduces edema that commonly causes bowel obstructions. Some patients may also receive tailored parenteral nutrition bags, delivered intravenously, to support gastrointestinal functioning.

In the last weeks of life, patients tend to experience some degree of delusion, seizure, or other agitation. This can result from decreased brain function, high doses of opioid medications, or unanticipated change in routine or caregivers. Some patients and their families may choose to allow this to play out naturally, while others have provided directives for sedation in these cases. Patients should be checked to ensure that there is no underlying cause for the delirium, such as infection. If not, their opioid dosage may be tapered, or they may receive a sedative such as midazolam. However, this is a controversial practice as some research indicates that mixing opioid and sedative medication, even though they may provide the most comfort for the patient, can be the direct cause of patient death.

Finally, **cannabinoids** and medical or recreational marijuana (where legal) are commonly used as part of palliative care methods to relieve a number of symptoms. Cannabinoids and marijuana can relieve pain, muscular tension, and nausea along with increasing appetite and thirst in patients. Since it can effectively relieve these symptoms simultaneously, small dosing can stave off a number of larger health issues, such as constipation that results from not eating or drinking enough.

Non-Pharmacologic

In the context of palliative and hospice care, **non-pharmacologic interventions** are delivered with the intention of relieving chronic conditions without medicine. These often address emotional, mental, psychosocial, or spiritual symptoms that patients experience with a terminal diagnosis. For example, many patients worry about leaving loved ones. They may find comfort in group therapy sessions with their family members that allow all participants to share their feelings, find feasible solutions, and relieve each other's perceived burdens. Talking with spiritual counselors may help patients relieve emotional and spiritual concerns relating to the purpose of their life, the point of their existence, and what may come after dying. Creative therapies, such as art therapy, music therapy, or journaling, can help patients reduce overall stress.

Non-pharmacologic interventions can also help patients with physical concerns. **Bowel stenting** can help patients with bowel obstruction without the need for stronger medications or bowel surgeries. Dietary changes can also support gastrointestinal functioning, relieve nausea, and reduce inflammation within the body that might cause pain or fatigue. Additionally, massage, stretching, and gentle physical mobility exercises can help patients with moderate pain relief, overall stress reduction, and promote a positive mood. Yoga, meditation, controlled breathing techniques, and tai chi are shown to promote overall relaxation in both hospice patients and their caregivers. A number of studies indicate that acupuncture has been shown to relieve pain in cancer patients specifically. Patients who are relieved of muscular tension and feel generally relaxed are less likely to be in pain or feel nauseous.

Non-pharmacologic interventions can also be extremely simple in nature, such as ensuring that the patient has a comfortable bedroom environment, access to entertainment (such as a television or radio in the room), or favorite books that can be read. Small creature comforts can go a long way in ensuring a positive daily quality of life for a patient.

Practice Quiz

1. Which of the following cancers is NOT commonly linked to hereditary factors?
    a. Breast cancer
    b. Non-polyposis colon cancer
    c. Cervical cancer
    d. Ovarian cancer

2. Which of the following statements correctly identifies the function of tamoxifen in the prevention of breast cancer?
    a. Tamoxifen reduces the risk of invasive breast cancer by 50 percent in postmenopausal women.
    b. Tamoxifen is more effective in premenopausal women.
    c. Tamoxifen is more effective as primary prevention and is not used in advanced disease.
    d. Tamoxifen is more effective against progesterone-positive tumors.

3. When do treatment-related secondary cancers tend to develop?
    a. During the first six weeks of treatment
    b. During the first year of treatment
    c. Within one month after initial exposure
    d. Within several years after initial exposure

4. Which of the following statements is consistent with disease characteristics that influence the selection and use of a screening test?
    a. The disease is associated with a projected survival rate of greater than five years after diagnosis.
    b. The test can produce positive results before physical symptoms of the disease are present.
    c. The disease must be widely disseminated in the population.
    d. Screening tests for genetically linked diseases are associated with greater specificity.

5. What is one way to support patients' caregivers during diagnosis and treatment?
    a. Encourage caregivers to create and maintain personal, meaningful self-care practices.
    b. Encourage caregivers to take on as many nursing duties as legally allowed in order to provide a sense of efficacy.
    c. Encourage caregivers to share any negative feelings they have with the patient in order to keep communication clear.
    d. Encourage caregivers to focus as much as possible on the patient's needs since they are the patient's primary support system.

See answers on the next page.

Answer Explanations

1. C: Cervical cancer is not linked to an inherited gene mutation. Breast and ovarian cancer, Choices *A* and *D*, are linked to inherited mutations in the BRCA1 and BRCA2 genes. Non-polyposis colon cancer, Choice *B*, is caused by inherited mutations in a group of genes affecting DNA repair.

2. A: Tamoxifen is effective in reducing the risk of breast cancer in at-risk postmenopausal women. It is not effective in pre-menopausal women due to the added estrogen burden. Tamoxifen is commonly used in advanced disease and is only effective against estrogen-positive tumors.

3. D: Treatment-related secondary cancers tend to develop within several years of initial exposure. Chemotherapy and radiation increase the chances of developing a secondary malignancy.

4. B: Screening tests are appropriate for conditions that can be identified and treated before symptoms of the disease are evident, which potentially improves patient outcomes, and in some cases, may prevent the development of cancer. Screening tests are not limited by projected survival rates. Screening tests assume a certain incidence of the disease in the target population; however, widespread incidence is not required for accurate testing. There is no published data to indicate that screening tests are more sensitive to genetic diseases.

5. A: Caregivers are susceptible to burnout, depression, and resentment. Ensuring that they take care of their own health enables them to provide better care for the patient. Meaningful self-care, or actions that help a person feel re-energized, can reduce fatigue, stress, and the intensity of negative emotions. Caregivers should never take on more duties than they feel capable of handling, especially complex nursing duties. However, if possible, they should avoid burdening the patient with their emotions since the patient is often overwhelmed as well.

Oncology Nursing Practice

Scientific Basis

Carcinogenesis

Carcinogenesis is the process by which normal cells are transformed into malignant cells, which are then capable of distant metastasis. Researchers estimate that 5 percent of human cancers are caused by viruses, an additional 5 percent are caused by radiation, and the remaining 90 percent are caused by exposure to chemicals. Lifestyle behaviors including smoking, exposure to second-hand smoke, and dietary habits account for a large part of this exposure; however, **occupational exposure** continues to be the second most common exposure to a variety of carcinogenic agents, including diesel exhaust and heavy metals. In addition, hormones are recognized as "promoters" of cancerous conditions that have estrogen receptors. There are three recognized steps of the process—initiation, promotion, and progression—and an intervening fourth step—transformation—is added by several sources. The **initiation stage** is characterized by irreversible and transmissible changes in multiple genes of a single cell that can result from a single exposure to the initiating carcinogen; however, it is most common for multiple exposures to occur prior to initiation. This damage can be cumulative, which serves to explain why an individual's risk for cancer escalates rapidly beyond the age of 65. The initiated cell becomes capable of autonomous growth, and, depending on the rate of cellular replication, may lay dormant for weeks to years, remaining histologically indistinguishable from the tissue of origin. The initial exposure to the carcinogen causes damage to the cellular DNA within hours of contact. Although the cell is capable of repairing the genetic material, if replication occurs before the repair is completed, the alterations become permanent. This explains why cells with rapid proliferation rates, such as the epithelial lining of the GI tract, bone marrow cells, and hair follicles, are susceptible to the adverse effects of chemotherapeutic agents.

Promotion of the initiated cell occurs as a result of continuous exposure to tissue-specific promoting carcinogens. A **promoting carcinogen** is characterized as a **complete carcinogen** when the promoting agent is capable of initiating and promoting the neoplastic process, while a **pure carcinogen** can only initiate, not promote, the neoplastic process. Promotion may result in cellular hyperplasia or an inflammatory process. An **incomplete carcinogen** may only be capable of a single step of one of the processes rather than functioning as an initiating or promoting agent. Transformation is sometimes identified as the interim period of carcinogenesis between the promotion of the initiated cell and the progression to a malignant cell. Progression is a complex sequence of events during which the initiated cell evolves to a malignant cell with the ability to proliferate and metastasize.

Immunology

Immunology is the study of the function of the immune system in health maintenance and disease. The immune system is comprised of multiple cell types that are distributed in all tissues of the body and lymphoid organs that function together to prevent tumor growth, repair cellular damage, and prevent and eradicate microbial infections. Under normal circumstances, the immune system differentiates and acts upon invading molecules and damaged self-tissues, but not normal host cells and tissues. As the "first responder," the immune system provides an essential biochemical and cellular barrier to infection. This response depends on the action of highly specialized B and T lymphocytes, including the long-lived memory cells that are capable of preventing or minimizing repeat microbial infection. Defects in the immune system may be caused by viral infections, malnutrition, or gene mutations, or they may be the result of cancer therapies. The resulting abnormal function causes the immune system to act upon and damage normal host cells and tissues. Advanced immunological studies provide new evidence that altered immune functioning is responsible for many disorders, including neurodegenerative, metabolic, neoplastic, and cardiovascular conditions.

The immune system is capable of detecting and destroying abnormal cells; however, cancer cells are able to block the surveillance of the immune system by altering the expression of cell surface antigens, including cell-surface proteins capable of inactivating the immune cells, and by triggering the release of immune cell suppressants by adjacent cells. Cancer immunology is focused on the development and application of immunotherapies, such as targeted therapies, chemotherapy, and radiation therapy, to treat multiple forms of cancer. In addition, current research is aimed at understanding why immunotherapies are not universally effective against a specific cancer. In other words, why is the treatment effective for some but not all patients with the same cancer? Presently, the study of immunotherapies is focused on increasing their ability to stimulate the action of the immune system and counteract the suppressant actions of the cancer cells.

Clinical Trials

Ongoing progress in the field of oncology relies heavily on the continued use of clinical trials. **Clinical trials** are a form of research in which human volunteers are evaluated and compared using one or more health-related variables to determine differences in efficacy and safety. Oncology nurses participate throughout the clinical trial process to support ethical and accurate outcomes.

Research conducted with human subjects is highly regulated by various global and regional laws and agencies. Internationally, researchers follow Good Clinical Practice (GCP) to maintain standards throughout all steps of the selection, conduction, evaluation, and reporting of human studies. In the United States, the Code of Federal Regulations (CFR) is utilized by the Office of Human Research as well as the Food and Drug Administration to regulate research practices locally. Every individual involved in human research has the utmost responsibility for maintaining these ethical and professional standards.

Clinical trials are organized by the type and phase of research being conducted. The five major types of clinical trials are prevention, screening, diagnostic, quality of life, and treatment. **Prevention studies** look at ways to prevent diseases from happening (e.g., development of HPV vaccine). **Screening studies** identify ways to globally evaluate the population for diseases to improve health outcomes for the public (e.g., frequency and age of onset for routine colonoscopy). **Diagnostic studies** evaluate how to detect specific illnesses before they become problematic (e.g., identification of tumor markers for specific tumor types). **Quality of life studies** identify ways to improve quality of life for individuals experiencing chronic disease (e.g., optimization of premedication regimen). Finally, **treatment studies** seek to identify new and better treatment options (e.g., development of targeted therapies).

Treatment studies are further broken down into trial phases. Phase I involves identification of general and maximum dosing, initial evaluation of safety, **pharmacokinetics** (how a medication processes, interacts, and is excreted from the body), and **pharmacodynamics** (how a medication functions and the impact it has on the body and disease process). Phase II summarizes the outcomes of Phase I and seeks to further evaluate safety and potential adverse effects or toxicity associated with the treatment. Phase III puts the study regimen (**variable group**) against the standard treatment (**control group**). Phase III trials are typically randomized, meaning that participants are placed sporadically into the control or variable group to increase the value of trial outcome data. **Blinding** is another technique that can be used by researchers to increase the validity of trial data by masking different information about study participants that could influence outcomes or conclusions. Examples of blinding include study participants not being told whether they are in the control or variable group, or researchers not being told whether study participants are hormone receptor positive or negative.

Oncology nurses participate in research processes at different stages and capacities. **Research nurses** are study coordinators who assist with enrolling participants, verifying and obtaining informed consent, ensuring timely completion of pre-trial requirements, ensuring ongoing following of protocols throughout the trial, and maintaining and reporting data. Oncology nurses may also be involved as the nurse administering the trial regimen in an outpatient clinic or inpatient hospital setting. No matter which setting or role the nurse is functioning within, the priorities of care are voluntary informed consent by the patient, strict adherence to treatment protocols, and continuous high-quality communication between the clinical and research teams.

Genomic and Genetic Testing

Molecular testing and genetics have become a major part of prevention, screening, diagnosis, treatment, and ongoing surveillance of cancer. In fact, these areas have led to the greatest advancements in oncology history. The identification of tumor-specific biomarkers and advances in DNA sequencing have resulted in the ability for researchers to develop more targeted therapies and recognize cancer earlier. Additionally, researchers have been able to identify at-risk patients and diagnose cancers at earlier stages with the goal of improved long-term health outcomes.

Most cancers develop sporadically as an **acquired mutation** occurring during the process of DNA synthesis. Mutations can occur at any time, but they become more likely to occur in different conditions or after exposure to certain substances (called **carcinogens**). The most common mutations that result in many types of acquired cancers are mutations of the tumor suppressor genes p53 and TP53, which function to regulate cell growth and death. **P53 mutations** are most associated with breast, colorectal, liver, lung, and ovarian cancers. **TP53 mutations** are associated with ovarian, breast, colorectal, head and neck, and lung tumors.

Cancer can also develop due to inherited genetic mutations, called **germline mutations**, that are passed from parent to offspring. **Hereditary cancers** make up approximately 5 to 10 percent of all cancer types. Genetic testing may be indicated for individuals with family history of cancer or may be performed following a cancer diagnosis to determine the type of cancer and whether the patient's family may be at increased risk. This type of genetic testing looks for specific genetic variants that have a known link to cancers or cancer syndromes.

For example, if there are genetic mutations in the tumor suppressor genes Breast Cancer Gene 1 (BRCA1) or Breast Cancer Gene 2 (BRCA2), there is an increased risk for the development of breast, ovarian, pancreatic, and prostate cancers. BRCA1 and BRCA2 are considered DNA repair genes; therefore, cancer risk is also increased since these genes will no longer recognize and fix errors that occur during DNA synthesis. These genetic mutations are often hereditary (called **Hereditary Breast and Ovarian Cancer Syndrome**) but may also be acquired sporadically during an individual's lifetime. Human Epidermal Growth Factor Receptor 2 (HER2), which is an oncogene that produces a protein associated with cell growth, can also become mutated and lead to uncontrolled cell growth. **HER2 mutation** is most associated with breast cancer, but it is also associated with gastrointestinal cancer as well as cancers of the ovaries, endometrium, bladder, lungs, and head and neck. Another group of oncogenes, **RAS genes**, functions normally to create proteins that regulate cell growth and death. When RAS is mutated, normal healthy cells can become cancer cells. Many pancreatic, lung, and colorectal cancers are associated with

RAS mutations. Lynch syndrome is yet another inherited mutation of one of the **mismatch repair** (MMR) genes that prevents DNA errors from being fixed, which will inevitably result in cancer. Lynch syndrome is strongly associated with colorectal cancer risk; however, it is also associated with increased risk for endometrial cancer as well as most other types of cancer.

Another way that molecular testing and genetics come into play in oncology is through tumor markers. **Tumor markers** are substances (often proteins) that are produced at a higher rate in the presence of certain cancers. They are used for screening, staging, monitoring, and treatment of cancer. Typically, tumor markers are measured using a blood specimen. Some examples of common tumor markers include the following: CA-125 (ovarian cancer), calcitonin (medullary thyroid cancer), beta-2-microglobulin (multiple myeloma, CLL, lymphoma), CA15-3/CA27.29 (breast cancer), CA 19-9 (pancreatic, gallbladder, bile duct, gastric cancers), CEA (colorectal cancer), CD19 (B-cell lymphoma and leukemias), CD20 (Non-Hodgkin lymphoma), fibrinogen (bladder cancer), estrogen receptor (ER) and progesterone receptor (PR) (breast cancer), immunoglobulins (multiple myeloma), prostate-specific antigen (PSA), and thyroglobulin (thyroid cancer).

Lastly, major advances in oncology within the past 20 years have increasingly made targeted therapies more widely available based on specific tumor types. These **biomarkers** are evaluated using tissue samples obtained via biopsy. They are used to determine treatments and continue to evaluate the efficacy of said treatment. Some of the common markers and their associated cancer locations are as follows: BRAF V600 (cutaneous melanoma, colorectal cancer, non-small cell lung cancer), DPD (breast, colorectal, gastric, pancreatic cancer), EGFR (non-small cell lung cancer), JAK2 (some leukemias), KRAS (colorectal and non-small cell lung cancer), NTRK gene fusion (solid tumors), and ROS1 gene rearrangement (non-small cell lung cancer).

Next Generation Sequencing (NGS)

Next-generation sequencing (NGS) is a highly advanced method of analyzing DNA and RNA fragments to determine information regarding gene activity, variations in genetic sequencing, gene behaviors, and genetic structuring. NGS allows genomic testing and research to obtain more cost-effective and accurate results. This ensures that proper analysis and disease insights can be obtained from the results acquired. NGS studies have been used to research a variety of disease processes, including infectious diseases, microbiomes, cancer, and genetic abnormalities. NGS has made it possible to analyze data regarding gene fusion, methylation, RNA editing, microbiome profiling, and targeted gene analysis. This data can be used in functional, pathway, and integrative analysis, which leads to advancements in diagnostic criteria, healthcare prognosis, treatments, and outcomes. NGS uses three main approaches to analyzing genomic data: targeted sequencing, whole exome sequencing (WES), and whole genome sequencing (WGS). Targeted sequencing involves analyzing the gene in a targeted area to obtain more specific data, including gene duplications, insertions, and deletions. WES is a broader approach that sequences the exome of the gene, where protein coding occurs in the genome. Most genome diseases are found in this area and, by sequencing the exome gene variations, can be analyzed. WGS is the most inclusive gene sequence in which an individual's entire DNA sequence and genome are analyzed. WGS can analyze both large and small whole genome sequences, making it a very comprehensive examination.

Site-Specific Cancer Considerations

Pathophysiology

Cancer is a large group of diseases that are commonly expressed as carcinomas, sarcomas, melanomas, lymphomas, and leukemia. The normal cells experience mutation due to one or multiple carcinogens, such diesel exhaust, radiation, or viruses. This results in changes in the cell membrane that inhibit the tumor-suppressing action of the normal cell and alter the cell surface antigens, which diminishes the immune response. The abnormal cell matures through the process already described and eventually manifests the following characteristics: abnormal cell structure; haphazard, uncontrolled cellular replication; and destructive invasiveness. **Malignant cells** cause harm not only by occupying space, but by invading adjacent and distant tissues, and although **benign tumors** can also cause harm by occupying space, the tumors remain encapsulated and do not invade surrounding tissues. In addition, oncology nurses understand that if a carcinoma originates in the breast and subsequently metastasizes to the brain, the tumor in the brain will resemble breast cancer since it is the original tumor type that has invaded distant tissues.

Once the normal tissue has been invaded, the malignant cells are able to create an extracellular environment that supports the growth of the tumor and facilitates ongoing metastasis by alterations in three processes that control normal **cellular proliferation**: density-dependent inhibition, cell-surface adhesion, and contact inhibition. The proliferation of normal cells depends on the level of growth hormones and the action of the cellular growth factors. When the **cell density** is sufficient for normal function, the levels of the hormones and growth factors decrease, which slows proliferation. Malignant cells continue to replicate because the cells are independently capable of producing sufficient growth factors even when hormone levels do not support growth. Normal cells create an orderly matrix that is supported by **cell surface adhesion** molecules; however, malignant cells are able to suppress these molecules, which allows the malignant cells to more easily invade normal tissue. When cells come in contact with one another, during normal cellular growth, replication is stopped according to the concept of **cell contact inhibition**; however, malignant cells do not respond to those signals. When a new tumor grows to a density of approximately one million cells, malignant cells are capable of initiating **angiogenesis**, which is the development of new blood vessels that support tumor growth and provide new pathways for metastasis.

Diagnostic Measures

A comprehensive physical exam is an essential first step in the diagnosis of cancer. Providers use the results of the exam to identify the appropriate diagnostic tests, which are intended to confirm the findings of the screening tests, provide direction for the therapeutic plan, and continue surveillance of recurrent or new disease. Diagnostic studies are often a variation of the screening test. For instance, a **screening mammogram** generally consists of two views—craniocaudal and mediolateral oblique—of each breast, while a **diagnostic mammogram** may use one or more additional views—spot compression and magnification views—to study an identified abnormality. In contrast, it appears that the most significant difference between a screening colonoscopy and a diagnostic colonoscopy is the issue of coding and reimbursement. Oncology nurses must be aware that the initial intent of the exam—surveillance of a previous condition, a history of current symptoms, or routine screening—may dictate the patient's responsibilities for payment. Depending on the location and form of the cancer, ultrasonography, CT scans, bone scans, MRI, nuclear imaging studies, and blood and body fluid analyses will be considered. In some instances, the definitive diagnosis can only be established by a **biopsy** of the malignant cells, which can identify the characteristics of the cells. Biopsy samples can be collected by shaving a thin layer of skin, by punching a core of tissue from the skin, by aspirating fluid and tissue from a superficial tumor with a fine needle or a coring needle, by an incisional or excisional biopsy, or by removing lymph nodes that are proximal to the malignancy.

In addition, tumor markers have been identified for many malignant conditions that may be helpful in monitoring the tumor burden or identifying a recurrence of the disease; however, in most cases, these markers do not provide definitive details about the primary disease. Some of the more common markers include carcinoembryonic antigen (CEA), cancer antigen 125 (CA125), prostate-specific antigen (PSA), and Estrogen Receptor Assay (ERA). **CEA** is a blood test that identifies the presence of an antigen that is associated with GI tissue malignancies. It is not specific for identifying a primary site; however, persistent elevations of this marker greater than 10 ng/mL are indicative of significant disease, and levels greater than 20 ng/mL are indicative of metastatic disease. Oncology nurses must be aware that cigarette smoking affects the accuracy of this test, and false-positive results are common in smokers. **CA125** is also a blood test that is useful for monitoring ovarian cancer, with levels greater than 35 U/mL considered positive. **PSA** is a blood test that measures an antigen that is present in prostate tumors. Oncology nurses understand that false-positives are common in individuals with **benign prostatic hypertrophy**, and the PSA level can also be falsely elevated if the test sample is drawn immediately after a rectal exam due to possible manipulation of the prostate gland. ERA identifies the presence or absence of estrogen receptors in a malignant tumor. This is an essential pre-treatment assessment because tumors that are estrogen-receptor negative do not respond to hormone therapy, while an estimated 55 percent of estrogen-receptor positive tumors can be effectively treated with hormone therapy.

Common Metastatic Locations

The ability to metastasize to distant tissues and organs differentiates malignant tumor cells from benign tumor cells and is responsible for the greatest harm to the patient. **Metastasis** is a sequence of events that allows the malignant cell to travel some distance and to establish a new tumor formation at that site. The most common sites of metastatic disease are the bone, liver, and lungs; however, predictable patterns of metastasis for individual forms of cancer have been identified. These patterns, identified in the following table, can serve as a blueprint for continued screening and early detection of metastatic disease.

Primary Site	Metastatic Site
Bladder	Bone, liver, lung
Breast	Bone, brain, liver, lung
Colon	Liver, lung, peritoneum
Kidney	Adrenal gland, bone, brain, liver, lung
Lung	Adrenal gland, bone, brain, liver, other lung
Melanoma	Bone, brain, liver, lung, skin, muscle
Ovary	Liver, lung, peritoneum
Pancreas	Bone, liver, lung
Prostate	Adrenal gland, bone, liver, lung
Rectal	Liver, lung, peritoneum
Stomach	Liver, lung, peritoneum
Thyroid	Bone, liver, lung
Uterus	Bone, liver, lung, peritoneum, vagina

The **metastatic process** is a sequence of events that begins when the malignant cell is able to penetrate the wall of a blood vessel or a lymph node at the site of the original tumor. The cell then travels through the blood vessel or the lymphatic vessel for some distance and eventually stops in a small vessel, penetrates the wall of the vessel, and enters the normal tissue or organ. The invading cells undergo cellular replication, evolve into a small tumor, trigger the process of angiogenesis, and create a vascular network to nourish the new tumor and facilitate the invasion of the surrounding tissues.

Staging and Histological Grading

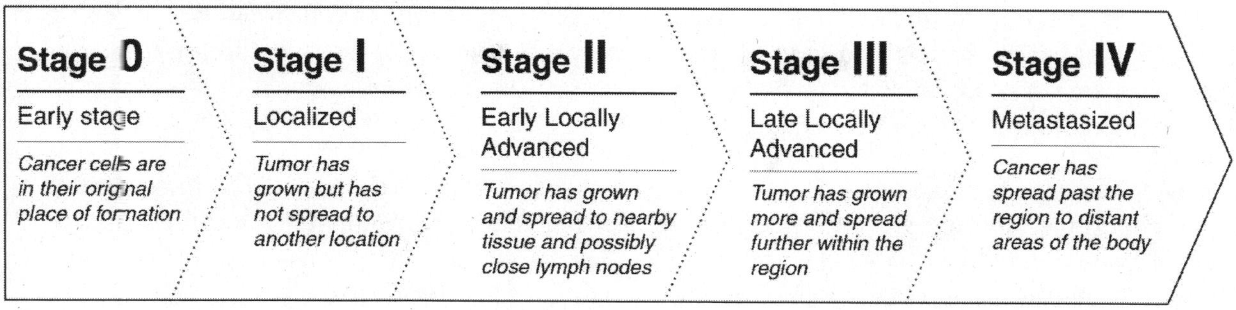

Malignancies are staged according to the tumor size and the presence or absence of lymph node involvement and metastasis. The **TNM system** is used to standardize the reporting of the patient's disease. The "T" classifies the size of the tumor from no tumor detectable to tumor in situ, or T1–T4. The "N" classifies lymph node involvement from N1 or N2—not able to identify or no nodes identified—to N3, which signifies the number of involved nodes. The "M" classifies the presence or absence of distant metastasis from not able to detect metastasis to no metastasis identified to M1, which indicates the presence of distant metastasis.

Tumor cells are also graded in terms of the degree to which the cellular structure deviates from the originating cell structure. **Well-differentiated** cells that more closely resemble the cell of origin are associated with a more favorable prognosis because the cells tend to grow and metastasize more slowly. The source of the original cell structure cannot be identified in **poorly differentiated** tumor cells which means that their behavior will be unpredictable and most likely harmful to the patient. These standardized details are used to develop an individualized plan of care based on treatment results from similar cancers and to predict the prognosis and possibility of recurrence or recovery. The scores of this general **grading system** range from GX (grade cannot be determined) to G4 (undifferentiated), which correlates with a high-grade tumor. This grading system is essential to the treatment of certain cancers including breast cancer, prostate cancer, primary brain tumors, and soft tissue sarcomas.

In addition, there are several condition-specific grading systems that compare the patient's tumor with different categories of normal cells. The **Nottingham Scale** is used in the diagnosis of breast cancer to compare tubule structure, size and shape of the nucleus, and the number of proliferating cells. The **Gleason scale** is used to grade cellular structure of a prostate tumor and is reported according to the similarities between the normal cells and the tumor cells. The **Byrne scale** is used to classify oral squamous cell carcinoma.

Prognosis

The **prognosis** is an estimate of the likely outcome of a cancerous condition and is the sum result of multiple factors related to that cancer, including the type, location, staging, histological grade, and evidence of metastasis. Additional factors that influence the prognosis include the patient's age, baseline health status, and individual response to therapy. The prognosis of individual cancer types varies widely, with the 5-year survival rate of stage I pancreatic cancer estimated at 12–14 percent, contrasted with the identification of some forms of leukemia as chronic diseases. The prognosis may be expressed in terms of survival rates, and oncology nurses must be knowledgeable about the various statistical models in order to assist patients in understanding their disease. Cancer-specific or disease-specific **cancer survival** is defined as the percentage of patients with specific cancerous conditions who did not die from the disease within a stated time frame, which is usually five years. In contrast, **overall**

survival is defined as the percentage of patients with the same disease who do not die from any cause within the stated time frame. **Relative survival** is not specific to the type of cancer but is an estimate of the percentage of individuals who survive a stated interval of time from diagnosis. Disease-free or **recurrence-free survival** refers to the percentage of patients who have no evidence of disease for a stated period of time following treatment.

Colorectal cancer prognosis depends on the stage at diagnosis, which is determined by the extent of tumor penetration through the bowel wall, as well as lymph node involvement. For localized disease, 5-year survival can be as high as 90 percent, but only 39 percent of patients are diagnosed at an early stage. Stage IV disease has a 5-year survival rate of less than 15 percent.

Lung cancer is often diagnosed at advanced stages, leading to poor prognosis. For **non-small cell lung cancer** (NSCLC), the overall 5-year survival rate is 26 percent, with localized and regional disease more favorable than distant disease. In **small cell lung cancer** (SCLC), the overall 5-year survival rate is 7 percent. Positive prognostic factors include less than 5 percent weight loss prior to diagnosis, female gender, and good performance status.

Prostate cancer prognosis is heavily influenced by the grade of the tumor. The 5-year survival rate of a grade 1 tumor is 60 percent, with grade 4 tumors being 5 percent. Localized and regional disease has a 5-year survival rate of near 100 percent, whereas distant—or metastatic—disease has a survival rate of 31 percent. Seminal vesicle involvement at diagnosis is an important, unfavorable prognostic indicator.

The **breast cancer** 5-year survival rate for all stages is 90 percent, with localized disease being 99 percent, regional 86 percent, and metastatic 29 percent. Poor prognostic factors include lymph node involvement, larger tumors, higher-grade tumors, hormone receptor-negative cancer, and invasive tumors.

Bladder cancer prognosis is influenced by stage and grade. Stage 0 has a 5-year survival rate of ninety-eight percent, while stage IV has a rate of fifteen percent. Most metastasis will occur within four years of diagnosis, with the majority appearing within one year. Poor prognostic factors include poor differentiated tumors, large tumors, and multiple tumors.

For **head and neck cancers**, the 5-year survival rate is 68 percent for oral cavity and pharynx cancers, 61 percent for laryngeal cancer, and 98 percent for thyroid cancer.

Upper gastrointestinal cancers have favorable prognoses when diagnosed in early stages and completely resected. However, the esophagus has no serosa (outer lining), so any tumor extension can spread rapidly. Additionally, stomach cancers are rarely diagnosed in early stages. The overall 5-year survival rate for **esophageal cancer** is 20 percent and for **stomach cancer** is 32 percent.

Leukemia prognosis varies based on type. **Acute lymphoblastic leukemia** (ALL) has a 5-year survival rate of 40 percent in adults, with males having a worse prognosis, along with those who have white blood cell counts greater than 50,000 at diagnosis. **Acute myeloid leukemia** (AML) has a 5-year survival rate of 24 percent despite over 65 percent of adults achieving complete response after induction therapy. **Chronic lymphocytic leukemia** (CLL) has a 5-year survival rate of 83 percent and a 10-year survival rate of 59 percent. **Chronic myelogenous leukemia** (CML) prognosis depends on the stage of disease and response to treatment, but 5-year survival rates are around 85 percent.

Lymphoma is broken into Hodgkin and Non-Hodgkin lymphoma. **Hodgkin** has a cure rate of over 80 percent with combined radiation and chemotherapy treatments. However, patients are at greater risk of other primary cancer types later in life. Newly diagnosed patients are given a prognosis according to the **International Prognostic Score**, which considers cell type, presence or absence of B symptoms (such as night sweats and weight loss), spleen involvement, and the number of node sites involved. **Non-Hodgkin** is split into low-grade or high-grade lymphomas. Low-grade can have a survival rate of over 20 years without aggressive treatment. High-grade is more aggressive, and the 5-year survival rate is over 60 percent.

Cervical and uterine cancers have similar 5-year survival rates. For localized disease, the 5-year survival rate is nearly 100 percent, but it drops to less than 60 percent if there is localized lymph node involvement and less than 15 percent for metastatic disease. In **cervical cancer**, adenocarcinomas have a worse prognosis than squamous cell. Poor prognostic factors for **uterine cancer** include older age, lymph node involvement, large tumors, and non-endometrioid histology. High estrogen receptor levels have a positive impact on prognosis.

Ovarian cancer prognosis has a 5-year survival rate of 48 percent. Localized disease has a 93 percent survival rate; however, it is usually diagnosed in an advanced state. Prognosis is determined by stage, histologic type and grade, and residual bulk of tumor after surgery. Positive prognostic factors include younger age, good performance status, absence of ascites, and a cell type other than mucinous or clear cell carcinoma.

Testicular cancer has a 5-year survival rate of 95 percent for all stages. Prognosis is initially determined by tumor markers and bulk of disease. If tumor markers are low and there is low volume of disease, it is considered favorable risk. If tumor markers are high or there is high volume of disease, it is considered unfavorable.

Kidney and ureter cancer has a 5-year survival rate of 76 percent. Prognosis correlates to cell type, with clear cell tumors having a more favorable prognosis. Poor prognostic factors include advanced age, male gender, poor performance status, elevated platelet counts, low hemoglobin, elevated serum calcium and lactate dehydrogenase levels, and elevated C-reactive protein levels.

Pancreatic and biliary cancers have a 5-year survival rate of 15 percent for stage I cancer and less than 1 percent for stage IV disease. Favorable factors for **pancreatic cancer** include a tumor that is resectable and confined to the head of the pancreas, shorter duration of symptoms, and low-grade tumor.

Melanoma prognosis is related to the stage of the tumor at diagnosis and is dependent on thickness and whether ulceration is present. Localized disease has a 5-year survival rate of over 95 percent, whereas distant metastatic disease has a 16 percent survival rate. It is considered an aggressive disease with high potential for metastasis and recurrence.

Brain and other neurological cancers can be either of a primary or secondary tumor. They are either benign, meaning they may be nonmalignant but still have the potential to cause significant issues depending on the location, or they are malignant, meaning they are aggressive or fast growing. Poor prognostic indicators include age and performance status. Whether the **brain cancer** is a primary CNS tumor or a secondary tumor, survival is considered to be in the range of months versus years.

Classification

Carcinomas are the most common form of cancer and originate mainly in the skin, breast, lungs, and pancreas. **Sarcomas** arise from connective and supportive tissues, including bones, tendons, cartilage, muscles, and fat, and are more common in younger individuals. Sarcomas most often present with bone pain and a tumor on the bone. **Myelomas** originate in bone marrow plasma cells, which are responsible for the production of serum proteins that are necessary for antibody formation. Leukemias also arise from the bone marrow and result in the production of excessive amounts of immature white cells that are not capable of combatting infection. **Leukemias** can also cause alterations in red cell production, which results in altered clotting of the blood, fatigue, and anemias. The three different forms of leukemia are identified by the cells involved: granulocytic leukemia is related to immature white cells, lymphatic is related to alterations in the lymphoid blood cells, and polycythemia vera is related to the red blood cells. **Lymphomas** are solid tumors that begin in the nodes and vessels of the lymphatic system and also in the stomach, breast, and brain. There are two forms of lymphomas—Hodgkin lymphoma and non-Hodgkin lymphoma—that are differentiated by the presence of the diagnostic **Reed-Steinberg cells** in Hodgkin lymphoma. Due to the complexity of the disease, there are also "mixed types" of cancer that manifest some combination of these basic forms of the disease.

Performance Status

Performance status assessment is a vital part of cancer prognosis and treatment. Performance status is used to assess a patient's ability to live independently and perform normal activities of daily living (ADLs) without assistance. This assessment is used to predict how the patient will react to treatment regardless of age or cancer type. ADLs include simple tasks such as ambulation, bathing, and eating or drinking. There are two assessments that are commonly used to determine performance status: the Eastern Cooperative Oncology Group (ECOG) assessment and the Karnofsky assessment. ECOG assesses patients on a scale of 0–5, with 0 being completely independent with no restrictions, 1 indicating some restrictions in strenuous activities, 2 being the ability to complete ADLs but not strenuous or nonstrenuous activities, 3 indicating limited self-care ability, 4 meaning the patient is completely disabled, and 5 indicating death. The Karnofsky assessment scores the patient on a scale of 0–100, with 0 being deceased and 100 being fully active. These scales are very important in determining which treatment plan is utilized as well as the quality of life expected following treatment. Performance status assessments are also commonly used as clinical trial exclusion criteria to determine if a patient is a viable candidate for the trial medication or treatment. Typically, patients with a 0–1 score on the ECOG assessment or over a 70 on the Karnofsky assessment are good candidates for clinical trials. Due to the severe side effects of most cancer medications, it is important to determine the patient's performance status to monitor their overall prognosis and outcomes.

Scope and Standards of Practice

Professional Practice Evaluation and Accreditation

Professional Practice Evaluation

Personal and collective growth in the field of nursing requires ongoing evaluation of professional practice. This occurs on individual, group, organizational, and global levels throughout the field of nursing. Performing this necessary critique identifies strengths and weaknesses and allows for ongoing advancement of the profession.

General areas of evaluation can focus on many performance aspects. Aspects of **professionalism** (e.g., appearance, behavior, communication, and leadership style) can be addressed as well as the level of adherence to applicable standards or policies. Another performance category could be related to growth and development, including completed continuing education or advanced certification (e.g., becoming an Oncology Certified Nurse). Other areas of evaluation include engagement with professional organizations, committees, quality improvement projects, or community involvement. Additionally, contributions to the field of nursing or healthcare (e.g., professional writing or political involvement) can be considered.

On a personal level, nurses perform self-reflection and planning to determine how they feel about their performance and potential areas for improvement. They can formulate professional goals and plan the development necessary to achieve those goals. At a team or organizational level, nurses also receive feedback from peers and leadership. **Peer feedback** identifies how colleagues perceive the performance of their coworkers. **Leadership feedback** often provides a more global view of performance through comparison of personal performance to averages of larger groups (e.g., the unit, hospital, or region). Organizations also receive feedback in the form of surveys from employees as well as the organization's customers. Each level of evaluation provides opportunities to examine growth pathways and formulate development plans.

Upon identifying an opportunity for improvement, it is critical to follow up with a plan for development. Goals should be specific, time-bound, and identify resources necessary to achieve the goal. On an organizational level, this can include referencing education materials, enrolling in professional or organizational groups or counsels, or breaking goals down into smaller steps. Lastly, re-evaluation must occur at regular intervals to follow up on previous goals. This provides external accountability for completing the steps and achieving the stated goals.

Accreditation

Oncology nurses often work with multiple accrediting agencies. First, their education usually must come from a regionally accredited university. Next, oncology nurses typically work in healthcare facilities that are accredited for safety, regulation, and quality. **The Joint Commission** is an independent, highly reputed, non-profit accrediting agency that focuses specifically on quality in healthcare. To be accredited by the Joint Commission, an organization must meet stringent benchmarks and undergo continuous monitoring to ensure they continue to meet these high standards. These standards include 250 practices that focus on patient satisfaction, environmental safety, hygiene and cleanliness, medical error prevention, disease control, provider credentialing, patient safety, security of personal information, and so on.

Beyond standards that support their education and workplace, nurses are likely to become familiar with standards that pertain to their daily operating procedures. The Commission on Cancer is an accrediting program run by the American College of Surgeons that specifically upholds standards for cancer programs. Its standards focus on patient-centric care, advocacy, emotional support and counseling, survivorship, reducing health outcome disparities, and other factors that encompass cancer patients and their families holistically and as interdependent units.

The Joint Commission is a globally recognized accrediting body from whom healthcare organizations seek evaluations and **accreditation** for quality of care. Oncology care sites operating within these organizations must comply with the same standards of care as any other care site in order to seek or maintain accreditation through The Joint Commission. Largely, this encompasses adherence to applicable local and federal laws as well as the development and following of policies and procedures. Additionally, all members of an accredited organization must comply with current **National Patient**

Safety Goals®, which set forth specific steps to reduce patient harm (e.g., infection control, fall reduction, and decreased medical errors).

In addition to standard accreditation through The Joint Commission, the organization also currently provides additional disease-specific certification for organizations specializing in treatment of brain tumors and lung cancer. Programs seeking these advanced certifications must offer comprehensive coordination and execution of care. They must utilize the highest standards of practice in the diagnosis and treatment of these cancers, while also holding staff to a higher standard of credentialing and ongoing education.

Outpatient oncology practices seeking to maintain high quality patient care practices also utilize the **Quality Oncology Practice Initiative** (**QOPI**). This program allows practices to self-report quality measures and receive scoring and evaluation in comparison with other participating oncology practices. Additionally, organizations can seek certification, which provides opportunities for earning points for submission for the **Merit-based Incentive Payment System** (**MIPS**). Quality standards focus on concepts such as timely testing and diagnosis, appropriate treatment planning and documentation practices, holistic management of patient complaints and side effects, and thorough patient education.

Yet another organization that provides healthcare accreditation is the American Nurses Credentialing Center (ANCC) Magnet Recognition Program®. This program provides a foundation and guidance to organizations seeking **Magnet designation®**, which denotes that they maintain the highest standard of nursing care. The focus of the program is to guide and support organizations to put processes and structures in place to support high quality outcomes. This includes concepts such as transformational leadership, professional development, opportunities for growth, excellent practices, promoting innovation, and the use of current evidence to support care. These principles are maintained in all care sites, including oncology care areas.

Collaboration and Communication

Collaboration

Oncology is a highly complex field that requires a high degree of collaboration between specialties and disciplines in order for patients to receive timely and appropriate care. The nature of cancer is that any delay in diagnosis or intervention can be costly to patient morbidity and mortality; therefore, efficient coordination of care is critical. One way that organizations facilitate this is by developing processes and policies to improve care coordination for oncology patients. One example of this is oncology-specific care sites which house laboratory, radiology, pathology, infusion centers, pharmacies, and other oncology resources in one location. The goal is to streamline services and improve patient experiences and outcomes. Additionally, care coordinators (often nurses or social workers) can help ensure that patients move through the system with minimal disruption. **Care coordinators** assist patients in understanding their care plan, ensuring that necessary procedures and appointments are scheduled and completed, processing and reporting critical results, voicing and addressing their needs, and finding available resources.

Another way that collaboration is utilized in oncology is through interdisciplinary involvement. Cancer is a systemic disease that requires collaboration between disciplines to ensure the best possible outcomes. For instance, oncologists collaborate with pathologists, surgeons, and radiologists to coordinate cancer treatments. **Referrals** may also be made to dietary/nutrition, physical therapy, psychiatry, psychology, integrative medicine, sleep medicine, palliative care, hospice, and other supportive services for patients during their cancer treatment. Pre-existing conditions or the development of toxicities related to treatment may require collaboration with other specialties such as endocrinology, gastroenterology, gynecology, or dermatology.

Yet another way that collaboration can occur is by way of second opinions or peer review. A patient may request a second opinion, or a provider may recommend patients for second opinions. This often occurs if the referring provider knows of another provider or organization that has further specialization in the type of cancer or circumstances the patient is experiencing. Tumor boards, care team meetings, and peer review are other ways that oncologists collaborate to improve outcomes. These peer meetings provide space for healthcare providers to compare approaches and review options for challenging or rare cases.

Communication

Effective communication is a critical aspect of providing high-quality oncology care. Appropriate communication (verbal, nonverbal, and written) ensures timely delivery of care, promotes positive health outcomes, and improves patient experiences. Additionally, treatment and patient conditions are highly susceptible to change and require precise assessment, documentation, and communication to maintain patient safety. Lastly, there are legal, professional, and ethical implications to consider regarding maintaining appropriate communication within the healthcare system.

To effectively coordinate care and provide efficient progression from diagnosis to treatment, healthcare professionals must be able to share information quickly and effectively. One way this is accomplished is by using clear and concise policies, protocols, and order sets. Clarity is key to ensuring that all members of the care team understand their roles in the process. Additionally, written process flows and patient education materials help patients and caregivers know what to expect as they move through the process.

Another aspect of effective communication is utilization of **electronic medical records** (**EMR**). These systems facilitate enhanced interdisciplinary communication throughout the care continuum by making pertinent patient information immediately available to care providers, decreasing errors in limiting handoffs of information, and increasing efficiency in eliminating the need to fax or call results to connected providers. **Patient portals** enhance patient access to their health information and patient-provider dialogue. EMR in-system messaging, alerts, and safety guardrails allow interdisciplinary providers to communicate quickly, provide more efficient care, and decrease errors in communication.

Oncology nurses are often the frontline caregivers working directly with patients throughout their cancer journey. For this reason, it is important that nurses understand how to effectively communicate. This requires clarity as well as timeliness of delivery. Within the interdisciplinary team, this fosters efficiency and safe delivery of care. With patients and families, effective communication encourages patient-provider connection and trust as well as improved patient experience and outcomes.

There are several ways oncology nurses can ensure effective communication within the care team as well as with patients and families. Standardized communication tools like **SBAR** (situation, background, assessment, and recommendation) provide caregivers with a concise and structured way to deliver complex information quickly to other providers. These tools can be useful in shift handoffs or when updating providers after a status change has occurred. Care team meetings are another way for interdisciplinary teams to communicate effectively about treatment plans.

During patient interactions, developing a trusting relationship ensures that patients feel comfortable sharing information with providers. Nurses can build trust with patients by using **active listening** techniques, such as sitting rather than standing during discussions, maintaining eye contact, using verbal cues (e.g., "I understand" and "Tell me more about that"), summarizing speaker's statements, asking clarifying questions, and using non-verbal cues (e.g., nodding, uncrossing arms, leaning toward the speaker, and having relaxed posture).

Culturally Congruent Care

Culture impacts every aspect of an individual's life. In the context of oncology nursing care, cultural experiences and beliefs shape the way patients and their families view cancer, cancer treatment, end-of-life and palliative care, grief, decision-making, the healthcare system, healthcare professionals, learning, priorities, and communication. Additionally, complex individual and systemic differences in cultural beliefs, prejudices, and biases lead certain groups to experience worse health outcomes. **Culturally congruent oncology care** considers and respects individual differences, enhances patient experiences, promotes equity in healthcare delivery, and improves overall outcomes of care.

Despite ongoing advancements in cancer detection and treatment, certain cultural groups continue to experience worse outcomes. For instance, Black and African American people have disproportionately higher rates of morbidity and mortality for many types of cancer. Death rates for breast cancer, cervical cancer, and prostate cancer are significantly higher for Black and African American people as opposed to White people. American Indian and Alaskan Natives have higher rates of death from kidney, liver, and intrahepatic bile duct cancers. Other **disparities** are evident in cancer incidence in rural versus urban areas; furthermore, higher education tends to decrease mortality rates for certain cancers. The reasons for disparities such as these are extremely complex; they relate to factors such as barriers to healthcare (e.g., education, financial status, and resource availability) or other lifestyle differences (e.g., diet, substance abuse, genetics, and environmental exposure). Additionally, systemic racism can contribute to chronic stress, distrust toward the healthcare system, mistreatment by healthcare professionals, and underrepresentation in health research. All of these factors impact health outcomes for **vulnerable populations**.

Cultural beliefs also shape the way patients and families process and respond throughout cancer diagnosis, treatment, and development. **Spiritual beliefs** about healing and disease can have a significant impact on treatment decisions and coping. Beliefs about conventional versus alternative medicine can also impact treatment decisions. Ethnic and familial cultural beliefs about healthcare decision-making, caregiving, resource allocation, isolation practices, and communication can also impact cancer care.

Myths and taboos can be yet another area where culture impacts care and may result in the withholding of information, treatment refusal, or delays in seeking care. Some examples of myths related to cancer include cancer being contagious or spread if operated upon. Some cultural taboos create difficulty when discussing topics of sexuality and reproductive organs. Additionally, cultural beliefs around communication of physical and/or mental health issues may pose challenges due to withholding of information. Oncology nurses serve as advocates and educators to assist patients and families to navigate these sensitive topics to improve patient outcomes.

Oncology nurses can further develop their cultural competency in many additional ways. One of the first steps is examination of personal beliefs and values. **Biases** and values are largely subconscious beliefs that impact how people interact with the world. They are dictated by the beliefs and values of our influences (e.g., family, friends, communities, religious and political groups, race, social class, ethnicity, sexual orientation, and disabilities). It takes intentional ongoing practice to recognize and critically reflect on one's personal beliefs.

Next, individuals must develop open, non-judgmental curiosity about the cultural beliefs of others. This includes an awareness of cultural differences as well as formal cultural education. Nurses should seek to educate themselves on how biases lead to disparities in health and healthcare delivery. It is also important for oncology nurses to seek cultural knowledge about individual patients by asking open-ended questions about beliefs, not making assumptions, and actively listening without judgement. These practices foster relationship-building and trust with patients and improve care for populations at risk of experiencing healthcare disparities.

On a systemic level, culturally congruent oncology care utilizes practices and resources to support individualized care. To begin, having **diversity** in hiring and promotion practices encourages more equal consideration and representation in business practices. Language resources, such as communication boards and interpreter services, can also support culturally sensitive care. Financial services can remove barriers to equal provision of healthcare services. Intake and assessment questionnaires can help identify cultural and spiritual practices that could potentially influence care. Staff training and continuing education is yet another way that organizations support culturally congruent care.

Occupational Health and Safety

There are unique **environmental safety** concerns to consider within oncology. Many cancer treatments that are highly effective at disrupting and killing cancer cells also impact healthy cells as well. Therefore, oncology nurses and other healthcare professionals within the specialty must take considerable steps to ensure the ongoing safety of patients, the public, and staff.

Safe Handling

In addition to the ethical imperative to promote safety, oncology practices are held to legal and professional standards of safe operation. Standards are issued by organizations such as the Occupational Safety and Health Administration (OSHA), Oncology Nursing Society (ONS), the National Institute for Occupational Safety and Health (NIOSH), and the United States Pharmacopeia (USP) Chapter 800. These organizations develop and maintain safety guidelines and operational standards for individuals handling chemotherapy and any other **hazardous drugs** (HD).

Many chemotherapy (and some immunotherapy) medications are considered potentially hazardous to humans, even at low doses of exposure. NIOSH designates HDs based on findings of impact on one or more of the following: risk for cancer (**carcinogenicity**), risk to fetus (**teratogenicity**), risk of reproductive toxicity, risk of organ toxicity (at low dose), and risk of damage to DNA (**genotoxicity**).

Safety measures begin with safe handling and preparation of HDs. To begin, any healthcare professional who participates in the handling of chemotherapy and biotherapy products (receiving, preparing, administering, or discarding) must receive appropriate training. For oncology nurses, this means chemotherapy and immunotherapy education prior to administering chemotherapy medications to patients. Nurses must also receive ongoing continuing education to maintain safe handling knowledge. Medications considered to be hazardous are prepared in designated pharmacy workspaces, under a special biological safety cabinet, and with the direction of specially trained and licensed pharmacy personnel (e.g., pharmacist, pharmacy technician, nurse, or doctor). Disposal of any chemotherapy medication, residue, and materials used in preparation and administration is highly regulated to prevent HDs from unintentionally entering the environment as waste.

Personal Protective Equipment (PPE)

Use of **personal protective equipment** (**PPE**) is another way that staff protect themselves from accidental exposure to HD. At minimum, two pairs of chemotherapy-rated gloves should be worn when handling any potentially hazardous drug or material used to prepare or administer an HD. This includes handling of bottles and packaging as well as patient body fluids for 48 hours after receiving an HD. One pair of chemotherapy-rated gloves is required to handle intact oral chemotherapy pills. Disposable, single-use, chemotherapy-rated gowns are also to be worn when handling HDs. Eye and/or face protection are worn when there is a risk for splashing (e.g., when initiating and discontinuing treatment medications).

In the event of an HD spill, additional safety measures are taken to control and clean the spill and limit exposure to the staff and public. Two pairs of chemotherapy-rated gloves, a chemotherapy-rated gown, eye and face shields, a respirator (i.e., N95), and shoe covers should be utilized to protect oneself when cleaning a spill. Additionally, **spill kits** must be immediately available in areas where HDs are being administered, and they should be utilized to assist with large spill cleanup. Instructions within the spill kit should be followed, as well as any applicable policies and procedures within the organization. Lastly, the use of **closed system transfer devices** (CSTDs) for the preparation and administration of chemotherapy can help prevent spills altogether.

Radiation safety is another point of consideration for oncology healthcare professionals. Sources of radiation in oncology can be sealed (e.g., brachytherapy pellets) or unsealed (e.g., intravenous radioisotopes). Sealed sources are secured to prevent unintentional release before their intended use. Unsealed sources can be any form (powder, liquid, gas) that requires a container to prevent it from causing exposure. Regardless of the type of radiation used, however, those working with radiation must take measures to prevent prolonged exposure. Ways to manage exposure include the use of dosimeter badges to measure the level of exposure staff receive during their shift. Exposure is limited by minimizing the amount of time and putting as much distance as possible between oneself and the source of radiation. Additionally, shields (e.g., lead apron or drapes) can provide additional protection from radiation exposure.

Patient Advocacy and Ethical Considerations

Advocacy/Moral Agency

The American Nurses Association (ANA) provides this definition of nursing practice: "The protection, promotion, and optimization of health and abilities; prevention of illness and injury; facilitation of healing; alleviation of suffering through the diagnosis and treatment of human response; and advocacy in the care of individuals, families, communities, and populations." The ANA also addresses the importance of advocacy in its Code of Ethics, specifically in Provision 3: "The nurse promotes, advocates for, and protects the rights, health, and safety of the patient." The ANA Code of Ethics further states: nurses must advocate "with compassion and respect for the inherent dignity, worth, and uniqueness of every individual, unrestricted by considerations of social or economic status, personal attributes, or the nature of health problems."

Advocacy is a key component of nursing practice. An **advocate** is one who pleads the cause of another; and the nurse is an advocate for patient rights. Preserving human dignity, patient equality, and freedom from suffering are the basis of nursing advocacy. Nurses hold a significant role that gives them the opportunity to care for patients in every way: meeting their needs, addressing concerns, and working to achieve positive outcomes. Additionally, they aid in communicating with physicians while and serve as a guide through the complexities of the medical system. Nurses educate the patient about tests and procedures, while maintaining awareness of how culture and ethnicity affect the patient's experience. Throughout the process, nurses strictly adhere to all privacy laws.

Advocacy is the promotion of the common good, especially as it applies to at-risk populations. It involves speaking out in support of policies and decisions that affect the lives of individuals who do not otherwise have a voice. Nurses meet this standard of practice by actively participating in the politics of healthcare accessibility and delivery. They are educationally and professionally prepared to evaluate and comment on the needs of patients at the local, state, and national level. This participation requires an understanding of the legislative process, the ability to negotiate with public officials, and a willingness to provide expert testimony in support of policy decisions. The advocacy role of nurses has the potential to address the needs of the individual patient, society, and members of the nursing profession.

In clinical practice, nurses represent the patient's interests through active participation in the development of the plan of care and subsequent care decisions. Advocacy, in this sense, is related to patient autonomy and the patient's right to informed consent and self-determination. Nurses provide the appropriate information, assess the patient's comprehension of the implications of the care decisions, and act as patient advocates by supporting the patient's decisions. In the critical care environment, patient advocacy requires the nurse to represent the patient's decisions even though those decisions may be opposed to those of the healthcare providers and family members.

Professionally, nurses advocate for policies that support and promote the practice of all nurses regarding access to education, role identity, workplace conditions, and compensation. The responsibility for professional advocacy requires nurses to provide leadership in the development of the professional nursing role in all practice settings that may include acute care facilities, colleges and universities, or community agencies. Leadership roles in acute care settings involve participation in professional practice and shared governance committees, providing support for basic nursing education by facilitating clinical and preceptorship experiences, and mentoring novice graduate nurses to the professional nursing role. In the academic setting, nurses work to ensure the diversity of the student population by participating in the governance structure of the institution, conducting and publishing research that supports the positive impact of professional nursing care on patient outcomes, and serving as an advocate to individual nursing students to promote their academic success. In the community, nurses may collaborate with government officials to meet the needs that are specific to that location.

The nurse must function as a **moral agent**. This means that the nurse must be morally accountable and responsible for personal judgment and actions. Nurses who practice with moral integrity possess a strong sense of themselves and act in ways consistent with what they understand is the right thing to do. **Moral agency** is defined as the ability to identify right and wrong actions based on widely accepted moral criteria. The performance of nurses as moral agents is dependent on life experiences, advanced education, and clinical experience in healthcare agencies. Moral agency can often be difficult to decipher when managing complex patient situations. When ethical dilemmas arise, such as handling end-of-life and refusal of treatment cases, the care team must work together to make the best care decisions possible with the patient in mind.

The role of moral agent requires nurses to have a strong sense of self and a clear understanding of the definition of right and wrong; however, nurses must also be aware that these perceptions of right and wrong will be challenged every day. The nurse can expect to encounter difficult situations where the moral action related to the patient's right to self-determination is opposed to the moral action with respect to competent patient care.

Ethical Considerations

Oncology nurses rely on ethical principles to guide decision-making in difficult circumstances. It is a firm values-based foundation that can be applied to any situation, along with applicable legal and standard-of-care considerations to make sound decisions. Ethics can be particularly helpful when moral dilemmas arise.

Historically, the general principle of **ethics** in healthcare has been to do the most good and to do no harm. The Hippocratic oath, a Greek medical text, was introduced in approximately 400 BC and is still recited in some medical school graduation ceremonies today. It declares that physicians shall always benefit patients to the extent possible and shall never harm or abuse patients. This basis of ethics is sometimes referred to as the consequentialist view and is associated with the principles of **beneficence** and **nonmaleficence**. The **Nursing Code of Ethics**, maintained by the American Nurses Association, outlines additional principles that guide nursing practice, specifically. In addition to the principles of nonmaleficence and beneficence, it conveys the imperative that nurses respect and advocate for patient rights to education and self-determination (**autonomy**). Additionally, it speaks to the charge for nurses to seek fair and appropriate distribution of resources (**justice**) and to always be honest in interactions (**veracity**).

Within the field of oncology, nurses embody these ethical values in their daily practice. Dilemmas can occur, however, when there seems to be no "good" outcome to be achieved, or when there seems to be conflicting values between members of the team, the patient, or their loved ones. Some common dilemmas include disagreements related to end-of-life decisions; issues where the patient disagrees with family wishes but does not speak up; delays or withheld treatments due to inability to pay; or conflicts between patient's cultural beliefs and the nurse's personal values. In all situations, the nurse is called to advocate for the patient above all else. This is achieved by ensuring that patients receive appropriate education, respecting the patient's wishes, and supporting the patient as much as they can to achieve their wishes. This requires the nurse to be aware of their own personal beliefs and not allow those to impact the way they provide care.

Additionally, for ethical dilemmas that are larger in scope and implication (e.g., the healthcare team feels it is unethical to continue life support for a patient and the family disagrees with the decision), hospitals must have processes in place for review and decision-making. These ethics committees provide consultation for specific situations to ensure representation, applicable policy-making, support, and ongoing staff education.

Self-Care

Self-care is a crucial part of maintaining a healthy personal and professional life as an oncology nurse. Oncology is an emotionally taxing field, in addition to the physical and mental demands placed on nurses. Oncology nurses are at significant risk for experiencing compassion fatigue and developing burnout. Research has shown that insufficient self-care practices contribute to both.

Caregivers can experience compassion fatigue in response to the distress of others, and as a result, they may feel overwhelmed and have difficulty coping. **Compassion fatigue** occurs because of a lack or deficit in the ability to separate oneself from the emotional experiences of others. It can manifest itself as emotional overwhelm, feelings of emotional detachment, or difficulty providing care for oneself and for others. **Burnout** is an adjacent state that is caused by chronic and total exhaustion (mental, physical, and emotional). Burnout symptoms can include fatigue, brain fog, depression, low frustration tolerance, and poor emotional control.

The key to addressing and preventing compassion fatigue and burnout is through self-care and building resilience. Self-care requires balancing personal needs with one's responsibilities to others. **Resiliency** is the ability to effectively respond, adapt, and grow in response to adversity. Ways to promote self-care and resilience include development of skills in the areas of emotional regulation, stress management, communication, and boundary setting. Additionally, it requires a holistic approach to preserving and maintaining personal wellness through mental, physical, emotional, and spiritual health activities.

Several evidence-based strategies have been shown to have a positive impact on self-care and resiliency. One way is by building compassion for oneself as well as gratitude. Strategies to achieve this include practicing positive self-talk, accepting that all humans (including oneself) make mistakes, treating oneself like a loved one or friend, writing or voicing things one is thankful for, and practicing mindfulness. **Mindfulness** refers to accepting reality in the moment without making judgements. Physical strategies for maintaining self-care include taking breaks, eating regularly, moving one's body, being outside, maintaining good sleep habits, maintaining social relationships and support systems, and journaling.

Self-care is unique to the individual. Perceptions have a tremendous impact on a person's reality; therefore, each nurse must develop a practice that feels fulfilling, healthy, and manageable for them. Development of personal self-care and resiliency strategies can be performed on one's own, but many hospital organizations are also developing programs to address the growing rates of compassion fatigue and burnout experienced by their staff. Nurses may participate in these programs, and they may also seek professional help through mental health and counseling services to support and facilitate self-care.

Standards of Care

Oncology nursing is a specialized field that goes beyond general nursing. Cancer diagnoses are complicated and unique; no patient will be treated the same way. The ONS first defined the **scope and standards of oncology nursing** in 1979 and has revised these regularly since then. The most current statement is available in full on the ONS website.

The scope of oncology nursing includes both traditional and non-traditional roles. Oncology nurses may work in administrative, research, or clinical positions; some may work in all three over the course of their careers. They may work in different areas of cancer, such as with only patients who have the same type of cancer, cancer prevention, or with survivors. Oncology nurses may provide support to family members, serve as a liaison to other resources (such as financial information or social agencies), or they may oversee patients who are in clinical trials. Some oncology nurses may work purely in healthcare administration or as educators. Even oncology nurses in traditional clinical roles have a variety of duties with which they may be tasked. Some nurses may focus purely on screening certain types of cancer (e.g., breast cancer in women over the age of 40), while others may focus on palliative and hospice services for terminal cancer patients.

The type of work and the demographic with whom they work can vary vastly between two oncology nurses. Depending on the type of work they hope to do, nurses may have different educational and career paths. All registered nurses (RN) can choose to work in oncology settings, but to progress more deeply in the oncology field, additional training is often needed. While a graduate degree is needed to work as an Advanced Practice Registered Nurse (APRN), this distinction opens many professional doors for nurses, such as serving as a nurse practitioner. Those who do not pursue the APRN distinction but pursue graduate-level education, such as a master's or doctorate degree in a relevant field, will have the opportunity to manage large teams of nurses or oversee clinical research.

The ONS offers certification programs that prepare and test nurses for specialized oncology competencies. The main certifications offered include Oncology Certified Nurse, Advanced Oncology Nurse Practitioner, Certified Pediatric Hematology Oncology Nurse, Certified Breast Care Nurse, and Bone and Marrow Transplant Certified Nurse. These distinctions show a commitment to expertise in the general oncology field as well as in certain specialized areas of cancer.

Finally, nurses across all aspects of the oncology field commit to standard ethical and professional standards. These include respect, compassion, and inclusivity toward patients and their families; commitment to offer the best, safest, and most beneficial medical solutions and care to the patient; to advocate for and make decisions that are in the patient's best interest; to invite the patient to engage and collaborate in his or her medical care; to adhere to best practices, high professional and ethical standards, and continuing education; and ultimately, to practice in a way that promotes oncology nursing as a valuable and necessary field.

Critical Thinking

Critical thinking is a skill that comes from experience (both successes and failures). The nurse-to-be can be the smartest person in the classroom, making perfect scores on every test, but will not be able to provide quality care without using critical thinking. Common practices for using critical thinking in nursing include the following:

- Using self-regulation
- Practicing problem-solving
- Analyzing and interpreting information
- Making appropriate inferences
- Using the nursing process

Self-Regulation

Self-regulation is a responsibility of every nurse. To self-regulate, the nurse must first fully understand their individual scope of practice (federal, state, and agency regulations). Practicing within the established scope of practice, the nurse's goal is to provide effective, safe, and ethical care practices.

Problem Solving

Problem-solving skills are essential in the practice of critical thinking. Using critical thinking to recognize the problem is important, but the nurse must also cultivate the mindset of finding potential solutions. Problem solving can be seen formally in care plans, but the nurse will need to understand the importance of putting this into practice.

For example, say a patient is prescribed digoxin, and the nurse is due to administer the medication. The nurse with critical thinking skills will check the heart rate prior to administering the medication. Upon further assessment, the heart rate is 40 bpm. The nurse with problem-solving skills will recognize that this medication should not be administered, and the medical provider should be contacted for further orders.

Analysis, Interpretation, and Making Inferences

Additional key practices in critical thinking include analyzing data, interpreting results, and making inferences based on that interpretation. Why is the patient's heart rate 40 bpm? That would be the question the nurse needs to analyze, and they could find that information by looking through past vital sign trends, medications, comorbidities, and procedures. It is important for the healthcare team not to stop at just recognizing the problem and solving it, as that does not likely prevent the problem from happening again. Analyzing the data gives the nurse the information to interpret and then allows them to make clinical inferences based on the results.

For example, if the previously mentioned patient was also taking ivabradine, an HCN channel blocker for progressing heart failure, the nurse could infer that the combination of ivabradine and digoxin is the culprit of the patient's bradycardia. The following is a breakdown of the critical-thinking process in this scenario:

- Analyzing the medication administration record
- Interpreting the results
- Inferring that the synergistic effect of the medications can cause the problem

This process of critical thinking allows the medical team to either closely monitor the patient on both medications or make a medication change to acknowledge the problem.

Nursing Process

While the nursing process is an accumulation of the previously discussed components of critical thinking, the nurse will need to understand the cycle of the nursing process. Below is a visual to demonstrate the steps of the **nursing process**.

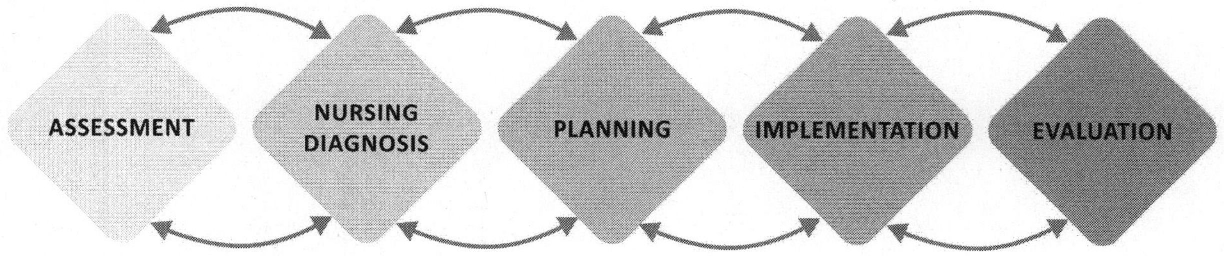

It is important to note that the cycle of the nursing process does not just move in one direction, and it may take multiple steps back to get to the solution. If the nursing diagnosis is no longer applicable, the nurse will need to go back to the assessment phase. Using this method of critical thinking gives the nurse an overview of the procedural process while also allowing for the flexibility needed in healthcare.

Documentation

The final step of assessment is the **documentation** of the findings. The oncology nurse is aware that safe patient care relies on accurate documentation that may or may not be shared in a larger provider network. Documentation is also required to meet reimbursement schedules for Medicaid, Medicare, and other private insurers. The assessment details, the subsequent interventions, and the patient's response to the interventions must be clearly evident and must be recorded in the appropriate EHR format.

A patient's chart is a legal record of assessments and care measures. Most facilities use an electronic health record, which with training provided during new employee orientation. Documentation may include timing related to observations, interventions, and patient responses. There are various charting systems used by patient care facilities to document patient data. Documentation requirements will be dictated by facility policy and regulatory guidelines. Two methods—charting by exception and comprehensive charting—are used.

Charting by exception requires that only vital signs and abnormal findings are documented. This charting method is somewhat controversial since a great amount of information about the patient is usually left out. It is sometimes argued that this is the safer way to chart, as only what is deviant from normal is noted, and thus, there is less room for documentation errors. The normal is assumed, unless otherwise noted. This method also saves time, as less information needs to be documented, leaving more time for patient care.

Some facilities prefer a **comprehensive method** of documentation, charting everything about the patient—normal and abnormal—in a very thorough manner. This way, when the patient's chart must be reviewed, especially in the case of a safety incident (e.g., a pressure sore develops or a patient falls), all details surrounding the event should be present in the medical record. This method is effective if all information is properly charted, although it can be quite time-consuming and take away from patient care time.

Documentation provides a defense for healthcare workers and patients in the case of patient incidents to show what was done for the patient. There is an adage that says, "If it wasn't charted, it didn't happen." The nurse needs to be mindful that the medical record is a legal document—a complete, thorough, and accurate documentation of care, according to facility policy.

Practice Quiz

1. Which of the following elements is most susceptible to the cytotoxic effects of chemotherapy?
   a. Endothelial lining of the GI system
   b. Cardiac myocytes
   c. Adipose cells
   d. Cells of the epidermis

2. In the absence of obvious bleeding, which of the following tends to be one of the earliest signs of colon cancer?
   a. Stomach pain
   b. Constipation
   c. Anemia
   d. Abdominal distension

3. The patient asks the oncology nurse to explain a pathology report. Which of the following choices is consistent with a tumor identified as T2, N2, M1, G2?
   a. A primary tumor of medium size with two positive lymph nodes, evidence of distant metastasis, and a moderately differentiated cell type
   b. A large tumor with positive lymph nodes that has spread locally and is well differentiated
   c. A tumor that is confined to the site of origin with positive lymph nodes and moderately differentiated cell type
   d. A small tumor with indeterminate node involvement, evidence of distant metastasis, and poorly differentiated cell type

4. When should oncology nurses develop relationships with patients?
   a. Before treatment begins
   b. During treatments when they first meet the patient
   c. After treatment and for all follow-up appointments
   d. Before, during, and after treatment

5. Which period of care is shown to be the most vulnerable to medical errors?
   a. Ten minutes into an operation
   b. Waiting rooms or time spent in a clinical room waiting for a provider
   c. Patient hand-offs
   d. The first follow-up appointment after discharge

See answers on the next page.

Answer Explanations

1. A: Rapidly dividing cells are more susceptible to chemotherapy because there is less time for the cell to repair the damage done by mutation and carcinogens, which means that the abnormal characteristics are passed on or "inherited" by the next generation of cells. The "turnover" times for each of the identified tissues include: 2 to 4 days for epithelial cells of the GI tract, 10 to 30 days for the epidermal cells, and 8 years for the adipose cells. In addition, although cardiomyocytes were believed to be incapable of regeneration due to the existence of scar tissue following myocardial injury, recent research indicates that 0.5 to 1 percent of the cardiomyocytes are replaced each year.

2. C: Iron-deficiency anemia may be the first sign of colon cancer, often before there is any frank bleeding noted in the stool. Choices *A, B,* and *D* are incorrect because these signs typically present in later stages once a tumor has grown larger in size.

3. A: T2 indicates that a tumor of moderate size is present. N2 indicates that malignant cells are present in two proximal lymph nodes. M1 indicates that there is evidence of distant metastasis of the malignant cells. G2 indicates that the cells are moderately well differentiated.

4. D: Oncology nurses play a critical role in developing relationships with patients, their families, and their caregivers. This relationship begins at the onset of a diagnosis and continues throughout the duration of and after treatment. Although Choices *A*, *B*, and *C* are all part of the process, the nurse-patient relationship spans from the beginning of the diagnosis to post-treatment.

5. C: Patient hand-offs between staff members and other transition periods, such as shift changes, are most vulnerable to medical errors due to poor communication, multitasking, or other distractions. These medical errors can lead to poor patient outcomes, additional health complications, and resource waste. Most medical organizations now have standardized hand-off procedures (i.e. SBAR hand-off technique) to reduce errors during this vulnerable period.

Treatment Modalities

Surgical and Procedural Interventions

Cancer surgery can refer to many different surgical procedures depending on the type, location, and severity of the cancer. When a **laparoscopy** is performed, the surgeon uses a thin tube and a camera to create a small abdominal incision in order to detect and possibly remove abnormal or cancerous growths. **Laser surgery** may also be used to remove affected tissues with the use of a high-intensity beam of light. In some situations, a surgeon may opt to use liquid nitrogen to freeze and kill abnormal cells with the use of **cryosurgery**. For certain types of skin cancer, surgeons may wish to perform **Mohs micrographic surgery** by removing one layer of tissue at a time and examining the tissue under a microscope until all the cells in a particular layer appear to be healthy. **Endoscopies** are minimally invasive surgical procedures using a narrow and flexible tube inserted into the patient's mouth, rectum, or vagina in order to explore the inside of a patient's body.

Fine-needle aspiration and core needle biopsies are common types of **needle biopsies** in which the medical professional inserts a needle through the patient's skin in order to collect a sample of cells in the affected area. These samples are sent to a pathologist for examination and to either confirm or rule out a cancer diagnosis. **Radiofrequency ablation** is another minimally invasive surgical procedure that uses electrical energy coupled with heat in order to kill cancer cells. The surgeon guides a narrow needle through the skin and toward the cancerous tissue. High-frequency energy is then passed through the needle and causes the surrounding tissue to heat up, destroying the nearby cells. Radiofrequency ablation is not intended to be a primary treatment for the majority of cancers but is an option to consider for patients who are not good candidates for surgery. If precancerous cells have been detected, a surgeon may perform preventative surgery to remove these cells. This type of surgery is common with precancerous polyps in the colon for instance. For patients who are at high risk for developing cancer due to mutated alleles that are known to cause cancer, prophylactic surgery may be an option. In **prophylactic surgery**, an organ or gland is removed that doesn't yet show signs of cancer but may eventually become cancerous. Prophylactic mastectomy (the removal of one or both breasts) is an example of prophylactic surgery.

Diagnostic surgery is primarily performed to confirm or rule out the presence of cancer. During diagnostic surgery, the surgeon will either remove some (**incisional biopsy**) or all (**excisional biopsy**) of the suspicious tissue which will then be examined by a pathologist. **Staging surgery** attempts to learn the actual size of the tumor or tumors; additionally, it may involve the removal of some lymph nodes in order to ascertain whether or not the cancer has spread and, if so, how far. One type of staging surgery is referred to as a staging or pathological laparotomy. Laparotomies allow surgeons to closely examine the abdominal organs for evidence of cancer and, if found, remove tissue samples for further examination. Curative or **primary surgery** refers to the removal of a tumor as well as the removal of some of the surrounding tissue known as the "margin." In some situations, however, it is too dangerous to remove the entire tumor. If this is the case, oncologists may perform a **debulking surgery** which removes as much of the tumor as is possible. Some surgical procedures are highly invasive and may negatively impact the appearance or function of certain areas of a patient's body. In these instances, **reconstructive surgery** may be an option in order to restore the body's appearance or function. **Palliative surgery** refers to surgical procedures that aim to relieve some of the side effects caused by the cancer. This is generally performed for patients with advanced forms of cancer in order to improve their quality of life.

Oncology nurses play an integral part of any surgical procedure and maintain varying responsibilities before, during, and after surgery. Oncology nurses prepare the operating room, organize the necessary instruments, perform patient preparation, pass instruments to the oncologist, monitor the patient's vital signs, control bleeding, document, and verify the instrument count once the surgery has ended. Prior to surgery, oncology nurses explain the preoperative instructions to patients and answer any questions. Following surgery, they perform post-assessment tasks such as monitoring the patient's emotional and physical well-being, providing patient education, anticipating and managing symptoms, administering medications and fluids, performing cancer treatments, and collaborating with a diverse group of healthcare professionals to establish an individualized treatment plan.

Blood and Marrow Transplant

Blood and marrow transplants are used for the treatment of certain blood-related cancers, such as leukemia and lymphoma. Blood cells can come from the patients themselves, related donors, or unrelated donors. Umbilical cord blood can also be donated and stored in public and private umbilical cord blood banks. When patients require a blood and marrow transplant, they will typically first go through chemotherapy or radiation to eradicate or decrease the number of tumors and/or reduce the size of the tumor. The second step is the infusion of either bone marrow, peripheral blood stem cells, or cord blood. **Bone marrow** refers to stem cells collected directly from bone marrow, as opposed to peripheral blood stem cells which are collected directly from the bloodstream. **Cord blood** refers to the blood that remains in the portion of the umbilical cord that has been cut after birth as well as the remaining blood in the discarded placenta. This blood is rich in hematopoietic (blood-forming) stem cells and contains red blood cells, white blood cells, platelets, and plasma.

Autologous blood and marrow transplants involve the collection of blood from a patient that will be given back to that same patient when required. Drawbacks associated with this form of transplant involve a shorter shelf life of the collected blood than blood collected from a donor, possible human error, and bacterial contamination of the blood. **Allogeneic blood and marrow transplants** involve the collection of blood from a donor that is then given to the patient when required. Allogeneic donors can be relatives of the patient or not related at all. Risks associated with this form of transplant involve the possible transmission of viral infections such as hepatitis, the human immunodeficiency virus (HIV), the human T-cell lymphotropic virus, and more recently, Creutzfeldt-Jakob disease (vCJD).

Before a transplant can take place, the nursing staff will educate and prepare the patient, relatives, and caregivers regarding the procedure as well as the possible side effects and complications during and post-surgery. The nursing staff should be prepared to answer questions and help the patient prepare for surgery as well as understand not only the risks involved, but also the short-term and long-term survivorship issues.

Prior to a patient's arrival at a hospital or transplant center, the nursing staff will have engaged in a comprehensive educational session with the patient, relatives, and caregivers. Part of the pre-op educational process also involves a comprehensive assessment as well as a detailed medical care plan including the following:

- Assessment
    - Patient's comprehension of the time commitment and overall transplant process
    - Patient's current symptoms from previous therapies or disease(s)
    - Patient's current coping ability and emotional support system

    - Patient's current pain
    - Patient's current blood product requirements
    - Patient's sedation preference during procedures
- Teaching
    - Length of time for work-up, mobilization, and transplant process
    - Potential late effects and survivorship issues
    - Role of caregiver and logistics of care coordination
    - Confirmation of family and/or friend caregiving plan
- Communication and collaboration with referring physician's office
- Confirmation of financial clearance
- If applicable, confirmation of a housing plan
- Creation of medical care plan
- Maintain working knowledge of proposed transplant plan for patient

Additionally, there must be a comprehensive pre-transplant evaluation process for both patients and prospective donors. For the patient, this will likely require a series of tests, including blood tests, a chest X-ray, a Positron Emission Tomography (PET scan), a Computed Tomography (CT scan), pulmonary function tests, a bone marrow biopsy, heart tests, and more. Likewise, the prospective donor will have to undergo a series of tests. In addition to being screened to help prevent transmissible diseases, donors will undergo a series of blood tests, a chest X-ray, lab tests, an EKG, and more. All of these tests are in place to rule out any potential problems before the surgery and avoid possible complications following surgery. Even with these pre-transplant tests, the patient is still at risk for certain complications. One such complication is **graft-versus-host disease (GvHD)**.

GvHD occurs when the T cells (specific types of white blood cells) from the donated bone marrow or stem cells attack the patient's body cells. There are two types of GvHD—**chronic GvHD** (cGvHD) and **acute GvHD** (aGvHD). aGvHD typically presents in less than one hundred days post-surgery and may manifest itself in the form of a skin rash or blisters on the skin, stomach upset, nausea, vomiting, diarrhea, bloated stomach or stomach pain, and/or symptoms of jaundice. Although aGvHD symptoms may only be temporary and can resolve after treatment, the patient may have long-lasting effects. cGvHD tends to begin more than one hundred days post-surgery but can also develop many months or even years after surgery. Patients suffering from chronic GvHD may develop skin rashes, joint and muscle pain, dry eyes, blurred vision, difficulty opening the mouth, coughing, shortness of breath, problems with digestion, as well as genital dryness, rash, and pain. One of the current methods for treating either form of GvHD is to prescribe immunosuppressive and antimicrobial drugs. However, this leaves the patient vulnerable to bacterial, viral, and fungal infections.

Before patients undergo a stem cell or bone marrow transplant, the nursing staff will discuss the risks of developing GvHD as well as the survivorship issues affecting patients who develop this disease. Generally speaking, anywhere from one out of five patients, to as many as four out of five patients may develop at least some degree of GvHD. The following is a list of some of the factors that increase a patient's chances of developing GvHD:

- Patient's and/or donor's age (the older the patient and/or the donor, the greater the risk)
- Non-related patient and donor
- Patient and donor not of the same sex
- Male patients who receive a donation from a female who has been pregnant in the past
- Mismatch of HLA (human leukocyte antigens)

Nurses work to educate patients, relatives, and caregivers regarding the specifics of the disease and prepare them regarding the disease's possible progression. If the patient presents with a mild form of GvHD, the disease has the potential to be better managed and last for a shorter period of time. Furthermore, mild cases of GvHD may in fact benefit the patient, since the attacking T-cells will likely also attack any remaining cancer cells. This is referred to as the **graft-versus-disease effect**. However, the more severe the disease or the longer the symptoms are left untreated, the more life-threatening it becomes.

When caring for affected skin in patients with GvHD, the nursing staff may use topical steroids as well as oil-based creams and lotions, but hydrating the skin should be of primary importance. If the patient goes outside, a high SPF sunscreen should be applied, and the patient should be covered to minimize sun exposure. For treatment of affected eyes, nursing care involves eye bathing, swabs, regular eye drop application, lubricant application, steroids, antibiotics, punctal plugs with or without the application of artificial tears, and eye-draining control. Mouth care may involve mouth washes in order to keep the mouth clean, application of artificial saliva, chewing gum introduction to encourage saliva production, and the assessment of other medications which may be inadvertently increasing dry mouth. Nursing staff may also be involved in the collection of stool samples to monitor the liver, assisting the patient with mobility to and from the bathroom, aiding in daily hygiene practices, and establishing and monitoring a proper nutritional plan. There are some suggestions that certain forms of **complimentary alternative medications and treatments (CAMs)** may also benefit patients and relieve pain, such as yoga and acupuncture.

Radiation Therapy

Radiation Therapy Basics

Radiation therapy techniques span well over a century with impressive advances in the past few decades. From traditional radiotherapy techniques and external beam radiation, to 3D conformal radiation therapy, image-guided radiation therapy, helical-tomography, proton beam radiation therapy, radioactive seed implants, and more, oncologists and healthcare professionals who specialize in oncology continue to discover breakthroughs in cancer treatment.

Since there are currently more than two hundred known types of cancer that originate in different locations within the body and manifest in unique ways, cancer treatments likewise vary in order to effectively treat each type. When patients are first diagnosed with cancer, they may arrive to the first office visit with mixed information or contradicting advice that they have received from well-intentioned loved ones or from their own research. It is very important that the oncology nurse and healthcare practitioners listen carefully to patient concerns and provide the most current information on the disease, available treatment options, and risk factors. Oncology nurses may begin by explaining basic cancer education topics in order to help the patient develop the necessary knowledge to make informed decisions. When it comes to radiation oncology, patients may be particularly concerned with side effects and how these will be managed. Oncology nurses play a fundamental role in educating and preparing the patients for what lies ahead, creating an effective treatment plan, and managing and monitoring the patient's progress.

Tissue Damage and Treatment Following Radiation Therapy

Although modern advances in radiation therapy have resulted in a reduction of damage to surrounding tissue, damage still does occur. Damage to blood vessels may limit the blood supply and negatively impact a patient's ability to heal. Bleeding—particularly in the rectum, small bowel, and bladder—is another common side effect after radiation treatment. **Hyperbaric oxygen** (HB02) has proven to be very effective in the treatment of tissue damage, especially for the affected jawbone, but may also be used to treat tissue damage in the brain, muscles, and soft tissue in the face and throat. By regenerating blood vessels and repopulating damaged tissue with new stem cells, HB02 remains the most commonly used treatment for tissue damage following radiation therapy. Some other common side effects after radiation therapy involve soreness of the mouth, mucositis, odynophagia or dysphagia (which greatly impair a patient's ability to swallow), nausea, vomiting, diarrhea, dermatitis, hair follicle damage, and more. Although oncologists may prescribe some pain medications such as lidocaine and doxepin, ibuprofen and other anti-inflammatory medications may also help to relieve pain. In addition to oral medications, some treatment therapies that have proven to alleviate side effects include application of topical medications, gentle cleansing, saltwater rinses, consumption of ice chips, and use of lozenges. Advising patients to avoid various mouth irritants, such as smoking, alcohol consumption, and acidic foods, and reminding patients about consistent, proper oral hygiene should also factor into a comprehensive care plan.

Radiation Safety

Although there is always a risk when exposed to radiation, the medical team takes great care to only suggest radiation therapy when the potential benefits greatly outweigh the risks. When treating cancer, the medical team ensures that only a necessary amount of radiation is used to target and eradicate cancer cells. Unborn babies, children, and adolescents are among the most vulnerable when it comes to radiation exposure due to their rapid growth and their higher sensitivity to radiation. As young adults age however, body tissue sensitivity decreases. When it comes to gender, female breasts are more sensitive to radiation than that of their male counterparts, and females are at a higher risk of developing lung, breast, and thyroid cancer from radiation exposure. However, the main factors that influence risk remain the level of and frequency of radiation exposure.

Continuum of Care and Management of Special Population

When it comes to the continuum of care for cancer survivors, certain challenges must be overcome. After a patient receives a diagnosis and treatment for cancer, the specialized team will continue to monitor that patient's progress for a set period of time. However, the expectation is that the patient's medical care will gradually shift back to the primary care provider. If the patient was a child or adolescent at the time of the cancer diagnosis, the gradual transition from pediatric care to adult care poses even further challenges and involves a high level of coordination and collaboration. Not all primary care providers are well equipped with the knowledge and skillset to effectively manage the medical needs of cancer survivors, who may require interventions to help them maintain a certain quality of life. Providing education on lifestyle changes that impact their quality of life, such as diet, drug, and alcohol consumption, self-exams, regular medical checkups, and annual mammograms, remains an ongoing concern for the need to develop more comprehensive and long-term medical plans for cancer survivors.

Systemic Therapy

Chemotherapy

Types of Chemotherapy

Chemotherapy refers to the medications administered to patients in order to destroy the cancerous cells and is especially administered to patients whose cancers have spread. These medications can be administered intravenously or with the use of a catheter directly placed into a large vein in the chest or arm. Chemotherapy medications can also be given orally in the form of a pill, a capsule, or a liquid, and can be administered directly into the spinal canal. If a main artery has been identified as a main blood supply to the tumor, specialized medication can be directly injected into an enclosed area, such as the chest, stomach, or a muscle, and even into the bladder. In some instances, chemotherapy medication may be presented as a topical cream, a gel, or an ointment. What form of chemotherapy a patient uses depends on the patient's age and general health, the type and stage of the cancer, current medications being taken, current or past radiation treatments, the patient's blood cell count, and many other factors that warrant consideration. The goal of chemotherapy is to cure, control, or palliate. Chemotherapy may completely eradicate the cancer cells, in hope that they will not return, but whether or not a patient is truly cured may take years to determine. Shrinking or halting the growth and spread of a tumor, so that the patient can feel better and live a more productive life, is another goal of chemotherapy. However, if the cancer is more advanced and widespread, chemotherapy may then be used to ease symptoms and improve the patient's comfort level.

Patient Education and Preparation

Oncology nurses help to prepare patients ahead of chemotherapy. Some patients will only need chemotherapy for a few minutes during each session, but others may be required to undergo a few hours. It is important that the patients are advised to eat a healthy meal ahead of these longer sessions. The staff should educate the patients, family members, and caregivers on what to expect during and after treatment, as well as how to ensure they are employing safe practices. A patient undergoing chemotherapy should be advised to keep their vaccines up to date and may want to consider receiving a flu shot, since individuals receiving chemotherapy are at a higher risk of developing serious complications should they contract the flu. Patients will have a compromised immune system during chemotherapy and should therefore be at a safe distance from anyone who is sick. Since the medications used in chemotherapy may inadvertently end up outside the patient's body (e.g., by way of vomiting or open sores), the patient and caregivers should ensure proper hygiene and regular handwashing. During—and for 48 hours after—chemotherapy sessions, patients should flush the toilet twice each time upon use and close the lid ahead of flushing to limit splashing. Whether the patient is a male or female, sitting on the toilet will limit inadvertent splashing as well. The toilet seat should be cleaned after each use, and the patient should wear throw-away gloves each time that should then be immediately discarded. When drying hands, it is recommended to use paper towels that can be discarded. Caregivers are advised to wear two pairs of gloves if and when in contact with the patient's body fluids, and the patient's clothes, bedding, and personal items should be washed separately from other household items.

Additionally, the nursing staff should discuss some of the possible short and long-term risks associated with the use of chemotherapy, such as the following: fatigue; easy bruising; loss of appetite; nausea and vomiting; hair loss; changes in weight; changes in libido; fertility complications; constipation; diarrhea; irritation, pain, and sores in the mouth, tongue, or throat; and nerve or muscle numbness and pain.

Management of Chemotherapy-Induced Side Effects

The oncology nurse's role in monitoring and managing a patient's well-being during chemotherapy treatment cannot be understated. Two areas of assessment—the patient's physical well-being and psychological well-being—need to be regularly employed and findings need to be recorded. Should any of the symptoms noted raise a red flag, the oncology nurse needs to report these findings right away, as they could be life-threatening complications.

One such life-threatening complication is **neutropenic sepsis**. Should the oncology nurse detect a fever while treating the patient, immediate attention is required. The patient may also present with breathlessness or diarrhea, which are less severe in isolation but could be life-threatening should they appear together. An immediate administration of a broad-spectrum antibiotic may be required, along with a full "septic workup" to determine the cause of the symptoms. This antibiotic administration may be enough to stabilize the patient; but if not, the patient may go into **septic shock** and require full resuscitative measures. By sharing both verbal and written information regarding the early signs and symptoms of neutropenic sepsis, oncology nurses strive to develop and reinforce educational awareness so that patients, family members, caregivers, and other health professionals know what to do and when to immediately seek medical care.

Other common side effects of chemotherapy treatment are nausea and vomiting, with symptoms ranging from mild to severe. Patient age, gender, concurrent medications, and diet all affect the severity of these symptoms. Since nausea and vomiting can greatly interfere with the patient's quality of life, oncology nurses aim to prevent these symptoms from occurring, but that is not always possible. Providing effective symptom management strategies, along with patient and caregiver education, remain of utmost importance. **Antiemetics**, drugs used to counter nausea and vomiting, are commonly prescribed in these cases, along with education on how to develop and manage a healthy diet. Patients undergoing chemotherapy should eat smaller portions several times a day, avoid greasy and strong-smelling foods, and ensure they are drinking plenty of fluids. Ginger has also proven effective for some patients and remains a common and popular intervention. Some CAM therapies, such as acupuncture, may also help to reduce the severity and frequency of nausea and vomiting.

Diarrhea, if left untreated, can be a potentially life-threatening side effect of chemotherapy and must be closely monitored. Since some patients may be reluctant to openly discuss this issue, oncology nurses play a vital role in introducing the subject by encouraging the patient to be open and frank. Additionally, education must be provided to the patient and caregivers on the potential health risks which may result from ongoing, untreated episodes of diarrhea, including renal failure, perforation, and serious infection. Educating the patient regarding a proper diet and regular hydration is also extremely important; however, should the diarrhea persist, some medications such as loperamide may be necessary.

Oncology nurses must also be very knowledgeable and prepared to handle signs and symptoms of peripheral neuropathy, stomatitis, and extravasation. Certain drugs used in chemotherapy treatments have the potential to cause peripheral nerve damage, affecting the patient's hands and feet. Oncology nurses must assess the patient's fine motor skills at every visit and ask pertinent questions regarding the patient's general mobility to search for clues. If there has been severe **peripheral neuropathy**, chemotherapy treatment may be interrupted. **Stomatitis**, a very common side effect of chemotherapy, refers to the painful inflammation of a patient's mucous membrane in the mouth. Preventative measures involve encouraging the patient to seek treatment for any dental issues before beginning chemotherapy and educating the patient on proper dental hygiene. Oncology nurses should also conduct an oral assessment at every visit. When chemotherapy is administered intravenously, there is a risk of the drugs leaking into surrounding tissue; this is called **extravasation**. Oncology nurses should have both the knowledge and the skillset necessary to minimize this risk and watch for signs in order to effectively manage this condition. In some instances, simply watching may be all that is necessary, but if the condition is more severe, the area might need to be flushed out and in the most severe cases, surgical intervention may be necessary.

Other side effects of chemotherapy involve alopecia, fatigue, hypersensitivity, and more. Educating patients on how to best manage these symptoms has been shown to be beneficial to the patient's quality of life and psychological well-being. Oncology nurses should watch for signs of depression, forgetfulness, anemia, and weight loss, and intervene when necessary. Should the patient present with allergic signs such as a sudden rash or skin irritation during a chemotherapy session, the treatment may be temporarily interrupted, and an antihistamine may need to be administered. Resuming treatment should only occur once the symptoms have completed disappeared. If the **allergic reaction** is severe, the patient may be suffering from stridor, bronchospasm, or angioedema, which require immediate medical attention and a possible full resuscitative support.

One important area of chemotherapy that deserves full attention is the risk of side effects to the healthcare team due to exposure. In particular, oncology nurses who work directly with the administration of chemotherapy need to take particular precautions to minimize this risk. Some exposure-related risks include the following: damage to the nervous system; acute and long-term reproductive damage affecting fertility; miscarriage; and the development of hematological malignancies, such as leukemia. Lowering the ratio of oncology nurses to patients should be a serious discussion. Other effective ways to minimize these risks include education on needle safety, the use of personal protective equipment, as well as safe practices in the disposal of drugs, tubing, needles, and other equipment used in chemotherapy treatments.

Biotherapy

Biotherapy employs the use of living substances to help fight cancer cells. These living substances can be found naturally in the body or may be made in the lab. Two common types of biotherapies are immunotherapy and gene therapy. With the use of cytokines (proteins that ameliorate cell communication), interferons, interleukins (which locate and kill cancerous cells while stimulating the body's immune system), specialized antibodies, or vaccines, **immunotherapy** employs the patient's own immune system to fight the cancer. The human immune system is essentially comprised of cells and organs. **White blood cells**—the infection-fighting cells—have a unique responsibility to target, identify, and destroy threats to the body's survival. In some instances, certain white blood cells (macrophages) will even surround and digest these invaders while stimulating the body's natural defense system.

In contrast, **gene therapy** is used if the disease is caused due to abnormal genes. In this case, a healthy functioning gene may be inserted into the body, the abnormal gene may be able to undergo repair, or modifications may be made to prevent the abnormal gene from causing further damage.

When other forms of treatment have proven unsuccessful, biotherapy treatment may be an option. It may be used to treat cancer as well as some of the side effects from chemotherapy and radiation.

Biotherapy may be used on its own or in conjunction with other forms of cancer treatment. Some of the most common types of biotherapies are described in the following table:

Type of Biotherapy	Genesis	Specific Purpose
Monoclonal Antibodies (mAB)	Produced in a lab	Mice are injected with cells of a specific type of cancer. The antibodies that the mice produce are then combined with other cells to create "hybrid" cells used to combat the cancer in human patients.
Interleukin (IL)	Naturally found in the human body but can also be synthesized in a lab	This form of therapy is generally used to fight against metastatic kidney cancer and melanoma.
Interferons (IFN)	Naturally found in the human body	This form of therapy is used to combat hairy cell leukemia, Kaposi's sarcoma, and chronic myeloid leukemia.

Like any cancer therapy however, biotherapy treatments do have certain risk factors. Depending on the type of biotherapy used, patients may experience a decrease in energy levels, limited concentration, low blood pressure, flu-like symptoms, kidney complications, skin irritations, fever, and joint issues among other side effects. Hospitalization may be required for more severe side effects, but in general, these symptoms are short lived and will likely subside on their own after treatment.

Immunotherapy

The immune system typically recognizes and controls abnormal or malfunctioning cells. Cancer cells can bypass this normal process by genetically camouflaging themselves from immune cells, facilitating deactivation of immune cells, or altering surrounding cells in order to change immune responses to the cancer cells. Immunotherapy is a type of biological treatment that improves the body's ability to identify, control, and destroy cancer cells.

Monoclonal antibodies (MOAs) are medications that have been developed in the lab setting using clones of B-cells from different sources (most commonly mouse and human cells). MOAs are made of protein markers (antibodies) that target cells with corresponding surface proteins (antigens). Some monoclonal antibodies, such as rituximab, function as immunotherapy agents by tagging cancer cells for immune system destruction. Blinatumomab is another cancer MOA which allows T-cells to get closer to cancer cells in order to recognize and eradicate them. MOAs are used to treat many different cancer types. Common side effects of this drug class include skin reactions (e.g., IV site reactions, hives); infusion reactions (e.g., sensitivity reactions, cytokine release syndrome); and flu-like symptoms.

Immune checkpoint inhibitors are another class of immunotherapy that prevent T-cells from being deactivated after binding with antigens on the surface of cancer cells. Common proteins targeted by immune checkpoint inhibitors are PD-1 (e.g., nivolumab and pembrolizumab); PD-L1 (e.g., atezolizumab and durvalumab); and CTLA-4 (e.g., ipilimumumab). This class of treatments is used to treat a wide range of cancer types. As with other immunotherapy treatments, side effects can vary from patient to patient; however, common side effects tend to include skin rashes, fatigue, and diarrhea. Additionally, immune checkpoint inhibitors can be associated with immune-related adverse events (e.g., skin inflammatory changes, diabetes, hepatitis, thyroid function changes, or myocarditis).

T-cell transfer therapy is a type of immunotherapy treatment that utilizes the body's own T-cells to better fight cancer cells. T-cells are harvested from the patient and sent to a lab where select T-cells are singled out and grown in massive numbers. Meanwhile, the patient is given chemotherapy and sometimes radiation therapy to suppress the patient's remaining immune system. Then, the lab-generated cells are reintroduced to the patient's circulatory system where they seek out and destroy cancer cells.

There are currently two types of T-cell transfer therapy: Tumor-infiltrating lymphocyte (TIL) therapy and CAR T-cell therapy. With **TIL therapy**, lab testing singles out which of the tumor-infiltrating lymphocytes respond the most effectively to the patient's tumor cells, and they stimulate those specific cells to grow for reintroduction into the patient's immune system. TIL has been successful in treating melanoma and is being studied for other uses, as well. TIL therapy can cause **capillary leak syndrome**, which results in leaking of fluid and proteins from circulation into the tissues; consequently, this can lead to severe hypotension up to shock and organ failure.

CAR T-cell therapy is a slightly different process where T-cells are modified to create the chimeric antigen receptor (CAR), which increases the T-cell's ability to detect and destroy the cancer cell. CAR T-cell therapies (e.g., axicabtagene ciloleucel and brexucabtagene autoleucel) are used to treat blood cancers, and researchers are in the early stages of exploring their efficacy in treatment of some solid tumors. Side effects of CAR T-cell therapy can be severe and vary widely depending on specific patient and cancer factors. Common reactions include **cytokine release syndrome**, which results in a massive release of cytokines into the circulatory system that causes a sensitivity-type reaction. Additionally, if CAR T-cells target healthy cells, there can be associated toxicities.

Cancer vaccines are yet another category of immunotherapy treatment that assists immune cells to recognize cancer antigens in order to effectively kill cancer cells. Cancer treatment vaccines (e.g., Sipuleucel-T) can be created using a patient's own tumor cells, antigens typical for a specific tumor type, or a patient's dendritic immune cells. **Oncolytic viruses**, which are designed to target and kill cancer cells while leaving normal cells unharmed, can also be considered cancer vaccines. T-VEC, an oncolytic virus used to treat melanoma, is based on the herpes simplex virus type 1 (HSV-1) and is directly injected into the tumor to multiply and cause **apoptosis** of the cancer cells. Once those cells burst, the oncovirus circulates to other cancer cells within the body. Common side effects of cancer treatment vaccines include flu-like symptoms or anaphylactic reactions. T-VEC has the potential to cause **tumor lysis syndrome** due to massive breakdown of cancer cells in the bloodstream. T-VEC can also cause systemic herpes infection.

Immune system modulators are a collection of treatments that increase the immune system's response to cancer cells. They tend to be used in the treatment of advanced stage cancers. **Cytokines** are one type of immune system modulator that stimulates different immune cells. Some cytokines, like **interferons (INFs)**, can be used to treat cancer by stimulating natural killer cells and dendritic cells to better recognize and control cancer cell growth. **Interleukins (ILs)** are another type of cytokine that can treat cancer by increasing the total white blood cell count, resulting in improved response to cancer cells. Cytokine medications can commonly cause flu-like symptoms and allergy-type reactions. Bacillus Calmette-Guerin (BCG), an immune modulator that is derived from the bacteria that causes tuberculosis, is instilled into the bladder to generate an immune attack on cancer cells. Common side effects associated with BCG use are urinary symptoms (e.g., dysuria, hematuria, and infection). Immunomodulatory medications (e.g., thalidomide and lenalidomide) are additional types of immune modulators that stimulate creation of IL-2 in the body, which prevents tumor blood vessel formation. Immunomodulatory medications have common side effects of blood clots and peripheral neuropathy. Immunomodulatory drugs have also been linked to severe birth defects if used during pregnancy.

Hormonal Therapy

Hormone therapy, also known as endocrine treatment, is used to treat or improve symptoms of cancers that use hormones to grow, such as breast and prostate cancers. Prior to initiating hormone therapy, it is important to determine the cancer type and stage along with the patient's comorbidities and performance status assessment. It is common to initiate hormone therapy alongside other cancer treatment options such as chemotherapy, radiation, and surgery. Hormone therapy has been found to be a successful adjuvant treatment that greatly reduces the risk of cancer recurrence following primary treatment with chemotherapy, radiation, or surgery. It has also been used as a neoadjuvant therapy to decrease tumor size prior to chemotherapy, radiation, or surgery. Hormone therapy can be administered orally, by injection, or by surgery. Surgery is typically done to remove hormone-producing organs, such as the testes in men and ovaries in women. Side effects are common with hormone therapy due to its interference with the body's typical hormone response or production. Side effects also vary with the gender of the patient. Common side effects in women include low libido, nausea, hot flashes, fatigue, and changes in menstruation. Men may experience enlarged breasts, fatigue, nausea, diarrhea, low libido, decreased bone density, and hot flashes. Frequent breast and axillary exams along with regular mammograms are necessary to ensure the correct amount and type of hormone therapy is being used for breast cancers. For prostate cancer, regular prostate-specific antigen tests should be taken to ensure levels are the same or lower to confirm the treatment is working adequately.

Localized Therapy

Intrathecal

Intrathecal chemotherapy may be used for cancers that are currently affecting or have a high chance of affecting the spinal cord or brain. Intrathecal therapies are characterized by medications that are injected directly into the cerebrospinal fluid (CSF), typically by lumbar puncture or Ommaya reservoir. Lumbar puncture is completed by placing the patient in a side-lying fetal position and using a small needle and syringe to inject the necessary chemotherapy medication. Ommaya reservoirs involve surgically placing a CSF reservoir under the patient's scalp, which can then be accessed multiple times for continued intrathecal treatments rather than repeating lumbar punctures each time. Intrathecal therapy is a targeted cancer treatment, which prevents the rest of the patient's body from being exposed to the chemotherapy agents. Cancers that may be treated with intrathecal therapy include lymphoma, leukemia, and malignant tumors that have spread into the spinal cord or brain. Side effects commonly include nausea, vomiting, fever, fatigue, and headache. Neurological effects such as increased confusion or changes in mood may also occur.

Intravesical

Intravesical therapies are typically used as an adjuvant therapy for early-stage bladder cancer. This type of therapy involves infusion of medications, such as immunomodulators and chemotherapy, into the bladder via a catheter to provide targeted treatment and limit systemic exposure. Surgical intervention such as a partial cystectomy and transurethral resection (TUR) is typically performed prior to the initiation of the intravesical therapy, which is then used to kill any remaining cancer cells after surgery.

Systemic chemotherapy is typically necessary for advanced-stage cancers, metastasis, and tumors that extend into the musculature. Common intravesical immunomodulators include interferons, interleukin-2, and tumor necrosis factor (TNF). Intravesical chemotherapy agents include doxorubicin, thiotepa, mitomycin, and epirubicin. Medication distribution and effectiveness during intravesical therapies can be affected by factors such as hydration status, urine volume, urine pH, and urothelium integrity. Therefore, it is vital to use the correct amount and concentration of medication to ensure that it is within the therapeutic range. Treatment success rate typically depends on how the cancer cells respond to the medication as well as the distribution and effectiveness of the medication.

Targeted Therapies

Targeted therapy involves the administration of a class of drugs that works to prevent the cancer from growing or spreading by targeting specific genes and/or proteins. Since these genes and proteins are found within the cancer cells or within the cells linked to cancer growth, they are commonly used in conjunction with chemotherapy and other treatments.

There are many different types, shapes, and sizes of cancer cells. One of the most significant challenges facing targeted therapy is developing drugs that target these unique cell characteristics as well as learning how these cells grow, divide, and spread. Some forms of targeted therapy inject small-molecule drugs directly into the cancerous cells, whereas monoclonal antibodies are not small enough to enter into the cells. Instead, they attach themselves to the outer surface of these specifically-targeted cells. Risks to the patient include a cancerous cell developing resistance to the drugs, diarrhea, liver complications, blood clotting, fatigue, skin irritation, and high blood pressure. The majority of these symptoms stop once the treatment ends; however, if necessary, there are medications that help to manage these complications.

Targeted therapies strive to destroy cancerous cells by targeting or tracking each cell's unique changes that allow them to grow and thrive. The more the healthcare profession learns about the hormones responsible for cancer production, the better the targeted therapies will work to starve the cancer of these necessary hormones. The following is a list of some of the current forms of targeted therapy:

- **Photodynamic Therapy**: With the use of a drug called a photosensitizer, photodynamic therapy has been shown as an effective method for destroying cancer cells and damaging blood vessels within these cells. There is evidence to show that this drug also activates immune system responses to attack the cancerous cells. **Photosensitizers** are administered into the bloodstream and are then absorbed by both the cancerous and normal cells. However, within one to three days, the majority of the drug leaves the healthy cells and remains in the cancerous cells. It is the light from this drug that is then released and produces a unique form of oxygen that works to kill the cancerous cells.

- **Signal Transduction Inhibitors**: These inhibitors work to prevent certain molecular activity that participates in **signal transduction**—the process in which a cell receives a specific signal which then sets off a series of reactions in order to produce the intended results. This interference prevents certain malignant cells from thriving.

- **Gene Expression Modulators**: One of the functions of the body's proteins is to control gene expression. When this function is modified, some cancers will be unable to survive.

- **Immunotherapy**: Immunotherapy works to stimulate the patient's immune system. It may even involve the introduction of manmade immune system proteins to strengthen the immune system's responses in combatting cancerous cells.

Immune Cell Therapy

Immune cell therapy is an adapted type of immunotherapy used for cancer treatment. External immune cells are used to supplement the patient's existing immune response as well as create new response pathways to fight against cancer cells. Immune cell therapy works to activate different immune cell types in the anti-tumor effort, such as macrophages, T lymphocytes, natural killer (NK) cells, and dendritic cells (DC). Depending on the type of cancer and stage, there are several low- and high-risk immune cell therapy medication options. Low-risk options include DC vaccine, cytokine-induced killer (CIK) cell therapy, tumor-infiltrating lymphocyte (TIL) therapy, and DC cell therapy. These are regarded as lower-risk options because they utilize the patient's own immune cells and response to fight cancer cells. High-risk immune cell therapies include chimeric antigen receptor (CAR) macrophages, T cell receptor T (TCR-T), including CAR-T, and CAR-NK therapies. These therapies are modified to utilize genetically modified cells, allogeneic cells, autologous stem cells, or xenogeneic cells to fight more specific cancer cell types.

Bispecific Antibodies

Bispecific antibodies (BsAbs) are highly effective medications due to the use of lab-made proteins, which can work in two ways at once. As a result of this dual ability, BsAb medications are considered to have higher efficacy and are often the chosen route for drug-resistant disease. Like immunotherapy, many types of BsAbs assist the immune response in fighting cancer cells. The bispecific antibody proteins are unique in that they can bind to the cancer cell and the immune cell at the same time. BsAbs are typically used to treat cancers of the lymphatic system or blood, such as lymphoma and leukemia, although some have been used for noncancerous disease processes such as hemophilia. BsAbs medications may be used in conjunction with other cancer treatments, such as chemotherapy, but are typically used after these other treatments have stopped achieving their desired efficacy. Dosages of these medications are typically gradually increased to decrease side effects and associated risks such as infections, cytokine release syndrome (CRS), and immune effector cell-associated neurotoxicity syndrome (ICANS). This medication is administered over the course of several visits, unlike other unlike other immunotherapies such as CAR-T cell therapy, which are typically given on only one occasion.

Oral Therapies

Oral chemotherapy is a cancer treatment option which utilizes medications given by mouth, such as those in pill or liquid form. This provides an alternative but effective treatment route to chemotherapy infusions or injections. Oral therapy can be employed to treat a range of cancer types, such as the use of etoposide for lung cancer and capecitabine for breast and colorectal cancers. Patient education should emphasize the importance of proper adherence to the treatment plan, including the right dose, timing, and specific considerations involved with medication administration. Other medications that the patient may be taking will need to be evaluated for potential drug interactions. Education must also include instructions on safe handling, storage, cleaning, and disposal requirements.

While some oral therapies may be used on a continuous basis, others are given on an intermittent schedule, with breaks in treatment to allow for healing from side effects. Like other routes of chemotherapy administration, treatment with oral therapy can result in unpleasant side effects such as mouth sores, nausea, diarrhea, and fatigue. Additionally, the resulting suppressed state of the immune system will make the patient more vulnerable to infection. Patients taking oral therapies should be monitored for compliance to ensure treatment success as well as with laboratory testing (e.g., CBC, kidney and liver function panels) to manage side effects.

Practice Quiz

1. A nurse s providing education to a patient on pembrolizumab. The patient asks how the drug acts to treat cancer. Which of the following is the most appropriate response by the nurse?

   a. "Pembrolizumab works by being absorbed into the cell and killing the tumor with radiation."
   b. "Pembrolizumab works by targeting cells that are in an active growth phase of division."
   c. "Pembrolizumab works by attaching to a receptor on a tumor cell and injecting a chemotherapy molecule into it."
   d. "Pembrolizumab works by enhancing the ability of the immune system to recognize and attack cancer cells."

2. A nurse is administering single-agent avelumab for a patient with metastatic urothelial cancer. Upon discharge, the nurse should reinforce education on all the following EXCEPT:

   a. Low blood cell counts may occur around seven to ten days post-infusion. Practice regular hand hygiene and call your team if you have a fever.
   b. Rash or itching may occur anytime during your treatment. Call your team if you begin developing rash, itching, blisters, or other skin changes.
   c. Diarrhea may occur anytime during your treatment. Call your team if you're having more than four loose stools in a 24-hour period.
   d. This medication can cause changes in your lungs. Call your team if you have a cough, shortness of breath, or chest pain.

3. A nurse is providing education to a patient receiving rituximab. The patient requests more information about this class of drug. Which of the following should be included?

   a. Monoclonal antibody therapies are most useful for reducing tumor burden.
   b. Monoclonal antibodies cause the immune system to create memory for future tumors.
   c. Monoclonal antibodies cannot be produced to target certain antigens.
   d. Monoclonal antibodies cannot have radioisotopes or chemotherapy attached.

4. A nurse is administering chemotherapy for a patient receiving doxorubicin. Which of the following is NOT true:

   a. Doxorubicin is an irritant, so a peripheral catheter may be used.
   b. A central line is recommended.
   c. Blood return should be checked every 2–5mL for an IV push medication.
   d. It can be infused peripherally through a large forearm vein.

5. A nurse is triaging a call from a patient who is being treated for metastatic kidney cancer with cabozantinib. The patient reports that their blood pressure has been elevated the past few days and had a reading this morning of 175/100, although they are having no symptoms. The nurse expects which orders from the provider?

   a. Continue cabozantinib and monitor blood pressure at home. Instruct the patient to call if their systolic blood pressure is over 190.
   b. Continue cabozantinib and refer the patient back to their primary care provider for management of hypertension.
   c. Hold cabozantinib and start antihypertensives.
   d. Direct the patient to the emergency room for further management.

See answers on the next page.

Answer Explanations

1. D: Pembrolizumab is a type of biotherapy that blocks the activity of a protein that prevents T-cells from recognizing and attacking cancer cells, allowing the immune system to more readily respond. Choice *A* refers to a radioligand therapy, Choice *B* refers to chemotherapy, and Choice *C* refers to an antibody drug conjugate.

2. A: By itself, avelumab is unlikely to cause myelosuppression or neutropenia. This type of precaution is more commonly seen with chemotherapies. Choices *B, C,* and *D* are common immunotherapy related side-effects. Patients should be counseled to call their care team if there are symptoms of immune-related side effects.

3. A: Monoclonal antibodies are immunoglobins that are engineered to bind to tumor-related targets and cause tumor lysis, activate apoptosis, or flag them for phagocytosis by other immune cells. This process makes them most useful for reducing tumor burden but will not result in significant immune memory for future tumors, making Choice *B* incorrect. Choice *C* is incorrect, as they can be produced to target antigens thought to be shared by tumor type. An example of this is rituximab, which targets a cell-surface receptor on lymphoid tumors. Monoclonal antibodies are either unconjugated or conjugated, meaning they have a radioisotope or chemotherapy attached to be delivered to the intended cell target, making Choice *D* incorrect.

4. A: Doxorubicin is classified as a vesicant. Vesicants are recommended to be administered through a central line. A peripheral catheter can be used, but blood return should be checked for at regular intervals and site selection is very important. Choices *B, C,* and *D* are incorrect.

5. C: Hypertension is a common side effect of cabozantinib and is unlikely to resolve without holding the drug or providing any necessary additional intervention. As the patient is hypertensive, they should start on antihypertensives and hold cabozantinib until blood pressure is better managed. Once the readings are lower, the patient can restart cabozantinib. Early intervention is recommended in order to reduce the time that the medication is held, so this symptom is best managed by the oncology team. A visit to the emergency room is unnecessary at this time, but the patient should be instructed to seek evaluation if their systolic blood pressure is over 200 or if they have symptoms such as headache, chest pain, or vision changes.

Symptom Management and Palliative Care

With over two hundred known types of cancer and multiple side effects associated with the treatment of each, symptom management is of particular importance to oncology nursing. Symptom management works to prevent the onset of these symptoms as much as possible. However, when these symptoms do arise, the focus shifts to minimizing the severity of symptoms, relieving the associated pain and discomfort, and striving to reduce or eliminate side effects to the extent possible.

Symptom management involves the management of both the physical and psychological side effects that may occur before, during, and after treatment. From educating patients on proper daily nutrition, exercise, and dental hygiene, to counseling patients presenting with anxiety, fear, and depression, symptom management is quite varied. Both palliative and curative care are vital in the development of individualized treatment plans for patients fighting cancer. Not only do issues such as pain management, fatigue, dry mouth, loss of appetite, shortness of breath, diarrhea, constipation, anxiety, and depression need to be addressed, some side effects may also require immediate medical attention (e.g., over-sedation and opioid-induced respiratory depression). Furthermore, oncology nurses must be careful not to neglect encouragement of meaningful discussions with patients and their caregivers. Evidence suggests that many patients are often reluctant to discuss certain side effects with healthcare professionals out of fear that their treatment may be interrupted or stopped altogether. If healthcare professionals do not incorporate a routine discussion with patients at every visit, some of these unreported side effects may become life-threatening. Built-in to every cancer treatment plan should be the assessment tools that oncology nurses intend to use to monitor the physical and psychological well-being of their patients, along with the steps to take when intervention is necessary. The more knowledge oncology nurses have regarding the physiology of pain, the pharmacology of analgesia, and the psychological and emotional factors associated with cancer, the more effective and appropriate the treatment goals will be for the patient.

Palliative care refers to any care that is provided to individuals experiencing a health or personal event that severely hinders their overall quality of life. Individuals receiving palliative care may or may not have a terminal medical diagnosis; however, their physical and/or psychological condition is usually severe. Palliative care intends to soften the severity of the recipient's conditions through physical, emotional, medicinal, and other comfort measures. The goal is to make the individual as comfortable as possible.

Anatomical and Surgical Alterations

Anatomy is the study of the structures of living organisms and is one of the branches of biology. Traditionally, this study required dissection but with advanced imaging technology such as X-rays, CT scans, and MRIs, specialists can study the anatomy with minimally invasive techniques. For patients with cancer, anatomical operations are used to diagnose as well as determine the severity of the disease.

Gross anatomy refers to the study of the structures within the body that can be seen without the use of a microscope, such as entire organs. In **microanatomy** (also referred to as histology), specialists study the cells and tissues of certain parts of the body that otherwise could not be seen by the naked eye. For patients with cancer, microanatomy allows specialists to view the behavior, size, and structure of cancerous cells and to better determine if the tumor has increased in size or the cells have divided and spread. Surgical operations for cancer refer to the complete or partial removal of the tumor. They may be performed to diagnose the cancer, ascertain the tumor's precise location, and determine whether or not it has spread. Surgical operations can also restore the appearance of areas of the body that have been altered, either due to surgery or complications of the disease, and relieve some of the debilitating side effects faced by patients with cancer.

Depending on the type and severity of the cancer, patients may experience **anatomical alterations**; some of these alterations may be temporary, but some may be permanent. During cancer treatment, patients may experience a temporary loss of appetite, which impacts their ability to maintain a healthy weight. As a result, these patients may lose a considerable amount of noticeable weight, affecting how they feel both physically and emotionally. Cancer treatment can also cause hair loss, changes to the texture and pigment of skin, as well as dental changes, all compounding the patient's ability to cope. Surgical alterations, such as a mastectomy or the removal of a limb, an eye, or other areas of a person's body, will likely—and greatly—affect the patient's self-esteem and overall emotional well-being.

Surgical cancer treatment can also result in **dermatologic alterations**. Surgical incisions typically result in scar formation related to the site and significance of the procedure. Surgical wounds range from small incisions (e.g., laparoscopic procedures) to very large surgical wounds [e.g., pancreaticoduodenectomy (Whipple procedure)]. Complicated wound healing can lead to more prominent, uneven scar formation. Factors such as very large or multiple wounds, presence of comorbidities (e.g., diabetes, obesity, malnutrition, or infection), exposure to tobacco smoke, and location of the wound can have significant influence on wound healing. Additionally, surgical procedures involving the resection of external structures (e.g., breast mastectomy, radical head and neck surgeries, surgeries involving sex organs, and skin cancer resection) can lead to profound anatomical changes. These types of alterations tend to cause significant distress and body image issues for affected patients.

Lymphedema

Lymphedema is the abnormal collection of fluid within subcutaneous tissue that occurs when lymph nodes are not functioning properly. Lymphedema can occur after surgical or radiation therapy for the treatment of cancer. Signs and symptoms are specific to the anatomical location and include swelling and changes in size of the affected area. Lymphedema at the head and neck region can result in voice changes, difficulty swallowing, or difficulty breathing. Care should be taken to avoid activities that could cause inflammation in the area below the affected lymph node(s) (e.g., venipuncture or restrictive clothing cuffs). Recommendations also include maintaining a healthy weight and strength training exercises to ensure proper blood flow and movement of lymph fluids. Compression clothing, compression devices, and lymphatic massage are additional interventions to support lymph drainage. More invasive treatment measures include laser therapy and surgical treatment.

Ostomy

Another surgical alteration associated with cancer treatment is placement of an **ostomy**, which is a surgically formed opening (**stoma**) in the skin. Surgical treatment of colorectal cancer is one example of a cancer treatment that can be associated with ostomy placement. Ostomies can be temporary or permanent, depending on the long-term treatment plan. They can be located at the ileum (**ileostomy**) or the colon (**colostomy**), allowing stool to bypass the distal colon and rectum to be excreted through the stoma. An adhesive pouch is applied to collect stoma output. Immediate postoperative stoma care includes monitoring the stoma for issues related to blood supply or signs of infection. Additionally, extensive patient education and support are required to introduce stoma care and application of pouching devices. Common ongoing issues associated with stoma use can include peristomal skin breakdown, often due to poor placement of the pouching device, and patient body image concerns related to social and sexual implications of ostomy placement.

Site-Specific Radiation

Radiation therapy is another treatment modality that can have side effects based on specific treatment areas. This occurs due to damage and scarring to surrounding healthy tissues as radiation is applied to the cancer site. Radiation to the pelvis, for instance, can result in side effects including incontinence, infertility, or sexual dysfunction. Radiation to the head and neck can lead to **xerostomia** (dry mouth due to reduction in saliva production) or hypothyroidism. Radiation to the chest and torso can result in permanent injury and scarring to the organs associated with the treatment site. For example, a patient undergoing radiation to the chest for breast cancer could sustain lung and heart tissue injury from the radiation therapy. Radiation injury to the lungs can result in the development of chronic lung disease, and radiation injury to cardiac tissue can result in long-term heart disease from damage to the muscle tissues, blood vessels, valves, and conductive tissue.

Vascular Access Devices (VADs)

Patients receiving intravenous chemotherapy and biotherapy/immunotherapy receive their treatment via a **vascular access device (VAD**). VADs can be peripherally (PVC) or centrally (CVC) placed venous catheters. The type and location of selected VAD depends on a multitude of factors, including the following: type of cancer, age of the patient, treatment plan, patient preference, and co-morbidities.

PIVs

Peripherally inserted intravenous catheters (**PIVs** or IVs) are short catheters placed under the skin into a vein and are used to deliver intravenous medications. PIVs are typically inserted into the hand or forearm and are intended for short-term use (typically three to five days). PIVs are often inserted by nurses at the bed or chairside. Oncology nurses must perform a thorough assessment to determine the appropriate size (gauge) of catheter and the most appropriate location for IV placement. Additionally, oncology patients should be evaluated based on degree of difficulty in placing a PIV. Risk factors for difficult IV placement include long-term IV chemotherapy history, which often results in changes to the vascular system that make IV placement more challenging. Additionally, advanced age, poor nutrition, dehydration, history of difficult IV placement, comorbidities (e.g., diabetes, heart disease, kidney disease, and anemia), and small vein diameter all impact the feasibility of peripheral IV placement. Patients who experience difficult IV placement have increased discomfort and pain as well as emotional distress related to IV placement.

Oncology nurses should assess, be able to recognize, and appropriately manage potential complications associated with PIV use. **Phlebitis**, which refers to inflammation of the veins, can be caused by traumatic PIV placement, rubbing of the catheter against the vein wall, or administration of irritants. It presents as redness, edema, pain, and warmth. Additionally, the vein proximal to the IV site may be indurated with red streaking along the vein. **Flare reactions** can also occur with PIV use due to irritant administration or local allergy-type response and appears as redness, streaking, and raised skin around IV site. This reaction can sometimes itch or may burn. **Infiltration**, which refers to leaking of IV fluid or medication into the surrounding tissue, is associated with swelling, blanching, coolness, and slowed IV infusion rate. Infiltration of medications considered to be an irritant will typically result in inflammation and irritation of the local injection site. Other chemotherapy medications categorized as vesicants can cause severe tissue injury and necrosis if they leak outside of the PIV (this is called extravasation). Prevention of infiltration and extravasation involves appropriate choice of IV location and size as well as initial and ongoing assessment. Additionally, for IV administration of **vesicant** medications, nurses should never administer these medications via infusion pump. IV patency should be checked frequently, as well, by assessing for free flow and blood return with aspiration.

Midline Catheters

Midline catheters are another type of peripheral catheter. Midline catheters are an alternative to peripherally inserted central catheters (PICC) and can remain in place for a month or as long as there are no complications. The difference between PIVs and midline catheters is that midline catheters are longer than 3 inches and are inserted into the upper arm (in the brachial or cephalic veins) rather than the forearm or hand. Placement is performed by specially trained healthcare professionals (often nurses) who use ultrasound to guide catheter placement. Catheter tip confirmation is not required, unlike with PICC placement. Due to the presence of an external line, there is an increased risk of infection.

PICC Lines

Peripherally inserted central catheters (PICC) feature a central line that is placed peripherally in the upper arm, neck, scalp (for infants), or lower extremity (for infants) with the guidance of ultrasound. A catheter is inserted to a length that is specific to the patient and long enough to terminate in the superior vena cava (SVC). Tip placement should be confirmed prior to use to minimize risk of arrhythmias, cardiac tamponade, or damage to heart valves related to mispositioning. Due to the external indwelling line, PICCs carry a risk for infection, and they also increase the risk of blood clot formation.

Ports

Implanted ports are yet another commonly used VAD for administration of oncology medications. Implanted ports are surgically placed devices that are completely under the skin and can remain in place as long as there are no complications. Ports are typically placed on the anterior chest wall and are accessed with special needles as needed. Implanted ports are then de-accessed when treatment is discontinued, leaving the patient with no external lines, which reduces the risk of infection. Implanted ports can remain accessed for one week before the needle and dressing need to be replaced. Risks associated with ports include blood clots and breakdown of skin (due to device rejection or improper access technique). Additionally, special care is required to ensure the line is flushed properly. Heparin flushes are often used, unless contraindicated, upon de-access. Disadvantages to this device are the high cost and the fact that placement, replacement, and removal require surgical intervention.

Pharmacologic Interventions

Pharmaceutical drugs (which can come in the form of tablets, liquids, patches, suppositories, and injections) that are prescribed to patients with cancer serve a number of purposes. **Antidepressants** may be prescribed to help patients cope with the stress and anxiety that often accompany a cancer diagnosis. **Opioids**, such as fentanyl and oxycodone, may be prescribed to manage and alleviate pain, while other medications are used to directly combat the disease. With regard to over-the-counter medications, aspirin is showing some evidence in its ability to prevent—and in some cases, lower the risk of—the development of certain cancers, in particular bowel, breast, esophageal, prostate, and stomach cancer. However, it is important to understand that there is no current conclusive evidence regarding this possibility. Furthermore, aspirin can also cause minor to severe side effects, such as asthma, stomach ulcers, and internal bleeding. In recent years, there have been staggering breakthroughs regarding pharmacologic interventions that combat cancer. One promising breakthrough is the vaccine known as Gardasil, which works to combat **human papillomavirus** (**HPV**) types 6, 11, 16, and 18 that are directly linked to cervical cancer. Since the FDA approved its use in 2006, the infection rate of HPV has been lowered by an astonishing 90 percent.

Oncology nurses should take great care in educating patients about the potential side effects, drug interactions, and contraindications of the medications they have been prescribed as well as those of over-the-counter medications. The more informed patients are about these medications, the more confident they feel in their battle against cancer.

Complementary and Integrative Modalities

Complementary and integrative therapies provide support to patients undergoing standard cancer treatments. The goal for treatment with complementary and integrative strategies is to improve quality of life and manage side effects of standard treatments. As opposed to alternative medicine, complementary and integrative interventions are not used to replace traditional treatment but to improve the patient's cancer treatment experience.

One category of complementary treatments are mind-body therapies. These treatments focus on the connection between our thoughts, intentions, breathing, and body movements. **Meditation** is a notable example of a mind-body therapy in which repetitive breathing and vocal patterns are used to manage stress. **Acupuncture** is another mind-body therapy which uses the insertion of very small needles at specific points on the body with the goal of improving health and quality of life. It is believed by its practitioners that acupuncture can help with complaints such as fatigue, pain, peripheral neuropathy, and dry mouth. Due to this modality being more invasive than other complementary treatment methods, patients with **neutropenia** (low white blood cell count) or **thrombocytopenia** (low platelet count) should avoid acupuncture. **Biofeedback** is yet another strategy that utilizes measuring devices to build connections between stress reduction techniques (e.g., breathing and meditation) and subconscious processes like heart rate and blood pressure. Art and music therapies are additional examples of mind-body interventions.

Biologically based practices are another category of complementary medicine that utilize natural substances to support wellness. Vitamins (e.g., vitamin B12, melatonin, and potassium) and supplements (e.g., protein and fiber) are biologically based treatments that can be utilized to support normal body functioning. **Medicinal cannabis** is an example of a botanical treatment used to manage cancer and treatment-related side effects like fatigue, pain, anorexia, and anxiety. Other botanicals include herbs and spices (e.g., ginseng, turmeric, and peppermint). Biologically based treatments have the potential for interaction with traditional treatment medications and should be evaluated by a medical practitioner before initiation.

Yet another group of complementary treatments are manipulative body-based interventions, such as reflexology and massage therapy. **Reflexology** is a combination of massage and the use of pressure to specific areas on the feet and hands that are considered to align with various parts of the body. Chiropractic therapy is another example of body-based therapy.

Energy healing interventions follow a belief system that energy flows within the body can be manipulated to improve health and wellness. **Reiki** is one form of energy work that uses the hands and intention to guide energy through a person's body in order to promote healing. **Therapeutic touch** is a similar process by which hands hover or lightly touch various parts of the body to facilitate feelings of well-being.

Alterations in Functioning

Etiology and Patterns of Symptoms

Etiology refers to the study of the cause and/or causes of disease. Cancer etiology is complex, with genetic, environmental, and behavioral influences. Growing awareness of the etiology of cancer provides many benefits such as: creating new strategies in cancer prevention, developing opportunities to improve public health awareness, strengthening safety standards, limiting exposure to known cancer-causing toxins, improving medical and surgical procedures, identifying at-risk individuals for early intervention, and educating individuals so that they may take an active role in reducing their risk of developing cancer. The following table details some common patterns of symptoms that individuals may experience, depending on if the cancer is acute (sudden onset); chronic (developed over a long period of time, metastasized, or returned); or late onset (in the final stages of cancer).

Patterns of Symptoms		
Acute	**Chronic**	**Late**
Sores that won't heal	Exhaustion	Extreme fatigue
Loss of appetite or loss of weight	Unexplained pain	Complete loss of appetite
Persistent fatigue	Bowel changes	Delirium
Unexplained bleeding or discharge	Loss of appetite or loss of weight	Drowsiness
Lump in breast	New lump in breast	Loss of bowel control
Lump in testes	New lump in testes	Loss of bladder control
Sudden change in shape, size, color, or thickness of mole, wart, etc.	Severe headaches	Extreme pain

Hematologic Alterations

The function of blood within the human body is quite diverse. Critical functions include oxygen delivery to all areas of the body, metabolic waste removal, infection prevention and hormone transportation, just to name a few. When these functions become altered, the body will experience adverse effects.

Chemotherapy treatment can adversely interfere with the hematologic function within the patient's body. It may cause bone marrow suppression, also known as **myelosuppression**. Since bone marrow is responsible for the creation of white blood cells, red blood cells, and platelets, serious side effects may occur. The patient may experience lower levels of red blood cells (**anemia**); lower levels of white blood cells (**neutropenia**), making the patient more susceptible to infection; or a decreased production in platelets (**thrombocytopenia**), resulting in abnormal coagulation.

Oncology nurses should pay close attention to the signs of any of these conditions and act accordingly:

Complication	Signs and Symptoms	Interventions
Thrombocytopenia	• Longer than normal bleeding times • Easy bruising • Large bruises	• Improve diet: include foods rich in B12 and folates • Include B12 supplements

Complication	Signs and Symptoms	Interventions
	• Several small bruises • Bleeding gums • Nosebleeds	• Decrease or limit alcohol consumption and sugary drinks • Stop taking pain medications, such as ibuprofen or aspirin, which thin the blood • Depending on the severity, a blood or platelet transfusion may be necessary
Neutropenia	• Diarrhea • Fever • Sore throat • Nasal congestion • Burning during urination	• Clean cuts immediately and often • Wash hands thoroughly and often throughout the day • Avoid large groups of people • Maintain proper oral hygiene • Avoid eating raw foods such as fish, seafood, meat, and/or eggs
Anemia	• Shortness of breath • Fatigue • Chest pain • Nausea and/or vomiting • Heart palpitations • Lightheadedness	• Eat a well-balanced diet • Get plenty of sleep • Rise slowly from a sitting or lying down position • In some cases, **ESAs (erythropoiesis-stimulating agents)** may be needed to stimulate the production of red blood cells

Immunological Alterations

The immune system of patients with cancer can be altered by the disease itself or by treatment side effects. Cancer cells work to evade the immune system and can inhibit the body's immune response to antigens, making the body more susceptible to other infections. Chemotherapy works by targeting rapidly dividing cells, which includes the skin, mucosal linings, and the cells that become white blood cells. This causes patients to be at high risk for life-threatening infections during their treatment period. Immunotherapy and biologic therapies work to stimulate the immune system to be able to detect and target tumor cells. This can cause the immune system to attack its own tissues, resulting in immune-mediated side effects.

Important nursing considerations include education of the patient surrounding risks of an altered immune system. For patients receiving chemotherapy, this includes education around hand hygiene, avoiding crowds and people who are ill, and proper food safety. These precautions are especially important during the **nadir period**, which occurs when a patient's blood cell counts reach their lowest point during each treatment cycle. Should they have symptoms of infection such as fever or chills, they should be treated urgently. For patients receiving immunotherapy, it is important to counsel them on the recognition of **immune-mediated side effects**, including rash, colitis, and pneumonitis. In mild cases, these symptoms can be managed with supportive treatment. For rashes and itching, this includes lotions, ointments, and antihistamines to minimize both damage to the skin and creation of entry points for infection. Colitis management includes antidiarrheals, dietary changes, and oral or IV hydration. If immune-mediated side effects are severe, high doses of steroids may be required. While a patient is receiving steroids, immunotherapy treatment will be paused; therefore, early identification of adverse effects and supportive management are preferred, when possible, to prevent the need to interrupt therapy due to initiating steroids. Patients who are at the end of their treatments should be counseled on avoiding illness and maintaining immunizations as recommended, since they are at an ongoing risk of increased complications if they become sick.

Gastrointestinal Alterations

Disease burden and treatments such as chemotherapy, immunotherapy, and radiation can impact the GI system, commonly causing mucositis, nausea, vomiting, diarrhea, and constipation. For all symptoms, patients and caregivers should be educated on when to seek urgent or emergent medical evaluation.

Mucositis is the inflammation of the mucosal lining of the mouth and GI tract as a side effect of chemotherapy or radiation treatment. In moderate to severe cases, a patient can develop painful ulcerations that can impact nutrition and become potential sources of infection. Nurses should assess changes in eating or drinking and examine the oral cavity for redness, swelling, ulceration, or white patches. Interventions include analgesics to relieve severe pain, preventative oral hygiene, and regular saltwater rinses.

Nausea and **vomiting** are two of the most feared side effects of treatment for patients with cancer. It is important to assess the two separately, as nausea is not always accompanied by vomiting and vice-versa. Assessment should include inquiries around pattern, severity, accompanying symptoms, and dehydration. Pharmacologic management includes antiemetics and education on administration schedule. Nonpharmacologic management includes dietary strategies such as small, frequent meals, avoiding spicy or fried foods, and relaxation techniques.

Diarrhea is defined as more than three unformed stools in 24 hours. Although diarrhea is a common side effect of treatment, it can also be the result of an infectious process. It is important to assess changes from baseline, pattern of diarrhea, and associated symptoms such as blood in the stool, bloating, cramping, gas, and dehydration. Pharmacologic interventions include antidiarrheals, and patients should be counseled on dietary modifications, such as the **BRAT diet**.

Constipation is passing fewer than three stools per week or having difficulty passing stool. Patients should be asked about changes from baseline and their definition of constipation. Nurses should assess for presence of bowel sounds and passing of gas; inspect the abdomen for symmetry, distention, bulges, or visible peristalsis; and inquire about abdominal fullness or bloating, accompanying nausea or vomiting, use of laxatives, and current diet. Interventions focus on optimization of laxatives and stool softeners, as well as counseling to increase dietary fiber, oral fluids, and activity.

Genitourinary Alterations

Urinary incontinence is an involuntary loss of urine and can be caused by disease, surgical interventions, radiation therapy, or chemotherapy agents that cause neurologic side effects. If there is new onset of urinary incontinence, the nurse should complete a thorough neurological assessment and assess for symptoms of infection. If there is no neurological or infectious cause, interventions include medications to improve continence and supportive care, such as toileting schedules and maintaining skin integrity.

Renal function is often impacted by chemotherapy and immunotherapy, but it can also be impacted by disease burden on the ureter or kidney. Assessment includes review of laboratory measures, such as creatinine, BUN, potassium, and sodium, as well as asking about flank pain, changes in urination, nausea, vomiting, or confusion. Interventions typically include hydration (oral or IV) and electrolyte replacement.

Integumentary Alterations

The skin, hair, nails, and exocrine glands make up the integumentary system. The skin is the largest organ of the human body and, as such, is the body's first defense against bacteria, fungus, and viruses that come in contact with an individual. When the skin is compromised, an individual is more susceptible to becoming sick. Alterations in the skin can involve anything from a scrape or an abrasion to a burn, a blister, or a surgical incision. If an individual suffers from specific allergies, the skin may react with a rash or even an inflammatory response. As an individual ages, the skin becomes thinner and loses more heat, causing difficulty in the body's ability to regulate its own temperature. Paying close attention to any alterations in the skin is of particular importance, as these changes may be telltale signs of potentially life-threatening conditions such as skin cancer. Abnormal growths, such as bumps, patches, or discolored moles, can be indicative signs of **skin cancer**. Receiving an early diagnosis and effective treatment are crucial to the individual's overall health and well-being. Some forms of skin cancer include **basal cell carcinoma** (BCC), **Actinic Keratoses** (AK), **squamous cell carcinoma** (SCC), and **melanoma**.

Alterations in one's hair may be due to a number of factors including the following: change in hormone levels (especially during puberty, pregnancy, and menopause); increased levels of anxiety; poor diet; medication intake; chemical treatments to the hair; thyroid gland issues; and male and female-pattern baldness (**alopecia**). When patients undergo chemotherapy and radiation to combat cancer, they will most likely experience a loss of hair, either just on their scalp or all over their body, including their eyelashes and eyebrows. Radiation and chemotherapy cause the immune system to attack rapidly dividing cells; since hair follicles are one of the most rapidly dividing cells in the human body, they are adversely affected by the treatment. In most cases, hair will begin growing back right away for patients receiving chemotherapy. However, for those receiving radiation, it may take months after the treatment has ended. Since a significant number of patients describe this side effect of treatment as very devastating to their emotional well-being, the medical community plays a vital role in helping prepare patients for this probable eventuality. Nursing staff can educate patients on how to care for the hair and scalp, along with sharing references for wig specialists and makeover artists who specialize in eyebrow and eyelash application. These interventions can help an individual to regain a higher level of self-confidence and lower possible levels of anxiety and depression. Examples of advice for proper hair and scalp scare include the use of mild shampoos and conditioners and wide-toothed combs. Teaching patients to avoid using hair dryers, curling irons, perms, and hair coloring treatments will help to reduce any further damage to the hair follicles.

Changes to the nails naturally occur as individuals age, but any significant changes either on the fingernails or toenails can also be symptoms of serious illnesses. Chronically brittle nails may indicate poor diet choices or may be caused by excessive use of chemicals that are negatively impacting healthy nail growth. Yellow and thickening nails may be indicative of lung issues, while brown, vertical stripes on the nail may point to a possible melanoma. Patients undergoing breast cancer treatment may experience changes to the color and thickness of their nails. Nursing staff should spend time educating patients regarding proper **nail care**, including keeping nails short, gently pushing back cuticles, wearing protective gloves when cleaning, avoiding nail polishes or using water-based polishes, and promptly reporting any signs of inflammation or infection.

The **exocrine glands** in the skin not only include sweat glands, but also sebaceous glands, which create and release the necessary oil to keep hair and skin waterproof. With the production of healthy mucous, sweat, tears, and wax, exocrine glands play a vital role in optimal human body function. Sometimes, these glands may become compromised and require medical attention. Compromised exocrine glands may be the result of a genetic condition, infection, an ulcer, an obstruction, or even cancer. Should an individual present with pain, swelling, excessive dryness to the dermis, fever, inflammation, or even an inability to cool down after exercise, this can indicate an issue with the exocrine glands that may require medical attention.

Respiratory Alterations

Pulmonary toxicities are caused by chemotherapy, radiation, or immunotherapies. With radiation, toxic effects are proportionate to doses received. Concurrent radiation therapy with chemotherapy increases the risk. During assessment, patients will often report dyspnea along with nonproductive cough, fatigue, fever, and pleuritic chest pain. Nurses can anticipate orders for imaging, such as a CT scan or X-ray. Pharmacologic interventions include steroids, cough suppressants, and antipyretics.

Pleural effusion is the presence of fluid in the pleural space between the lungs and chest wall. It can be from a malignant cause, indicating spread of disease into the pleura, or can be caused by a benign process such as congestive heart failure. Patients will note fever, tachypnea, cough, and chest pain. Upon auscultation, diminished or absent breath sounds, egophony, and pleural friction rub may be heard. Patients will often receive a chest CT for diagnosis, and a thoracentesis may be performed to remove fluid, ease symptoms, and determine the cause. Additional management strategies include education on ways to decrease symptom severity, relaxation techniques, use of assistive devices as needed for ADLs, and oxygen therapy as needed.

Cardiovascular Alterations

Many chemotherapy agents have **cardiovascular toxicities** as a side effect that can cause damage to the cardiac muscle, conduction system, valves, arteries, or pericardium. The effects can be seen acutely, usually within 24 hours, and as a late effect, usually over a year after completing chemotherapy. The risk of cardiotoxicities increases with a history of heart disease or cardiac dysfunction. Certain therapies, such as doxorubicin, have a higher risk for cardiotoxicities. Upon assessment, patients may report shortness of breath, chest pain, palpitations, periods of syncope, or weight gain. Nurses can expect patients to need an ECG to further evaluate heart rhythms or a **MUGA scan** to assess the heart structures and function. Pharmacologic interventions include prophylactic medications to protect the cardiac tissue with certain chemotherapies, as well as medications to manage effects such as hypertension. Nurses should educate patients on symptom reporting, along with heart-healthy diet and exercise.

Neurological Alterations

Individuals undergoing cancer treatment may experience neurologic complications. In fact, neurologic complications are some of the most common side effects following chemotherapy treatment.

Cognitive

Cognitive impairment is a commonly reported issue among patients undergoing cancer treatment. Often referred to as **brain fog** or chemo brain, patients can experience varying degrees of deficits in memory, processing, awareness, recall, and learning. These changes are often associated with initial diagnosis and treatment, but they can persist for several months or years after treatment ends. This can have a significant impact on quality of life as patients struggle to continue normal activities, such as working and caring for themselves and their families.

The factors that lead to **cognitive changes** are complex and are not clearly defined. However, research has suggested that several factors increase a person's chances and severity of changes in cognition. For instance, the presence of cancer itself can result in decline in cognition due to chronic inflammation and increased metabolic activity related to tumor proliferation. Additionally, cancer treatments such as surgery, chemotherapy, radiation, and bone marrow transplants can impact cognition during treatment and in the post-treatment period. Use of supportive medications, such as steroids and antihistamines, are known to potentially cause altered cognition as well. Additionally, some comorbidities (e.g., anxiety, depression, anemia, insomnia, pain, and hormone changes) can exacerbate cognitive changes due to cancer and cancer treatment. Lastly, the presence of primary or metastatic brain cancer has a substantial impact on brain function and cognition, depending on the size and location of the tumor(s).

Management of cognitive changes is focused on supporting normal body and brain function as well as maintaining safety. This includes encouraging adequate nutrition and hydration, gentle physical activity, and stress management. Patients can also participate in cognitive training through memory, processing, and learning activities. Journaling and organizational tools can improve quality of life as well. Lastly, cognitive behavioral therapy and management of comorbid conditions can aid in improvement of cognitive symptoms.

Neuropathies

Neuropathy is any disturbance of the nervous system, which can be caused by the disease itself or is often a side effect of chemotherapy and radiation therapy. **Peripheral neuropathies** present as numbness, tingling, or burning in the hands and feet that cause discomfort and impact mobility in severe cases. **Central nervous system neuropathies** may present as tremors, balance and coordination issues, weakness, or vision changes. Assessments should include a baseline neurological examination and reassessment at regular intervals. Pharmacologic interventions include analgesics, antidepressants, and anticonvulsants to help in managing painful peripheral neuropathies. Nurses should educate patients and caregivers on the following topics: potential neurological effects of new treatments; hand and foot care, such as protecting from cold, heat, and friction that patients may not notice due to lack of sensation; and collaboration with physical and occupational therapy.

Musculoskeletal Alterations

Musculoskeletal alterations include myalgias, arthralgias, and impaired mobility. While there can be direct causes, such as a brain or spinal cord tumor (resulting in impaired mobility) or chemotherapy treatment (resulting in joint pain), many musculoskeletal symptoms are caused by a **muscle-wasting syndrome** that is common in patients with cancer. Inactivity can lead to decreased muscle size, atrophy, and weakness. Assessments should include a physical examination for changes in muscle tone, strength, and mass; pain level; range of motion; and changes in mobility or motor function. Interventions may include analgesics to treat myalgias and arthralgias in order to encourage activity. Nurses should educate on active range-of-motion activities, safe ambulation practices, and use of appropriate assistive devices if needed. Referrals should be made to physical therapy, occupational therapy, and rehabilitative services as appropriate.

Nutrition

Maintaining a healthy weight requires the adoption of a balanced daily diet. Individuals are encouraged to eat more vegetables, fruits, and whole grains and lower their consumption of red meat, fats, sugar, alcohol, and even salt. However, for individuals who are being treated for cancer, this can be very problematic. When patients undergo chemotherapy and radiation treatment, they often require a high-fat, high-calorie diet in order to maintain their weight and lessen the risk of too much **weight loss**. If the mouth and throat are causing pain and discomfort, patients may opt for cool, thick foods such as ice cream to temporarily soothe this pain. Other factors that may adversely affect a patient's nutritional status include loss of appetite, persistent constipation or diarrhea, vomiting, dry mouth, changes in taste and smell, as well as dental and gum problems. When the nutritional status of patients is adversely affected, their overall response to treatment, quality of life, and rate of survival are all compromised.

Pain Management

Pain is a common symptom in patients with cancer. It is a personalized experience, so individual reports should be respected. Many patients experience cancer pain caused by tumors, diagnostic tests, and treatment. While **acute cancer pain** is typically due to a known cause and lasts less than six months, **chronic cancer pain** may have an unknown cause and persist longer than six months.

The prevalence of pain is higher in patients with head and neck cancer, breast cancer, and lung cancer due to chemotherapy, radiation therapy, and surgical side effects. Many patients with cancer are hesitant to discuss and treat their pain appropriately due to fears of being considered a problematic patient, that pain may be a symptom of worsening disease, and the potential of medication addiction or side effects. Culture plays an important factor in the reporting, expression, and treatment of pain.

A thorough assessment is critical in identifying and adequately treating pain. In older adults, it is important to assess for risk of falls, as most pharmacologic interventions can increase this risk. **Polypharmacy** is common, and the risk for interactions with pain medications is high. An assessment of the physical, psychological, social, and spiritual impacts of pain should be completed to determine the impact on normal activity. Pain should be reassessed regularly to understand whether interventions are appropriate.

Pharmacological interventions are the primary treatment for pain and should be tailored to the individual patient's needs and response. Non-opioids, such as acetaminophen and NSAIDs, should be used for mild pain. For moderate pain, opioids such as oxycodone and hydrocodone should be added. When pain is severe, opioid analgesics such as morphine and fentanyl are implemented to manage pain. If there is little relief from these interventions, other mildly invasive procedures such as radiation therapy or epidurals can be used for additional pain relief.

Nurses should provide education to patients and their caregivers on the medication administration schedule, side effect management, and safety precautions. Non-pharmacologic interventions such as heat, ice, stretching, and relaxation techniques should also be offered. Nurses should stress that if pain is not adequately managed or there are other concerning symptoms, patients should have a low threshold to contact their medical provider to ensure that there is not an impending serious impairment occurring, such as cord compression.

Practice Quiz

1. A nurse is preparing to administer ABVD chemotherapy to a 65-year-old female with Hodgkin lymphoma. The patient notes that she is anxious to receive this because she heard it causes extreme nausea and vomiting, and she tends to get queasy with car rides. The nurse notes all of the following to increase her risk for chemotherapy-induced nausea and vomiting EXCEPT:
   a. History of motion sickness
   b. Gender
   c. Age
   d. Anxiety or expectations

2. A nurse is providing pre-surgery education to a patient preparing to undergo a cystectomy with ileal conduit creation. Which of the following should the nurse include in the education?
   a. A bladder will be surgically constructed, and emptying of the bladder will occur through the urethra.
   b. A portion of the small bowel is connected to the ureters and brought through the abdominal wall to create a stoma. This results in almost constant urine production.
   c. An external collection device is not needed, but catheterization through the stoma will be required every 4–6 hours for emptying.
   d. External tubes will be placed through the back into the kidney to drain urine continuously.

3. A nurse working in an outpatient clinic receives a phone call from a patient currently undergoing treatment for testicular cancer. The patient reports new pain in his right arm at the site of his PICC, along with swelling and redness down his arm. He denies fevers, chills, or drainage at insertion site. The nurse reports the findings to the provider and expects to receive which of the following orders next?
   a. Compression sleeve
   b. Chest X-ray
   c. Blood cultures from PICC and peripheral site
   d. Venous ultrasound of right arm

4. A nurse is preparing to administer docetaxel to a 76-year-old man with prostate cancer. Which intervention can be implemented to reduce the risk of peripheral neuropathies?
   a. Ice gloves and booties
   b. A dose of gabapentin 1 hour prior to administration
   c. Encourage ambulation during the infusion
   d. Elevation of extremities during the infusion

5. A nurse is caring in the hospital for a 63-year-old female with advanced kidney cancer who is receiving daily radiation for treatment of spinal cord compression. Which of the following is a priority intervention for musculoskeletal health?
   a. Collaborating with physical and occupational therapy services
   b. Assessing for a specialty bed with a low air-loss pressure mattress
   c. Creating a regular toileting schedule
   d. A nutrition referral for high-protein meal and snack recommendations

See answers on the next page.

Answer Explanations

1. C: Younger individuals (under 60) have a higher risk for chemotherapy-induced nausea and vomiting (CINV). A history of motion sickness, hyperemesis with pregnancy, female gender, prechemotherapy anxiety or expectations, and postoperative nausea are among other risk factors for CINV, making Choices *A, B,* and *D* incorrect.

2. B: An ileal conduit is a type of urostomy created by implanting the ureters into a segment of the small bowel that has been brought through the abdominal wall. This creates a near-constant flow of urine and requires a collection device to maintain skin integrity. Choice *A* describes a neobladder, which is created surgically from the intestine and is relocated to the original bladder location. It allows for voiding through the urethra, although intermittent catheterization may be required. Choice *C* refers to an Indiana pouch, in which a reservoir is created from the large intestine and accessed through a one-way flap valve allowing for catheterization. Choice *D* describes a nephrostomy tube and is used when there is a blockage of urine between the kidney and bladder.

3. D: This patient is reporting symptoms concerning for deep vein thrombosis (DVT), including unilateral swelling, pain, and redness. Central lines (such as a PICC), active cancer, and active treatment for cancer are risk factors for developing a DVT. A venous ultrasound is done to determine whether a clot is present. Choice *A* is incorrect and is a more appropriate treatment for edema. Choice *B* would be appropriate imaging to visualize the location of the PICC or further evaluate the lungs for abnormalities. Choice *C* would be used if there was concern for infection. Since this patient does not have a fever, chills, or drainage from the insertion site, there is low suspicion for infection.

4. A: Cryotherapy can help reduce the incidence of peripheral neuropathies associated with docetaxel administration, although results are mixed. Choices *B, C,* and *D* have not been shown to be effective in prevention of chemotherapy-induced peripheral neuropathies.

5. A: After spinal cord compression, many patients have ongoing motor, strength, sensory, and mobility issues. A referral to physical therapy and occupational therapy helps to safely mobilize patients, assist with ADLs, and work to maintain muscle tone. While a specialty mattress may be needed, it is not a priority intervention, making Choice *B* incorrect. A regular toileting schedule can help prevent falls and maintain skin integrity; however, it will not help the patient with mobility and strength, so Choice *C* is incorrect. Choice *D* is also a necessary referral, but it is not a priority since it will not assist with mobility.

Oncologic Emergencies

Oncologic emergencies refer to life-threating conditions that occur as a direct result of the presence of cancerous cells or specific cancer treatments. Some of these situations could occur as a result of some other medical intervention (such as surgery), but oncologic emergencies specifically result as a secondary condition due to the presence of cancer.

DIC

Disseminated intravascular coagulation (**DIC**) refers to a situation in which blood clotting processes are disrupted. As blood cells begin to form clots, the body does not recognize when clots become too large or when too many have been formed. Therefore, it does not attempt to break them down. The extra clots may cause blockages or strokes. They may also damage red blood cells upon contact; this continues a feedback loop, as the body thinks it is further injured and creates more clots. This process also uses up the body's store of platelets, which are crucial to closing open wounds, faster than they can be replaced. In instances where the body needs to healthily clot and heal tissues, it becomes unable to do so. The wound does not heal and continues to bleed, which can lead to internal or external hemorrhage. DIC is a risk of any surgery and can also occur as a secondary condition to many different diseases. If DIC occurs in major blood vessels (such as arteries or deep veins), it is likely to result in tissue death, organ failure, or some type of permanent damage. Almost half of all DIC cases result in patient death. While trauma and trauma surgery patients are more likely to experience acute cases of DIC (instances that come on quickly as a direct result of traumatic or surgical wounds), cancer patients are more likely to experience chronic DIC (continuous clotting problems that have to be regularly monitored and treated). Both types of DIC in cancer patients can be triggered by the presence of tumors. DIC in cancer patients is primarily treated with blood transfusions or anticoagulants if the patient's system is able to handle medication; however, these procedures are often unsuccessful.

SIADH

Syndrome of inappropriate antidiuretic hormone secretion (**SIADH**) is characterized by issues relating to electrolytes and their balance in the body. It is the most common cause of hyponatremia, or a sodium deficiency that results in excessive water in the body. Hyponatremia is a common condition and can happen regularly in mild forms from routine activities, such as drinking too much water. When the body becomes unable to regulate water and sodium levels to bring them into balance (often due to a medical condition), swelling can become severe. SIADH is a disorder that affects the production and function of antidiuretic hormone (ADH), which is responsible for keeping the body's fluid levels and electrolyte levels in balance. ADH is secreted in abnormal amounts or frequencies, which impacts the circulation of water through the kidneys and ultimately results in an abnormally diluted amount of electrolytes in the body. SIADH may be caused by diseases that affect the hypothalamus, which produces ADH; pulmonary diseases; pharmaceuticals that affect the hypothalamus or kidneys; genetic disorders; and other acute conditions. However, a number of cancers result in abnormal ADH production and function, either due to tumor location (e.g., near the hypothalamus or kidneys) or the way they cause certain organs to act or fail. Small cell lung cancer, for example, is highly correlated with SIADH. Managing SIADH includes managing the causal condition, treating symptoms of hyponatremia with intravenous fluid and electrolyte solutions in order to disrupt the feedback loop, and utilizing steroid-based pharmaceuticals and vasopressors.

Sepsis

Sepsis refers to any instance of an infection in the bloodstream. It is a secondary condition to another infection in the body, but is most closely associated with infections of the lungs, kidneys, skin, or gastrointestinal system. Sepsis is most commonly triggered by *Staphylococcus*, *E. coli*, and *Streptococcus* infections. This may be due to the resistance that strains of these bacteria have developed to antibiotics; therefore, health care providers have a difficult time eradicating the strains from the patient's body. As the patient's body tries to treat and heal the infection, it may inadvertently create autoimmune responses that result in system-wide inflammation. Due to the large scale of inflammation, normal endocrine and neural transmitters fail to regulate internal processes normally. This may result in a high fever, tachycardia, and extreme shortness of breath. More severe symptoms of sepsis include little or no urine elimination, visible cognitive and neurological changes, pain, respiratory and cardiac problems, and changes in some biomarkers (e.g., blood cell counts, platelet counts, and lymph composition). Mild sepsis affects only the blood stream, whereas more serious cases may affect blood flow to vital organs and result in tissue death or organ failure. Cancer patients may be more vulnerable to sepsis, due to their compromised immune system when cancer is present and during treatment. They are more prone to infections overall, spend a large amount of time in hospitals, are more likely to have a surgery that may need time for the wound to heal, and may be older in age. These factors all increase the likelihood of not only contracting an infection, but also experiencing complications of sepsis. Sepsis is normally treated with continuous antibiotic dosing, IV fluids, blood transfusions, surgery, assisted ventilation, and/or dialysis.

Septic shock is a life-threatening outcome of untreated or unmanageable sepsis. Nearly half of patients whose case of sepsis escalates to septic shock do not survive. Cases of sepsis that are caused by antibiotic-resistant bacterial strains are most likely to escalate to cases of septic shock. A patient who is experiencing septic shock is exposed to infection in their blood stream and vital organs, especially the heart and lungs. This results in a dangerous drop in blood pressure, which often results in widespread organ failure, stroke, and/or death. Even in patients who recover, permanent organ damage may subsist. Septic shock is characterized by clotting issues, changes in biomarkers (e.g., excess blood waste and low platelet counts), severe electrolyte imbalances, kidney failure, and/or liver dysfunction. Septic shock often does not respond to standard protocols for elevating blood pressure, such as fluid and electrolyte replacement. Instead, it is treated with IV administration of antibiotics, fluids, and blood transfusions; vasopressors (to increase blood and fluid circulation); continuous insulin; and steroid-based pharmaceuticals. Additionally, extra medical care is given to any open wounds (such as post-surgery wounds) to ensure adequate healing is taking place.

Tumor Lysis Syndrome

Tumor lysis syndrome occurs as a result of cancer treatments, primarily in cancers of the lymph, bones, or blood. As tumors are broken down, the internal contents of cancerous cells are displaced into the body. Symptoms include significant changes in specific metabolic biomarkers and electrolyte imbalances in the blood, including increased potassium levels, decreased calcium levels, high nitrogen compounds, and high uric acid levels. The body becomes unable to filter and balance these products effectively. Mild symptoms may include nausea, while severe symptoms include seizures, heart arrhythmias, organ dysfunction, organ failure, and death. In cancer patients that are at high risk of developing tumor lysis syndrome (such as lymphoma patients), preventative measures should stringently be maintained throughout treatment, and patients should be continuously monitored after treatment for symptoms. Measures to prevent tumor lysis syndrome include IV fluid infusions during treatment, pharmaceuticals that regulate uric acid production, and/or solutions that help alkalize the blood and urine. If the syndrome develops, treatment will be tailored to the patient's specific needs. Based on the metabolic products that appear in the blood, patients will present with different conditions. Most commonly, patients show disruption in kidney function; therefore, dialysis is a common treatment protocol for this syndrome.

Hypersensitivity

Hypersensitivity refers to any allergic or other immune response that occurs toward an agent of any kind. This response, referred to as a hypersensitivity reaction, may appear as inflammation, fever, rash, swelling, or hives; in severe cases, these responses can lead to shock, loss of consciousness, or inability to breathe. Common agents that may cause hypersensitivity reaction include nuts, shellfish, latex, dairy, some fruits, insect venom, and numerous pharmaceuticals. Many cancer patients experience a hypersensitivity reaction in response to treatments such as chemotherapy. As cancer treatments are aggressive in nature, many patients may experience reactions such as extreme nausea, vomiting, hair loss, fever, rashes, and swelling. These reactions during treatment should always be monitored to ensure they do not progress to life-threatening levels. Typically, these symptoms will be managed in cancer patients by stopping treatment for a short period of time, diluting the dosage, changing to a different medication, and preparing for an emergency situation if necessary. Emergency situations are most commonly managed with medications containing epinephrine, dopamine, or vasopressors. Hypersensitivity reactions can be prevented by ensuring all allergen history is up to date and available in the patient's medical records. Some treatments may cause a reaction regardless, due to their aggressive nature. **Desensitization** protocols, in which the patient is exposed to therapy in progressively larger doses over time, may be used for these depending on the diagnosis and prognosis.

Anaphylaxis

Anaphylaxis refers to an allergic or hypersensitive reaction that has the potential to become fatal in a short period of time. When a person is exposed to an agent that causes anaphylaxis, the immune response is so extreme that it limits (or even shuts off) some functions of the body. This may include low blood pressure, which triggers a number of other effects (e.g., dizziness or poor circulation). Patients can also experience excessive, system-wide swelling which can result in airway constriction. Anaphylaxis is an emergency situation that requires immediate intervention. Patients who have known severe allergies may carry epinephrine injections to use in case they interact with an allergen. In cancer patients, routine treatment may cause anaphylactic reactions due to the aggressive nature of treatments. Consequently, all nurses should be well-versed in how to handle emergency situations based on each patient. This may require a more in-depth understanding of pharmaceutical interventions for anaphylaxis, the distinction between appropriate and inappropriate clinical reactions to cancer treatments, and stringent monitoring of patients after treatment to ensure there are no delayed reactions.

Hypercalcemia

Hypercalcemia refers to high concentration levels of calcium in the blood stream, which may indicate weakened or brittle bones. Additionally, calcium plays a vital role in cardiac and neural signaling; any imbalance can cause a disruption in systems relating to these processes. Disruptions relating to hypercalcemia may include presentations such as fatigue, heart arrhythmias, kidney stones, kidney failure, dementia, or lack of focus. Hypercalcemia occurs in approximately 20 percent of cancer patients and is a serious condition in this group. It most commonly appears in later stages of cancer and is associated with a high mortality rate. The presence of this condition commonly indicates that tumors have metastasized into the bones and can affect vital functions such as blood cell production and calcium reabsorption. Hypercalcemia is most commonly seen in patients with breast cancer, lung cancer, or myeloma. Upon diagnosis, hypercalcemia is most commonly treated with IV bisphosphonate, which inhibits further bone breakdown. Steroid- and nitrate-based medications may also be utilized. Additionally, if patients are receiving excess calcium from any sources (e.g. through diet or supplements), those should be immediately eliminated. Supplementation with phosphate and magnesium may also be needed, since the levels of these elements decrease significantly in hypercalcemic conditions and are crucial for intracellular and neural functions.

Cardiac Tamponade

Cardiac tamponade is considered an immediate emergency. It refers to a condition in which excess fluid pressure around the heart causes cardiac disruption, primarily restricting the ventricles from expanding fully. Cardiac tamponade results from an injury to or wound in the pericardium, the firm membrane that encases the cardiac muscle. As other fluid fills the sac, it results in a pressure differential and places excess weight onto the ventricles. This prevents the heart from delivering oxygenated blood into circulation, and ultimately can result in tissue death, organ disruption, organ failure, or a heart attack. In cancer patients, cardiac tamponade progresses gradually and is most likely due to cancer that has spread from elsewhere into the heart. It may also result from an underlying infection. Symptoms include visibly distended veins, high blood pressure, shortness of breath, chest pain, anxiety, and visible changes in consciousness. Oncology nurses should be aware of these symptoms, especially in high-risk patients, and have an emergency plan in place. Cardiac tamponade is managed through **pericardiocentesis**, a procedure in which a syringe is placed into the pericardium in order to manually draw out excess fluid. Due to the rate at which fluid can fill the pericardium, even through a small wound, both healthy and ill patients are unable to correct this condition without medical assistance. Additionally, patient activity is minimized or eliminated completely, and vital signs are stringently monitored until the pericardium heals. Medications which raise blood pressure may also be given. Overall prognoses for cardiac tamponade cases are positive when they are treated in a timely manner.

Spinal Cord Compression

Spinal cord compression occurs when weight or pressure is placed directly or indirectly upon the spinal cord. The spinal cord runs the length of the vertebral column and innervates large and small muscle groups in order for the body to move and feel sensations. Compression can occur anywhere along the spinal cord; the location of compression dictates how symptoms manifest. Mild symptoms may include numbness, pain, pressure, or tingling. While mild cases may cause discomfort, they can typically be managed with medications or manual therapies and do not usually prevent the patient from engaging in routine activities. Moderate to severe symptoms may include debilitating pain, complete loss of feeling or sensation in an area, a limp, or even paralysis. Spinal cord compression becomes more frequent as people age. The vertebral discs around the spinal cord are cushioned with a thick, viscous substance that prevents the discs from touching. With age, poor posture, repetitive motion, injuries, pregnancies, scoliosis, or surgeries, these intervertebral discs become worn. As a result, the positioning of the vertebrae may shift and place pressure on the cord.

In cancer patients, the presence of tumors or bone degeneration can cause spinal cord compression. Symptoms come on acutely and severely, whereas they result gradually in instances of normal aging or spinal curvature. Cancer patients may experience nerve pain, sharp muscular pain that feels electrical in nature, numbness or tingling in the extremities, and general loss of muscular coordination. **Cauda equina syndrome** is an emergency situation that can arise from severe compression of the lower (lumbar) spinal cord. It is characterized by acute loss of feeling and voluntary control in the lower half of the body, resulting in loss of bladder or bowel control, inability to walk well, and paralysis anywhere in the lower limbs. Sometimes this comes on suddenly, such as in the cause of a traumatic injury to the lumbar spine. In gradual cases, patients may first experience symptoms (e.g., uncomfortable pain or sciatica) before the compression becomes severe. Therefore, patients who develop these symptoms should immediately be evaluated in order to ensure they will not progress in severity. Spinal cord compression can be treated with anti-inflammatory medications; steroid injections or medications; manual therapy (e.g., massage, physical therapy, or chiropractic care); or surgery. In cancer patients, surgical removal of the tumor is likely the main avenue for relief. Due to the proximity of tumors to the spinal cord, however, surgery may be complex.

Superior Vena Cava Syndrome

Superior vena cava syndrome results from obstructions to the superior vena cava, the primary blood vessel that carries deoxygenated blood from the upper half of the body to the heart. Virtually all instances of obstruction occur from cancerous tumors (although rarely the syndrome may result from aneurysms or infections). Most commonly, obstructions leading to superior vena cava syndrome are from lung cancers due to the close physical proximity of the lungs to the heart. The syndrome is not immediately life threatening but does have highly visible symptoms, including observable swelling and puffiness in the patient's face, arm, chest, and veins in the chest. Other symptoms include shortness of breath, wheezing, and excessive, unmanageable coughing. In patients with cancers that may cause the syndrome, these symptoms come on quite gradually and increase in intensity as tumors increase in size. Superior vena cava syndrome is primarily treated through steroid medications to decrease inflammation and relieve pressure around the vein. Fluid monitoring and adjustment may also be used to create systemic pressure in the cardiovascular system that allows better circulation through the superior vena cava. While the syndrome itself is easily managed and not typically considered a primary cause of death, most patients who experience it are likely to die in under three years. This finding is correlated with the types of cancer that influence the presence of the syndrome, as they are all highly aggressive types.

Increased Intracranial Pressure

Increased intracranial pressure refers to increased pressure inside the skull and around the brain. It mostly commonly occurs due to an increase of cerebrospinal fluid, a fluid that surrounds the brain and spinal cord. At normal levels, it serves as a cushion for the brain and spinal cord along with playing a fundamental role in the amount of blood that travels to the brain. When cerebrospinal fluid levels become too high, usually due to brain injury, tumor, or aneurysm, the pressure can severely damage brain tissue. Symptoms of increased intracranial pressure include headache, nausea, vomiting, loss of cognitive functions and abilities, high blood pressure, confusion, vision problems, unresponsive eye and pupil movements, seizures, fainting, and coma. Any presence of an intracranial tumor will cause increased compression and pressure inside the skull. Additionally, the presence of tumors in other locations of the body, such as near the spine or nerve endings, have the potential to affect blood flow to and fluid levels relating to the brain. **Lumbar punctures**, where spinal fluid is extracted, can both diagnose increased intracranial pressure as well as slightly relieve the pressure. Other treatments include utilizing a lumbar shunt to drain more fluid than a puncture is able to or draining fluid directly from the skull. In the presence of intracranial tumors, the pressure is likely to need continuous monitoring unless the tumors are removed or greatly reduced in size. Without treatment, increased pressure in the skull can lead to brain damage, permanent coma, or death. In patients with advanced brain cancers, these results may occur even with treatment.

Obstructions

Bowel and urinary tract obstructions are side effects of a number of different cancers, including stomach, colon, rectal, ovarian, and prostate. **Bowel obstructions** occur when the intestines are compromised in a way that prevents the normal flow of digestion through the bowel or when tumors are located near nerves that control bowel functions. Symptoms include constipation, nausea, vomiting, and visible bloating or abdominal distention. Treatment may include an enema, stenting or surgical removal of parts of the bowel, or tube feeding. Some patients with severe cases may need to have a colostomy, where waste is eliminated through the abdomen into a bag that must be regularly changed. In these cases, the bowels have lost complete ability to function, and this is the only way to provide relief to the patient. In **urinary tract obstructions**, a blockage (e.g., tumor or kidney stone) prevents urine from leaving the body. Without treatment, this can lead to kidney damage and infection, with an increased possibility of sepsis. Symptoms of urinary tract obstructions include pain and decreased urination. Treatment may include hormone therapy to reduce tumors that are in reproductive areas, stenting the urinary tract in the area of obstruction, or dialysis in severe cases.

Pneumonitis

Pneumonitis refers to inflammation of tissues in and of the lung. This term is primarily used to indicate non-infectious lung inflammation. It is characterized by dry cough, shortness of breath, fever, and fatigue. Appetite and weight may also be affected. A number of cancer treatments may cause pneumonitis, such as chemotherapy drugs which can cause widespread inflammation. Since radiation treatments can cause localized tissue injury, radiation near the lung (e.g., to treat lung cancer, breast cancer, or the lymph nodes) may cause pneumonitis. This is more likely to occur in patients who specifically have lung cancer or other lung diseases, such as emphysema. It is also important to note that the condition usually has a delayed onset, occurring weeks after treatment begins, and often results in a misdiagnosis of pneumonia. When treatments are finished, symptoms of pneumonitis usually subside. In late-stage cancer cases that require regular chemotherapy dosing and radiation treatments near the lungs, chronic pneumonitis may result in permanent lung damage. This occurs due to scarring and loss of elasticity that happens as a result of the lungs remaining chronically inflamed. Patients may also develop pulmonary fibrosis or chronic obstructive pulmonary disease as a secondary complication to their cancer diagnosis. As a result, treatment may be paused if pneumonitis develops until symptoms subside (if it is not detrimental to the patient's overall prognosis). Pneumonitis in cancer patients is most commonly treated with steroid medications, oxygen therapy, assisted ventilation, and surgeries to remove tumors when possible.

Extravasations

Extravasation refers to any instance where an entity moves beyond its normal and usual parameters of containment. In cancer patients, this term is most commonly used to describe how and when cancer metastasizes. Cancerous cells begin as a single tumor or contained mass. When they spread, they begin by invading the cells and tissue directly adjacent to the primary mass. From here, they enter the blood stream, are circulated throughout the body, and leave the blood vessel to invade cells at another site. This act of leaving the blood vessel is the point of extravasation. Often, this is how cancer that originates in one area often spreads to the lymph nodes, lungs, or stomach, as these are all critical sites of blood circulation For cancer to spread in this manner, it requires changes in the structure of the cellular walls that allow the cancerous cells to exit the vessel, enter a new area, and take hold. It also requires the cancerous cells to be strong and aggressive enough to withstand this process. This often occurs on a micro-level that is not easily detectable until a new tumor is detected through medical imaging or the presence of new symptoms. Consequently, the surgical removal of a primary tumor does not mean the cancer is unable to spread; instead, the spread simply may not yet be detectable. However, surgical removal of cancerous tumors is normally the first line of defense in patients unless the surgery is too risky. Specific proteins support cancerous cells in this journey, and new research aims at denaturing or inhibiting these proteins in order to make the process of extravasation more difficult for the cells. It is also important to remember that not all cancer that metastasizes is considered advanced or untreatable cancer. Often, these can be treated through radiation or chemotherapy the same way the primary tumor would have been treated. Furthermore, the patient may still go into remission or have a decent quality of life with treatment. However, certain sites (e.g., the lungs or in the bones) make treatment extremely difficult and prognoses typically become worse with these cases.

Immune-Related Adverse Events

Immune-related adverse events are a collection of side effects associated with the use of immune checkpoint inhibitors. **Immune checkpoint inhibitors** function by removing natural balancing mechanisms to increase the activity of immune cells. This enhances the ability of T-cells to recognize and eliminate cancer cells. However, the same mechanism that encourages the immune system to eradicate cancer cells can also lead to unintended autoimmune-like side effects. The most common sites of immune hyperactivity are the gastrointestinal tract, the skin, and the endocrine system. Neurological, cardiac, and pulmonary immune-related adverse events are less common, but they tend to be more serious and sometimes fatal.

Each group of side effects presents with a variety of symptoms and treatment options. Examples of gastrointestinal manifestations include nausea, vomiting, diarrhea, and epigastric pain. Initial treatment includes symptom management, systemic steroids, and immune system modulators. Joint and skin symptoms include rash, itching, joint pain, swelling, and warmth. Treatment includes NSAIDs and antirheumatic medications for joint pain, topical steroids, and topical antihistamines. Skin toxicities are the most common and rapidly developing immune-related adverse events. Endocrine toxicity can result in type 1 diabetes, changes in thyroid function, adrenal insufficiency, or hypophysitis (inflammation of the pituitary gland). Endocrine manifestations tend to be permanent, unlike other immune-related toxicities. Management of endocrine toxicities involves hormone replacement. Additional toxicities include hepatitis and acute interstitial nephritis. Kidney toxicity may result in initiation of dialysis.

Neurological adverse events can include encephalitis, meningitis, Guillain-Barre syndrome, and myasthenia gravis. Treatment may require admission to intensive care unit, systemic steroids, plasmapheresis, immunoglobulins, or immune modulator treatment. Neurotoxicity occurs at a rate of approximately 1 percent. Cardiac adverse events include myocarditis, acute coronary syndrome, arrhythmias, and congestive heart failure. Cardiac toxicity represents the second highest fatality rate with immune-related events, though rare. The presence of cardiac adverse effects necessitates discontinuation of immune checkpoint inhibitor therapy. Immune-related pneumonitis represents the highest rate of fatality among immune-related adverse events. History of lung disease and history of radiation therapy to the chest increase the risk of developing pulmonary toxicity. Treatment includes steroids, immune modulators, and discontinuation of immunotherapy.

Cytokine Release Syndrome (CRS)

Cytokine release syndrome (CRS) is a life-threatening adverse reaction to immunotherapies, such as bispecific antibody therapy and CAR-T cell therapy. CRS is characterized by a massive cytokine release into the bloodstream due to the activation of multiple immune cell types, such as B cells, macrophages, NK cells, and T cells. This activation then leads to systemic inflammation with the potential for organ failure and mortality. The condition initially presents with flulike symptoms, which occur within two weeks following immunotherapy treatment and rapidly advance into severe inflammation causing organ disfunction. CRS often mimics presenting symptoms of other conditions, such as macrophage activation syndrome (MAS) and opportunistic infection, as well as meeting the systemic inflammatory response syndrome criteria for sepsis, which may complicate diagnosis. Diagnosis of CRS typically relies on the patient's history of immunotherapy and laboratory studies along with physical and biomarker assessments. High cytokine levels are a hallmark sign of CRS, particularly when TNF-α, IL-6, and IFN-γ are elevated. Elevated CRP and ferritin show high inflammation and are also indicators of CRS. The severity of CRS has been shown to be linked with the level of tumor burden the patient is experiencing, with a higher tumor burden level equating to a higher severity of CRS and inflammatory response. Treatment of CRS is highly reliant on early intervention and diagnosis to prevent the worsening of symptoms and prognosis. When CRS is caught early, treatment may solely consist of supportive measures. American Society for Transplantation and Cellular Therapy (ASTCT) criteria are used to determine the level of CRS as well as the required treatments. Grade 1 can often be treated with IV fluids and antipyretics. Grades 2 and 3 typically entail changes in immunotherapy to tocilizumab to help control moderate to severe CRS cases. Grade 4 often requires tocilizumab along with a corticosteroid.

Immune Effector Cell Associated Neurotoxicity Syndrome (ICANS)

Immune Effector Cell Associated Neurotoxicity Syndrome (ICANS) is a reaction following the administration of CAR-T cell therapy. ICANS is a common but dangerous side effect of CAR-T cell therapy in which cytokines become elevated in the bloodstream and, in severe cases, lead to permeability of the blood-brain barrier. Symptoms will typically present between five days and three weeks following CAR-T cell therapy treatment and may involve confusion, tremors, seizures, aphasia, cerebral edema, and possibly cerebral hemorrhage. ICANS can sometimes be confused with CRS due to the similarity in elevated cytokine levels. Diagnosis typically follows a complete history and physical assessment along with an MRI to rule out possible CRS. Many cases of ICANS may be managed with corticosteroid therapy or even resolve on their own. Higher disease burden, prevalence of CRS, and low platelet counts put the patient at an elevated risk of developing severe ICANS. The Immune Effector Cell Encephalopathy (ICE) score is used to assess patients receiving CAR-T cell therapy twice daily for neurological function, including assessments for writing, language, and orientation. ICE is scored on a 10-point basis, with 10 being no impairment to cognition and 2 or fewer indicating that the patient should be transferred to the ICU for intensive care.

Venous Thromboembolism

Venous thromboembolism (**VTE**), which includes **deep vein thrombosis** (**DVT**) and **pulmonary embolism** (**PE**), occurs when a blood clot mobilizes in the bloodstream and leads to obstruction of a blood vessel. This condition is more common in cancer patients due to complex factors including cancer-mediated hypercoagulability, venous stasis, and injury to the endothelium. VTEs are one of the top causes of death among patients with cancer.

Among cancer patients, there are many contributing factors that compound the risk for the development of VTE. These include personal or family medical history of VTE, heart failure, or obesity.

Advanced stages and certain cancers carry higher risk for the development of VTE (e.g., pancreas, lung, uterus, stomach, and brain). Treatment-related risk factors include surgery, treatment with certain medications (e.g., erythropoiesis-stimulating medications, platinum-based chemotherapy, l-asparaginase, hormone therapies, and antiangiogenic medications), and presence of central venous catheters. Additional risk factors include the presence of infection, immobility, and bulky tumors which can cause venous stasis.

Care related to VTEs begins with screening and prevention. Oncology patients should be initially screened for risk of VTE development and reassessed periodically throughout treatment. Patient assessment and prevention strategies should include monitoring for signs and symptoms of VTE, infection prevention, and thrombus prophylaxis as indicated (e.g., exercise, passive/active range of motion, anticoagulant therapy, antiembolism stockings, and intermittent pressure devices).

Patient education should include recognizing signs and symptoms of VTE, which include pain or tenderness, swelling, local erythema, and warmth. DVTs are typically found in the lower (most commonly) or upper extremities. PE, on the other hand, typically manifests as dyspnea, chest pain, cough, and tachypnea. If a DVT is suspected, standard diagnostic confirmation often involves a D-dimer blood test and duplex ultrasound imaging. Other diagnostic tests can include venography with contrast, magnetic resonance imaging (MRI), or computed tomography (CT) scan. PE is typically diagnosed via computed tomographic pulmonary angiography (CTPA) or ventilation-perfusion (V/Q) scan. Other diagnostic tests for PE include pulmonary angiography or MRI.

Treatment of confirmed VTE involves oral, subcutaneous, or intravenous anticoagulant therapy. Ongoing monitoring for recurrence of VTE as well as anticoagulant-therapy-associated bleeding are essential, as well. Chemotherapy-induced thrombocytopenia increases a patient's risk for bleeding complications. Lastly, some patients may require placement of an inferior vena cava (IVC) filter along with anticoagulant therapy to provide additional prevention of further events.

Practice Quiz

1. A nurse is administering the first dose of ipilimumab/nivolumab to a 49-year-old female with advanced melanoma. The patient calls the nurse 5 minutes into the infusion to report an itchy spot on her arm. Which of the following is the next step for the nurse to take?
   a. Stop the infusion and call for assistance.
   b. Slow the infusion rate and notify the provider.
   c. Ask the provider for orders for a steroid cream.
   d. Reassure the patient that rash and itching are an expected side effect.

2. A nurse is reviewing the chart of a patient with ovarian cancer who is in DIC. Which lab value is indicative of this?
   a. Increased fibrinogen level
   b. Increased platelet count
   c. Increased thrombin time
   d. Decreased D-dimer assay

3. A nurse in an outpatient infusion clinic is preparing to administer etoposide and cisplatin to a 45-year-old male with testicular cancer. Upon taking vitals, the nurse notes his temperature to be 100.5°F, blood pressure 92/63 mmHg, heart rate 102, and respiratory rate 20. Upon assessment, the patient notes nausea, fatigue, and muscle aches. The nurse anticipates the following orders and understands which to be the priority action?
   a. IV antibiotics
   b. Urine culture
   c. Antipyretics
   d. Blood cultures

4. A nurse on an inpatient oncology unit is caring for a patient with ALL (acute lymphocytic leukemia) who received cycle 1, day 1 chemotherapy earlier today. The nurse knows to watch which lab values closely?
   a. ANC
   b. Sodium
   c. Hemoglobin/hematocrit
   d. Potassium

5. A nurse working in an outpatient clinic receives a phone call from a 57-year-old male with non-small cell lung cancer (NSCLC). He notes that he must be coming down with a cold because he started having a headache, nasal stuffiness, a nonproductive cough, shortness of breath, and facial puffiness when he woke up this morning. He notes the symptoms have improved some since he's been awake and moving around the house. The nurse should do which of the following?
   a. Recommend that the patient begin taking an antihistamine such as Benadryl.
   b. Instruct the patient to present to the emergency room for evaluation and CT.
   c. Ask the patient to continue to monitor at home until their planned visit with the physician in three days.
   d. Ask the patient to monitor for fever and recommend taking OTC cold and flu medication.

See answers on the next page.

Answer Explanations

1. A: Itching that presents during the first few minutes of an infusion, with or without the presence of hives, is concerning for a hypersensitivity reaction. The nurse should stop the infusion and request help from another nurse for management. Choice *B* is incorrect, as the rate should not be adjusted without the order from a provider. Choice *C* is incorrect, as the reaction will escalate if the infusion continues to run. Choice *D* is incorrect; although a rash and itching can be a side effect from this regimen, it will not begin within a few minutes of the infusion, and this is more likely related to a hypersensitivity reaction.

2. C: Disseminated intravascular coagulation (DIC) is a disorder that causes abnormal coagulation. It can lead to organ damage by inappropriate development of clots and hemorrhage due to consumption of platelets and coagulation factors. Lab results will typically see decreased fibrinogen levels, decreased platelet counts, increased thrombin and prothrombin times, and increased D-dimer assay; therefore, Choices *A, B,* and *D* are incorrect.

3. D: The patient is showing symptoms concerning for sepsis and needs to be treated quickly with IV antibiotics. However, blood cultures need to be drawn prior to administration of antibiotics, making Choice *D* the correct option. Choice *B* may be ordered but does not need to be collected prior to administration of antibiotics. Choice *C* may be ordered for symptom relief but will not treat the underlying infection.

4. D: Due to their diagnosis, this patient is at high risk for tumor lysis syndrome (TLS), which is usually seen 12–72 hours following the initiation of cytotoxic therapy. It is caused by the destruction of cancer cells and leads to the leakage of cellular contents into circulation. The patient should be closely monitored for hyperkalemia, hypocalcemia, hyperphosphatemia, and hyperuricemia. Blood counts and sodium levels are not substantially impacted by TLS, making Choices *A, B,* and *C* incorrect.

5. B: This patient is showing signs of superior vena cava syndrome (SVC syndrome) and, based on the rapidity of onset, should be directed to the emergency room for diagnosis with a CT and emergent treatment of the obstruction. Patients with NSCLC and SCLC are at high risk of SVC syndrome. Choices *A, C,* and *D* do not reflect the urgency of the situation and will not address the underlying cause of symptoms, making them incorrect.

Psychosocial Dimensions of Care

Nursing care goes beyond simply providing physical medical aid. Oncology patients are often undergoing complex medical situations that can be a matter of life or death; they also may be under nursing care for extended periods of time. Nurses, especially in the field of oncology, must be equipped to also provide mental, emotional, and social support to their patients in order to care for all aspects of the patient's wellness. Nurses are often the patient's primary advocate for receiving comprehensive, quality care.

Cultural, Spiritual, and Religious Diversity

The nursing profession sees patients from all cultural, spiritual, and religious walks of life. Cultural norms, spiritual beliefs and practices, and religious faith often strongly influence how patients manage and cope with cancer diagnoses and treatment.

Therefore, accounting for and catering to these differences provides a holistic perspective of care from which patients feel acknowledged, understood, and satisfied. It is important to not assume a patient's beliefs, or to assume that a patient's beliefs match that of his or her family's. Rather, compassionate inquiries should be made into both the patient and the family's personal beliefs and how they relate to the patient's diagnosis and treatment. Patients and their families should be warmly encouraged to communicate their needs and desires for care as it related to their personal beliefs. When providers display an attitude of acceptance and willingness to shift protocols of care to accommodate personal beliefs (as long as it is still medically safe to do so), it can help the patient feel more comfortable with the nursing staff. Cultural, spiritual, and religious values may affect a patient's treatment preferences, type of support system, emotional and mental response to diagnoses and treatments, and decisions regarding the end of life. Most hospitals also employ the services of different spiritual and religious guides to support the different practices of a diverse patient group.

Altered Body Image

Both pediatric and adult oncology patients may struggle with issues relating to **body image** while undergoing treatment and after treatment ends. Cancer treatments such as chemotherapy may cause weight loss, while some oral pharmaceuticals may cause weight gain. Surgical procedures to remove cancerous tissues (such as a mastectomy) may cause permanent physical changes for the patient, while removal of cancerous organs may cause permanent functional changes. Coping with these changes can be a long and difficult process. Patients may feel depressed, shocked, a loss of identity, or experience low self-esteem in response to physical changes. Nurses can help to ease the burden for patients by communicating as much as possible about the scope of treatment and how it may affect the patient's physical appearance. This may allow the patient to mentally prepare for changes, as well as seek out potential solutions that may help them cope after treatment is over. For example, patients who lose a limb due to surgical treatment may seek out information about getting a prosthetic limb, including costs and adjusting to its use. Nurses can serve as a resource for providing this type information as well as connecting the patient to others who have experienced the same scenario and are willing to provide support. It is also important to remember that the patient's family members may need help adjusting to the patient's altered body image, as well. For example, children may feel anxious or scared when seeing a parent who has lost a large amount of weight due to their illness.

Learning Preferences and Barriers to Learning

Patient education is a critical part of empowering patients to make informed decisions and be actively involved in their health care. Additionally, patient health education after they have received a serious diagnosis may be the most intensive health education that the patient has ever received. Therefore, it is important that nurses have a comprehensive understanding of the different styles in which people learn and barriers they may face. People primarily learn best through auditory, visual, or kinetic learning techniques; often, an integrated approach provides the best educational value. **Auditory education** techniques may include having a conversation with the patient, providing a relevant podcast for the patient to listen to, or holding an open lecture on a specific health topic. **Visual education** techniques may involve the use of charts, 3-D models, printed materials, pictures, or a presentation. **Kinetic education** techniques allow the patient to apply the material in a hands-on way, such as by practicing injecting a medication into a mannequin before trying to do so at home. Barriers to patient learning may include a lack of interest or the inability to take their health status seriously, poor literacy or comprehension skills, or an inability to attend educational sessions (e.g., due to lack of transportation or childcare). Other barriers may involve the healthcare provider. For example, the healthcare provider must ensure that they are communicating in a way that is easily understandable to the patient rather than using complex medical lingo. They also must ensure that they create a warm environment and build a relationship with the patient, so that the patient feels comfortable discussing topics he or she doesn't understand. Patient discomfort or unwillingness to discuss topics with the healthcare provider, due to embarrassment or shame, is a barrier that can be easily prevented.

Social Relationships and Family Dynamics

A cancer diagnosis goes beyond the individual patient. It has a strong impact on their close friends and family members, creating an integral effect on these relationships. Friends and family members may be called on for caregiving duties, which may be easy to do at first but may become more exhausting over time. The romantic relationship and roles of responsibility between partners may shift significantly as one partner becomes ill. Children may need to provide care for parents, or parents may need to learn how to split time caring for a child with cancer without neglecting the needs of their healthy children. Overall, these changes can lead to feelings of guilt or emotional burden, which can be overwhelming as the patient also tries to manage his or her physical health. These changes can also lead to feelings of depression, exhaustion, stress, resentment, overprotectiveness, hopelessness, or anger in caretakers. Navigating these emotions, sharing duties, asking for support, and seeking healthy ways of self-care can be coping tools for friends and family members of the patient. Above all, allowing space for **open communication** can help set expectations that maintain healthy social relationships and family dynamics during the course of the patient's treatments. Friends and family members can seek new ways to maintain friendship, uphold intimacy, and share positive experiences with the patient as treatment continues.

Coping Mechanisms and Skills

Coping mechanisms and skills refer to any actions, thought patterns, or behaviors a person undertakes in order to manage a perceived stress or threat. These can be positive, healthy resolutions that lead to increased resiliency and ability to manage adverse events. Alternatively, coping mechanism can be negative, unhealthy resolutions that introduce new stressors, decrease resiliency, and harm oneself or others. Positive coping mechanisms include **adaptive mechanisms** (that introduce positive behaviors into the situation); **behavioral mechanisms** (that change negative behaviors into positive ones); and

cognitive mechanisms (that change negative thinking patterns into positive ones). Examples of positive coping skills may include reframing one's perspective, altruistic or philanthropic gestures, crying, meditating, and exercise. Negative coping mechanisms include **attack mechanisms** (when someone projects his or her stressors into an attack on another); **avoidance mechanisms** (when someone undertakes behaviors to avoid the stressor); and **self-destructive mechanisms** (when someone purposely does something that harms oneself physically, emotionally, socially, or mentally). Examples of negative coping skills include substance abuse, showing aggression to others, misbehaving, and repressing feelings. **Defense mechanisms** can be positive or negative; these typically refer to any action a person takes immediately in response to a triggering stressor to protect his or her sense of self.

Support

Patient

Support groups provide a way for cancer patients and their families to connect with others that are experiencing similar challenges and emotions. Cancer is a unique and serious diagnosis; therefore, having empathy from others who truly understand the journey from diagnosis onwards can be an uplifting and morale-boosting influence. It allows patients and families to process their emotions with a community and share information on unique topics (e.g., lifestyle adjustments, financial concerns, and social changes as they relate to cancer). Support groups may grow organically, such as through friends who create an online social media support group and invite others to join, or they may be pre-established, such as at a medical facility. They may be informal and social in nature or may be led in a formal setting by a counselor or therapist. Support groups may also target specific audiences, such as the spouses of cancer patients. Not all patients may enjoy the context of a support group, depending on their personality and their diagnosis. Some may prefer to lead their lives as close to their pre-diagnosis life as possible, while others may simply want only their friends and family for support. If a patient is seeking out a support group and feels uncomfortable upon joining, nurses may serve as a resource to direct the patient towards another type of group that may be a better fit.

Caregiver

Caregivers of patients with cancer experience a variety of challenges and stressors. This role can be very overwhelming and isolating to a caregiver, and self-advocacy can be difficult. For this reason, it is important for oncology providers to advocate for and provide proper support to caregivers. Challenges they may experience include effectively managing the complex needs of the oncology patient while continuing to care for themselves. A well-supported caregiver tends to lead to more positive patient health outcomes, decreased risk of abuse or neglect, and less physical and emotional complications from burnout.

Caregiver support begins with education to assist caregivers in providing physical care needs to the patient. Consultation in the office, written materials, online videos, and virtual or live classes can be provided to support ongoing care training needs. Palliative care referral can assist patients, as well as caregivers, with support and resources. Additional caregiver resources include support groups for social connection, referral for counseling or psychiatric support, and involvement of extended family to share caregiving needs. Oncology providers can assist caregivers and patients with appropriate referrals and allocation of services for patients with home healthcare needs, as applicable. Additionally, patients receiving hospice care are also provided with respite services to provide caregivers with breaks.

Psychosocial Distress

It is common for most people to experience some form of psychosocial disturbance or alteration in response to a cancer diagnosis; this can even occur after they have been undergoing treatment for some time. These issues can affect close friends, family members, and caregivers as well. Seeking social or medical support systems to navigate a cancer diagnosis can provide some relief. Additionally, self-care techniques (e.g., adequate rest, exercise, massage therapy, quiet time, meditation, yoga, or other activities that promote refreshment) can ensure that both patients and caregivers are able to relax their bodies and soothe their nervous systems. This will allow them to cope with stress in a healthier way.

Emotional and Spiritual Distress

Anxiety

Anxiety is characterized by intense, uncontrollable periods of nervousness, fear, or panic. Acute anxiety may last just a few minutes, while chronic anxiety can last for weeks or longer. **Acute anxiety** is characterized by a sudden feeling of fear, feeling as though one is unable to breathe, an increased heart rate, sweating, dizziness, and nausea. **Chronic anxiety** may be characterized by constant worry focused on one or more topics, teeth grinding, insomnia, muscular pain, stomach problems, indecisiveness, and an inability to concentrate. Anxiety may be triggered by a traumatic experience, chronic stress, a neurotransmitter imbalance, and by some medications. Cancer patients may feel acute anxiety upon receiving their diagnosis and prognosis. They may feel worried about their next steps, what it will feel like to receive treatment, how their case will respond, finances, end-of-life decisions, and their loved ones. Even if the patient overcomes their cancer, they may develop chronic anxiety surrounding the possibility of recurrence, resulting financial burdens, or lifestyle and relationship changes that were a direct result of the disease.

Loss and Grief

Grief—the experience and response an individual has to perceived or actual loss—is an unavoidable part of oncology nursing. Patients, loved ones, caregivers, and communities can all experience varying degrees of grief in response to a patient's cancer diagnosis. Additionally, the manifestations of that grief can appear very different from person to person; therefore, it is important for oncology nurses to have a thorough understanding and compassion for the experiences of those in their care.

The experience of grief often begins at the very moment a patient suspects that something is wrong with their health. This may even occur before the first medical visit or confirmation of diagnosis, as the individual anticipates the potential loss that they imagine experiencing due to their illness. This phenomenon, called **anticipatory grief**, is experienced by patients and individuals close to the patient in anticipation of the patient's decline and eventual loss of life.

Oncology nurses can prepare to care for grieving patients and loved ones by developing an understanding of what grieving is and what it looks like. The most recognized framework used to understand the grieving process is the **Kubler-Ross Model**, which categorizes grief into the following five stages: denial, anger, bargaining, depression, and acceptance. Denial is an initial protective state that one experiences to manage the emotional pain of a loss. It can present as questioning, disbelief, or apathy. Anger is the next stage of grief in which the individual is now feeling the weight of the anticipated or actual loss, and they begin to experience spiritual distress from the situation. Bargaining can be an internal or external experience in which the individual attempts to negotiate on a spiritual level. In the realm of oncology, this may present during end-of-life conversations as patients or loved ones ask for additional treatment options. Depression is the stage of grief in which the individual is feeling a sense of hopelessness at the reality of the loss. This can present as tearfulness, voiced hopelessness, or withdrawal from normal activities. Lastly, acceptance is the stage of grief in which the individual acknowledges, reflects, and accepts the loss. It is important to note that grief is a complex, nonlinear, and individualized experience. Some individuals experience all stages. Others circle back through some or all of the stages as they process their grief. Still others may only experience some of the stages of grief.

The goal for the oncology nurse is to recognize signs of grief and promote emotional and physical safety. Nurses maintain a **therapeutic environment** by providing calm reassurance and privacy; using active listening, allowing opportunities for pauses rather than filling silences; reducing stimuli such as television or bright lights; and providing comfort items. Additionally, nurses may further support individuals through grief with referrals to supportive services (e.g., grief groups, mental health services, chaplain services). Nurses may also educate patients on topics such as the grieving process or coping techniques.

Depression

Depression is characterized by intense, prolonged feelings of sadness, hopelessness, and loss of interest in daily activities. Its severity can fall somewhere on a spectrum of mild to extreme symptoms. Mild cases may be short in duration or caused by a specific event, and the individual may return to normal after processing the event. **Mild depression** may cause some symptoms like sadness, fatigue, or an inability to concentrate, but these symptoms likely won't interfere with the daily functions of the individual's life. **Major depression** is extreme and lasts longer than two weeks, usually interfering significantly with the individual's normal routine. It often involves altered sleeping or eating habits; significant changes in energy; loss of interest in routine and pleasurable activities; suicidal thoughts; inability to focus; and/or poor memory and concentration. Medications (e.g., beta blockers and corticosteroids), changing seasons (e.g., winter in areas with shortened periods of sunlight), and vitamin and mineral deficiencies (e.g., vitamin D, B vitamins, and magnesium) can also contribute to depression. Almost all cancer patients will experience some level of sadness or shock after receiving news of their diagnosis; however, factors relating to their overall health and wellness, seasonal influence, nutrition, social support, details of their diagnosis and prognosis, and personal coping skills will influence the severity of their response.

Spiritual Distress

Oncology patients and caregivers commonly experience **spiritual distress**. Spirituality encompasses things which bring meaning and purpose to a person's life. Examples include religious beliefs and practices, meaningful relationships (e.g., children, family, pets, friends, and groups), communities, nature, art, music, career, hobbies, and other items deemed as sacred. Distress can occur when individuals attempt to find meaning and/or make sense of their cancer diagnosis or mortality alongside their spiritual beliefs. Distress can also occur when expressions of spirituality change or are limited (e.g., when physical decline or hospitalization prevents the patient from performing a spiritual activity or practice as usual).

Oncology nurses can assess and identify spiritual distress by recognizing the signs, such as anger, hopelessness, doubting previous religious or spiritual beliefs, or questions surrounding God, suffering, or the meaning of one's life. It is not uncommon for healthcare professionals to feel discomfort discussing spiritual topics with patients and families. Oncology nurses can address spiritual distress by listening with non-judgement and empathy. Use open-ended questions such as, "What things bring meaning to your life?", "What brings you comfort when life gets tough?", or "Do you consider yourself spiritual or religious?" Nurses can also serve as advocates to find ways patients can express their spirituality within the care setting. This may involve referral to chaplain services, modifying an environment for prayer or meditation, or facilitating ways for a patient to perform a spiritual or religious practice. These interventions can help patients work through difficult feelings and begin to form meaning and acceptance during their cancer treatment.

Loss of Autonomy

When people experience any type of chronic illness, their lifestyle is likely to significantly change. Illnesses limit the mental, physical, and emotional functioning an individual; even after the illness has been treated, there may be long-lasting effects that influence the patient's quality of life. Cancer patients usually undergo treatments that are physically taxing on the body. Side effects of treatment can include extreme fatigue, nausea, weight loss, hair loss, and physical weakness. During treatment and for a period afterwards, patients' lives change substantially in that they often cannot do activities that were a normal part of their routine prior to the diagnosis—such as managing their household, paying bills, gardening, working, walking, or other leisure, recreational, or social activities—and this can feel like a major loss of personal control. Patients may feel as though their mind and body have failed them, and this can be challenging for their sense of self and overall self-esteem. During this time, patients may become heavily dependent on family, friends, and other caretakers to manage their affairs since this can be an emotionally and mentally difficult task for the patient to handle. Allied health workers, support groups, and social services can help ease some of this burden for families and provide coping tools to help the patient navigate feelings of loss.

Caregiver Fatigue

Caregivers of patients undergoing cancer diagnosis and treatment can experience a tremendous amount of emotional, mental, and physical demand. They are experiencing and attempting to cope with the diagnosis of a loved one, managing their own lives, possibly managing the lives of additional loved ones (such as spouses and children), and providing physical and emotional support for the oncology patient. With this, caregivers can experience significant **caregiver fatigue**.

Oncology patients experience a high level of burdensome symptoms, including chronic pain, fatigue, weakness, nausea, vomiting, insomnia, diarrhea, constipation, dermatological changes, organ toxicity, depression, anxiety, and many others. Patients require varying degrees of assistance with daily activities, travel to appointments, and management of symptoms. Caregivers can experience distress related to the discomfort of the oncology patient. With advanced stage and terminal cancers, caregivers are also experiencing their own grief and distress at the decline and eventual loss of their loved one. Each of these factors contribute to a significant risk for caregiver fatigue and caregiver burnout. These conditions can lead to the development of emotional (e.g., anxiety and depression) and additional physical symptoms (e.g., insomnia, pain, autoimmune disease, and frequent infections).

Oncology nurses can address this by recognizing and intervening when the need arises for caregiver emotional and resource support. Strategies for support should begin at the point of patient diagnosis and include recruitment of multiple caregivers, if possible. Caregiver support classes and groups can also provide social and educational support. Additionally, educating caregivers on the importance of self-care strategies (e.g., healthy diet, exercise, stress management, counseling, and frequent breaks) can assist them in managing caregiver burden. Lastly, nurses may provide caregivers with recommendations for mental health services for additional support.

Crisis Management

Domestic Violence

Oncology nurses are trusted and highly involved members of the healthcare team. Due to this closeness to patients and their loved ones, they may become involved with management of patients in crisis. For example, adult patients may confide or seek help from nurses about **intimate partner violence**. Nurses may also be the first to identify signs and symptoms of domestic violence. Domestic violence can have physical, mental, emotional, financial, sexual, or social aspects. Obvious signs include physical injuries, often at different stages of healing (e.g., bruising, lesions, or fractures). Nonverbal signs from the patient include shaking, flinching, or aversion to touch. Partners may be overly protective and domineering, with behaviors such as refusing to leave the patient's side and speaking for the patient. Nursing management includes assessment at intake, provision of resource and emotional support, and ensuring patient safety. For suspected minor or elder abuse, nurses have an ethical and professional responsibility to objectively report to local authorities.

Suicidal Ideation

Another crisis that oncology nurses may need to respond to is **suicidal ideation**, which is the serious thought and planning of attempted suicide. Screening for suicide risk should be part of initial and ongoing assessment for all patients. Oncology patients, in general, have a higher risk for suicide. Moreover, oncology patients at higher risk for experiencing suicide ideation include patients in the first months of diagnosis; those with certain types of cancer (e.g., head and neck, lung, pancreas, prostate, testicular, or bladder); or patients with certain clinical factors (e.g., pain, fatigue, insomnia, poor support systems, or poor coping). In addition to positive verbalization of suicide ideation, nurses should be able to recognize more subtle warning signs. These include voiced hopelessness; feeling trapped or like a burden to those around them; increased risky behaviors (e.g., drug or alcohol use), erratic or agitated behavior; withdrawal or isolation; or reports of hallucinations commanding them to harm someone else or themselves. Nurses who suspect or confirm positive suicide ideation should seek emergency assistance according to organizational guidelines while always ensuring the safety of the patient. Suicidal patients should never be left alone, and the immediate environment should be as free as possible from items that could be used for self-harm.

Sexuality

Sexuality refers to the way people feel about themselves in terms of sexual needs, sexual desires, and physical intimacy. When patients receive a cancer diagnosis, this topic may not immediately come to mind, but is likely to emerge at some point during their care. Just as cancer and its treatment affects other physiological needs, such as appetite and sleep, it can affect a patient's sex drive, reproductive processes, and romantic relationships. If the changes are significant or disruptive, it can be an extremely stressful or depressing shift for patients and their romantic partners.

Reproductive Issues

Female patients should regularly be screened for **pregnancy** throughout cancer treatment, as many of the side effects from treatment are similar to symptoms of pregnancy (e.g., nausea and fatigue). Without screening, pregnancy may be overlooked and the patient may not receive adequate prenatal care for a viable pregnancy. Pediatric patients of both sexes may have **fertility issues** when they hope to conceive due to the presence of cancer in the body, the effects of radiation treatment on reproductive cells, and the long-term impact of drugs on reproductive and hormonal processes. When possible, patients should avoid becoming pregnant while undergoing treatment. Common **contraceptives** for long-term use include vasectomies in men and intrauterine devices, hormonal implants, or tubal litigation in women. Patients who are being treated for cancer in reproductive areas are advised to wait up to one year before trying to conceive in order to ensure tissues have regained full health and functioning. However, if a patient does not want to avoid pregnancy or is already pregnant upon diagnosis, precautions include ovarian and uterine shielding during radiation, reducing the use of radiation treatment, and changing chemotherapy medications to reduce toxicity to the fetus. Patients should be aware that this can be extremely physically burdensome to the parent carrying the fetus. However, according to the American Cancer Society, most cancer cases can be successfully treated during pregnancy and termination has not been shown to improve outcomes. In cases of aggressive or advanced cancer, healthcare providers should work with the patient to determine the best treatment plan with the greatest benefit to both the mother and fetus. In some rare cases of leukemia and melanoma, cancerous cells have been shown to pass from the mother to the fetus.

In the case of cancers that can safely be treated while a mother is pregnant, it is recommended that these patients take a break from treatment for approximately one to two months before delivery. Chemotherapy does not appear to affect the fetus in the second or third trimesters; however, the fetus is vulnerable to developmental delays if exposed to chemotherapy medications in the first trimester.

Sexual Dysfunction

Sexual dysfunction refers to the inability of a person to perform sexually. A cancer diagnosis and ensuing treatment is likely to affect patients both physically and psychologically; the degree of the impact will be dependent on the type of cancer, severity, patient's age, and their coping skills. Physical effects in both sexes may include an inability to maintain arousal, loss of pleasurable sensation, an inability to reach or feel orgasms, fatigue, and/or pain. Psychological effects in both sexes may include anxiety over having sexual intercourse (if the patient fears pain or discomfort), low self-esteem, feeling unattractive, being unsure of a romantic partner's feelings or desire, and/or a loss of interest or desire. If a patient is being treated for cancers in the reproductive areas, they may experience long-term physical sexual dysfunction even if the cancer is completely treated. Additionally, a patient's partner may have difficulty adjusting to the patient's new sexuality, even if they have been in a relationship for a long time. Physical therapists, psychologists, and sex therapists may be able to help patients and their partners return to normalcy.

Intimacy

Sexual intimacy can still be maintained between partners during and after a cancer diagnosis and treatment, though it may be different in nature. Intimacy is an important part of psychosocial wellness. It may involve a sexual relationship, but it also encompasses mutual respect and trust, sharing meaningful information and experiences, and physical touch that is not only sexual intercourse. Many patients and their partners experience increased intimacy as they face the challenge of cancer together. Intimacy can be maintained in the following ways: sharing feelings about the experience; supporting one another's desires, concerns, and fears throughout the journey; showing appreciation and gratitude for one another; and engaging in physical comfort (e.g., hugging, kissing, and hand holding). Partners can also maintain intimacy by reducing their sexual expectations or pressures toward one another and by nurturing any mutual desires that do arise. After treatment, a nurse, counselor, sex therapist, or allied health worker may help with redefining roles within the relationship, addressing concerns, and providing exercises that can help encourage heightened levels of intimacy. Patients and their partners should avoid emotionally and physically distancing themselves from one another during treatment, even if it seems uncomfortable to be together. This can decrease intimacy, reduce social support, and lead to extra, unnecessary stress for both partners during treatment and recovery.

Considerations for Sexual and Gender Minorities

Oncology nurses can advocate for patients of **sexual and gender minorities** by educating themselves as well as promoting inclusive practices within their organizations. Before approaching this topic, it is important to first perform self-examination; this involves reflecting upon any personal beliefs or biases surrounding gender and sexuality that could impact the provision of care for one's patients. Next, recognize that sexuality and gender experiences are highly individualized and nuanced. Patients have vastly different experiences, behaviors, temperaments, and beliefs.

Sexual and gender minorities often report experiencing adverse interactions within the healthcare system. These interactions can lead to an overall anxiety and distrust of healthcare professionals. They can present as anxious, scared, timid, or defiant. This requires patience, calmness, compassion, and confidence to commit to building a trusting patient-provider relationship. This also requires all members of the care team to be educated and respectful. One insensitive remark can be detrimental to the patient's trust. Organizations can help to build a sensitive culture by providing staff education, posting signage indicating sensitivity to gender and sexual minorities, and adding pronoun verbiage to name badges.

Another way to facilitate sensitive conversations is with the intake questionnaire and process. Question items may ask for information related to identification of preferred pronouns, gender assigned at birth, sexual identification, and specific concerns that could be sensitive or impact care delivery. These questions can open dialogue and further build trust between the patient and care team. Being aware of patient body language and comfort levels during intake can also assist with decreasing potential distress. Discussions about sexual anatomy can be highly distressing for some individuals and not for others. Therefore, asking open-ended questions allows the patient to feel more comfortable. Responses should always be respectful, non-judgmental, and relatively neutral.

Financial Concerns

Financial concerns are one of the top issues that cancer survivors experience. Even with medical insurance, paying for long-term, complex treatment can drain one's financial resources completely. Additionally, many individuals are unable to work during their treatment; time that is taken off may lead to loss of employer-sponsored insurance. The Centers for Disease Control and Prevention reports that in the United States, cancer survivors are more likely to be in debt or declare bankruptcy than any other demographic. Survivors who experience these types of financial burdens often end up skipping critical follow-up appointments, which ultimately may lead to poor health outcomes. Survivors who experience financial stress also report increased rates of depression and anxiety; additionally, their family members may have to work additional hours or extra jobs, and this can cause stress on the family unit.

Patients may feel uncomfortable bringing up financial difficulties and asking for assistance in navigating their insurance options or other financial resources. Nurses may be one of the first lines of information for patients in this situation; additionally, the rapport that nurses are able to build with patients may encourage them to share financial concerns. Nurses may be able to serve as an advocate for or liaison between the patient and the medical facility's financial department. They may also be able to work with social workers or other allied health workers to connect patients with public or private resources that offer financial aid (e.g., grants, charities, or government assistance), money management (e.g., in-house financial planner), or other services that support patients with fiscal concerns.

Employment

Survivors may run into issues relating to their employment. Depending on how long they have been out of work, some survivors may lose employment status as well as corresponding benefits, such as health insurance and short-term disability. Under the federal **Family and Medical Leave Act (FMLA)**, some employees are guaranteed 12 weeks of protected, unpaid leave where their employers must hold their position and pay. However, there are a number of complicated stipulations to this law, including the size of the organization, the length of the individual's employment, and factors relating to the need for using leave; survivors that do not meet the requirements are not guaranteed anything. This can be a stressful experience for employees who must miss work due to their illness or treatment. While cancer patients and survivors are protected under the federal **Americans with Disabilities Act (ADA)** if they work for certain types of private organizations, this provision and certain state-specific discrimination laws do not always protect survivors as intended. For example, employers may try to fire an employee who is consistently absent due to his or her illness, but cite some other reason for it. Survivors may face the additional stress of filing a lawsuit (which costs considerable amounts of time and money) if they feel they have been wrongly discriminated against by their employer. Finally, up to a third of cancer survivors report that they are simply unable to work after their treatment for reasons such as cognitive decline or physical disability. This can place a burden on their immediate family members and cause additional financial and emotional duress.

Insurance

If survivors have comprehensive and affordable medical coverage, they may only have to spend a small amount of money out of pocket. For many survivors, this may not be the reality. Typically, survivors will have private **medical insurance** through an employer (either their own, their spouse's, or their parents' if they are 26 years old or under). If they do not have an employer-sponsored option, survivors may choose to obtain health insurance through federal government programs or state health insurance marketplaces. Depending on income, survivors and their families may qualify for tax credits that help offset the cost of buying insurance through marketplace exchanges. However, paying health insurance premiums and deductibles may place a financial burden on survivors and their families if employment income is lost due to the diagnosis. Survivors may also have short and/or long-term **disability insurance** through their workplace or through an individual plan. This type of insurance can help offset the cost of employment income that is lost during treatment or if the survivor is unable to work after treatment has ended. Short and long-term disability insurance plans usually pay a percentage of the survivor's monthly earned income. Depending on the rate and the survivor's lifestyle and needs, this may be a difficult financial adjustment to make. Finally, survivors may struggle to find **term life insurance** after their diagnosis if they did not get a plan before they became ill. Term life insurance pays named beneficiaries a designated amount in the event that the policy holder dies. Since a cancer diagnosis is subject to secondary malignancies and increases the overall risk of poor health and death, life insurance companies may choose to deny policies to survivors or ask them to pay inflated premiums. Sometimes, experienced insurance brokers will be able to assist survivors in obtaining life insurance policies. Otherwise, many insurance companies require that survivors have been in remission for a specified number of years (depending on the form of cancer that they had) before they will issue a new life insurance policy to them or increase the beneficiary amount gradually as the survivor ages.

Resources

Patients with cancer experience exceptional challenges related to finances. Factors contributing to this burden include cost of cancer treatment; cost of healthcare services to manage cancer, side effects, and toxicities; added expenses related to health and disability needs (e.g., assistive devices, travel expenses to and from appointments, and dietary supplements); disruptions or losses in employment; and varying insurance liabilities. Patients and their families can struggle to maintain access to critical resources like food, housing, utilities, transportation, and medical needs.

Financial and resource burdens have a tremendous negative impact on patients and caregivers. Loss of financial security can lead patients to be unable to afford ongoing treatments and health-related interventions, which impacts treatment outcomes. Additionally, fear and actual loss of basic needs has been shown to manifest in symptoms that are psychological (e.g., anxiety and depression) and physical (e.g., fatigue, pain, insomnia, failure to thrive, and anorexia). These factors can greatly decrease quality of life and can negatively impact the success of treatment.

Oncology nurse navigators and social workers address these issues by facilitating resource allocation and education to help with financial concerns related to cancer treatment. Resources include referral for **patient assistance programs**, which are created and funded by various charities, groups, and businesses. Examples of assistance programs include medication patient assistance programs to address the high cost of cancer treatment for individuals with high personal liability or those who lack insurance coverage. Advocacy groups or charity organizations also offer transportation assistance programs that provide taxi, bus, gas reimbursement, or other transportation service vouchers for patients and families struggling to get to and from medical appointments. Some organizations also offer assistance to families and patients for hotel expenses incurred when travelling long distances for treatment. Additional resources include applicable government welfare programs (e.g., food stamps, utility assistance, and housing assistance) to address basic needs. Lastly, hospitals (particularly not-for-profit organizations) can set up funding and resources for patients determined to be in need (e.g., gift cards for gas or groceries, transportation vouchers, and hotel vouchers).

Practice Quiz

1. Which piece of federal legislation guarantees 12 weeks of protected, unpaid time off from work for certain employees?
   a. The Americans with Disabilities Act
   b. The Affordable Care Act
   c. The Consolidated Omnibus Budget Reconciliation Act
   d. The Family and Medical Leave Act

2. Which of the following is a common barrier to successful patient education?
   a. Poor literacy
   b. Lack of disease prevalence
   c. Lack of safe places to hold patient education sessions
   d. Patient ego

3. During which trimester are fetuses most vulnerable to developmental delays from chemotherapy that the mother is undergoing?
   a. First
   b. Second
   c. Third
   d. All of the above

4. Jenny has just found out that she has stage two pancreatic cancer. It is an unexpected diagnosis, and she is completely in shock. She schedules her follow up appointment to begin treatment, but then goes home and spends a full day enraged, often screaming out loud. The next morning, she wakes up and decides to meditate each morning, recite positive affirmations daily, and focus on three things each evening for which she is grateful. What is this an example of?
   a. Positive coping
   b. Negative coping
   c. Pavlovian response
   d. New Age wisdom

5. Which of the following is the typical order in which people experience the stages of grief?
   a. Acceptance, Bargaining, Anger, Depression, Denial
   b. Denial, Anger, Bargaining, Depression, Acceptance
   c. Anger, Denial, Bargaining, Acceptance, Depression
   d. Depression, Denial, Bargaining, Anger, Acceptance

See answers on the next page.

Answer Explanations

1. D: The federal Family and Medical Leave Act guarantees that some employees have 12 weeks of protected, unpaid leave for family and medical reasons. A number of stipulations to this act include that the organization granting leave must have 50 or more employees, the employee in consideration must have been employed for 12 months before asking for protected leave under the act, and the employee must ask for leave for certain medical conditions. Other rules may also apply based on the organization and employee.

2. A: Patient literacy plays a major role in understanding educational material, especially written handouts. Many healthcare providers rely on written materials, such as pamphlets and discharge papers, to provide patient education. When the patient struggles with literacy, these items may not be useful. If the patient fails to fully understand their diagnosis, treatment, and follow up instructions, they are more likely to be readmitted to the hospital. Therefore, healthcare providers should also offer to talk through the material with the patient in simple language. They can also ask if the patient prefers other forms of media, such as online videos. This can be done in an objective way, framed as asking for the patient's personal preference, in order to not potentially embarrass the patient. The other options are not accepted as common barriers to education.

3. A: Fetuses are vulnerable to developmental delays during the first trimester of pregnancy; no links have been shown during the other two trimesters. This may be due to the robust amount of brain growth that takes place specifically during the first trimester. Any teratogenic agents may inhibit new neural pathways or brain matter from forming.

4. A: These are methods of dealing with a stressor in a positive way. Positive coping mechanisms include behaviors such as reframing one's perspective, exercising, thinking positive thoughts, and focusing on healthy actions. Negative coping includes methods that are harmful to the self or the patient's environment. The other two options listed do not apply.

5. B: In order, grieving people typically progress through the emotions of denying the event, anger at the event, bargaining to bring the loss back, depression when they realize the loss cannot come back, and finally acceptance of the loss. Depending on the individual and the context of the loss, this cycle can occur slowly or rapidly. People may also relapse into previous stages before finally arriving at acceptance.

Practice Test #1

1. Which best describes the role of macrophages in normal immune function?
   a. To signal cell responses such as inflammation
   b. To recognize, ingest, and kill microbes
   c. To develop cell-mediated immunity
   d. To produce antigen-specific antibodies

2. How long does the period of survivorship last?
   a. From the time of an official cancer diagnosis by an oncologist until the patient's cancer goes into remission
   b. From the time of an official cancer diagnosis by an oncologist until the time of the patient's death, if the death is directly a result of the cancer
   c. From the time the patient completed treatment and cancer is undetectable until the time of the patient's death, regardless of the cause of death
   d. From the period of the first cancer treatment session to the second cancer treatment session

3. What solid tumor diagnosis can be treated with autologous stem cell transplant?
   a. Small-cell lung cancer
   b. Melanoma
   c. Testicular cancer
   d. Bladder cancer

4. What is the association between the presence of chronic inflammation and the risk of the development of cancer?
   a. Treatments associated with inflammatory diseases damage DNA.
   b. The inflammatory process exposes the individual to DNA-damaging chemicals.
   c. Chronic inflammation slows the process of initiation.
   d. The risk is greatest for inflammatory conditions of the GI system.

5. Which action performed by an oncology care site would best evaluate if they are meeting the requirements of their patient education program?
   a. Distribution of patient satisfaction surveys
   b. Staff polling to determine the current process
   c. Review of current standards of practice
   d. Discussion with community stakeholders

6. What is radiofrequency ablation?
   a. Minimally-invasive surgery that involves electrical energy coupled with heat to kill cancer cells
   b. The use of high-intensity beams of light to remove tissue
   c. The freezing and destroying of abnormal or cancerous cells
   d. Preventative surgery to remove cells that are precancerous

7. When providing patients with education related to preventing lymphedema following mastectomy with lymphadenectomy, which of the following would NOT be included?

a. Avoid strength training with the affected limb.
b. Use sunscreen when going outdoors.
c. Do not pick at fingernails or the surrounding skin.
d. Take care to control your weight.

8. The nurse is reviewing a patient's neutrophil count to assess if their results are within parameters to receive their next cycle of chemotherapy. The physician has provided orders to proceed as long as the patient's absolute neutrophil count (ANC) is above 1000 cells/microliter. The patient's total white blood cell count is 4.5 thousand cells/microliter. Their neutrophils are 15 percent. The nurse calculates the patient's ANC to be what?

a. 150
b. 300
c. 675
d. 3333

9. The nurse is caring for a patient for the first time. This patient has a history of ovarian cancer and is currently participating in a clinical trial for their chemotherapy treatment. The nurse notices that the administration guidelines for this patient's orders differ significantly from the monographs. What is the most appropriate action for the nurse to take next?

a. Administer the orders exactly as written.
b. Clarify the orders with the research nurse.
c. Follow the monograph for administration of the patient's medications.
d. Review how the previous nurse administered the patient's medications.

10. What is chemotherapy?

a. Medications administered to a patient in order to fight against cancer
b. The complete removal of cancerous cells through surgical procedures
c. A medical procedure known as helical-tomography
d. A medical procedure involving radioactive seed implants

11. Which of the following types of cancer has a relatively high correlation rate with secondary malignancies?

a. Hodgkin's lymphoma
b. Melanoma
c. Glioblastomas
d. Osteosarcoma

12. Which patient is at the highest risk for spinal cord compression?

a. 54-year-old female with stage IV breast cancer
b. 72-year-old male with stage III colon cancer
c. 55-year-old female with stage II bladder cancer
d. 74-year-old male with stage III prostate cancer

13. Patients undergoing chemotherapy and radiation treatment require what specialized diet?
   a. Low in fat
   b. Low in calories
   c. High in fat and calories
   d. High in fiber

14. Which complementary therapy would typically be contraindicated in a patient with chemotherapy-induced neutropenia?
   a. Acupuncture
   b. Aromatherapy
   c. Massage therapy
   d. Guided imagery

15. Which of the following statements is consistent with the autosomal dominant inheritance pattern as it relates to cancer?
   a. The parent and the child will both manifest the disease.
   b. The parent contributes the gene but does not manifest a cancerous condition.
   c. Both parents carry the altered gene.
   d. The child must inherit the mutation from both parents.

16. Monoclonal antibodies with the suffix of *-omab* are derived from which source?
   a. Human
   b. Rat
   c. Primate
   d. Mouse

17. The nurse is assessing a 44-year-old male patient with complaints of chest pain and shortness of breath. Examination by the nurse reveals distended neck veins and muffled heart sounds. The patient's blood pressure is 80/55. The nurse should suspect which of the following?
   a. Cardiac tamponade
   b. Abdominal aortic aneurysm (AAA)
   c. Cardiopulmonary arrest
   d. Cardiogenic shock

18. A nurse is performing an implanted port access and dressing change for the first time after the device was initially placed for daily home infusion therapy. The nurse teaches the patient that the needle and dressing should be replaced how often?
   a. Every day
   b. Every three days
   c. Every five days
   d. Every seven days

19. Which patient would have the highest risk of developing graft versus host disease?
   a. A patient receiving allogeneic stem cell transplant
   b. A patient receiving donor lymphocyte infusion
   c. A patient receiving cord blood transplant
   d. A patient receiving autologous stem cell transplant

20. Which of the following represents the most common form of leukemia diagnosed in children?
   a. Chronic lymphocytic leukemia
   b. Acute lymphoblastic leukemia
   c. Chronic myelogenous leukemia
   d. Acute myelogenous leukemia

21. Which of the following manifestations is considered to be a late sign of increased ICP?
   a. Mental confusion related to time
   b. Blurred vision
   c. BP of 170/40
   d. HR of 94 bpm

22. In planning care for a patient with acute renal failure, what imbalance does the oncology nurse expect to manage?
   a. Elevated GFR
   b. Decreased BUN
   c. Elevated calcium
   d. Decreased sodium

23. Which patients are generally prescribed opiates?
   a. Patients who are fighting an HPV infection
   b. Patients who are experiencing severe, unmanageable pain and discomfort
   c. Patients who have been diagnosed with acute anxiety and/or depression
   d. Patients who are at a high risk of developing cancer

24. Hypercalcemia is most commonly seen in patients with which types of cancer?
   a. Breast cancer, lung cancer, and myeloma
   b. Kidney cancer, lung cancer, and skin cancer
   c. Lung cancer, brain cancer, and spine cancer
   d. Stomach cancer, pancreatic cancer, and uterine cancer

25. What is a key difference between sepsis and Systemic Inflammatory Response Syndrome (SIRS)?
   a. Sepsis only occurs in pregnant women, while SIRS affects all populations.
   b. Sepsis is more likely to occur immediately after radiation treatments, while SIRS is more likely to occur after chemotherapy.
   c. Sepsis affects only the blood, while SIRS affects only the brain.
   d. Sepsis occurs as a result of infection, while SIRS can result from infectious or non-infectious agents.

26. Which of the following is an analytical, process improvement tool that helps determine if all steps in a workflow are efficient and contributing something of use to the overall procedure?
   a. Gap analysis
   b. Value stream mapping
   c. PDSA cycle
   d. Step chart

27. A 32-year-old patient returns for follow-up after completing breast cancer treatment. The patient mentions that she works at a large retail chain as a cashier and is having difficulty standing for long periods due to permanent neuropathy she experiences as a result of chemotherapy treatment. She is concerned about her ability to continue working. Which federal law may support and protect the patient to negotiate reasonable changes to her work conditions and accommodate her medical concerns?
   a. Family and Medical Leave Act
   b. Americans with Disabilities Act
   c. Fair Labor Standards Act
   d. Occupational Safety and Health Act

28. The nurse is sitting with a patient who is receiving treatment for breast cancer. The patient mentions to the nurse, "My family and friends keep trying to get in touch with me, and I just don't want to see anyone. I don't really care about anything like I used to." Which of the following is the most appropriate response by the nurse?
   a. "This is something that everyone goes through."
   b. "That must be difficult. Have you talked to anyone else about how you are feeling?"
   c. "Maintaining support systems is really important, so you should really keep contact with your family and friends."
   d. "I know how you feel. I have experienced that feeling, too."

29. What procedure involves the insertion of a thin tube and a camera into the abdomen in order to detect and possibly remove abnormal or cancerous growths?
   a. Laparoscopy
   b. Laser surgery
   c. Endoscopy
   d. Biopsy

30. Doug is an oncology nurse working with a 50-year-old male patient with advanced skin cancer. Besides the cancer, he has no history of any mental, emotional, or physical health issues. As Doug begins to provide education relating to the diagnosis and the next treatment session, the patient begins to look very angry, and his eyes glaze over. As Doug is talking, the patient falls asleep. Doug tries again a few hours later, but the patient ignores him and begins to listen to music on his phone. When Doug asks if the patient would like to know any more about the treatment, the patient rolls away and grumbles under his breath. What should Doug do next?
   a. Accept that the patient is not interested in patient education and leave the patient alone.
   b. Assume his teaching methods are boring and spend some time figuring out how to make the material more interesting.
   c. Double-check the patient's health records to ensure there is no history of cognitive dysfunction.
   d. Speak with the patient's next of kin or caregiver to ask if he can share the patient education material with them.

31. A patient with metastatic non-small cell lung cancer (NSCLC) is receiving inpatient oncology care for new onset of chest pain, worsening cough, and shortness of breath requiring the use of supplemental oxygen. The patient is afebrile and has been receiving treatment with nivolumab and ipilimumab for approximately five months after completing radiation therapy. Which treatment-related complication is most consistent with the patient's symptoms and medical history?

a. Pneumonitis
b. Myocarditis
c. Cancer progression
d. Neutropenia

32. What is one common side effect of radiation treatment?

a. Overstimulation of the body's blood supply
b. Impairs the body's ability to produce protein
c. Overstimulation of hair follicles
d. Damage to tissue and blood vessels

33. Which term is used interchangeably with leukopenia, a condition in which the white blood cell count is lower than normal?

a. Thrombocytopenia
b. Lymphocytopenia
c. Neutropenia
d. Monocytopenia

34. Patients on the cusp of respiratory failure may exhibit which of the following early signs and symptoms?

a. Decreased respiratory rate
b. Unconsciousness
c. Cyanosis
d. Agitation

35. Which of the following is an intervention used when treating a person with a lower platelet count?

a. Use of ESAs (erythropoiesis-stimulating agents)
b. Stress the importance of avoiding large crowds to lower the risk of infection
c. Stress the importance of refraining from eating iron-rich foods
d. Stress the importance of consuming foods rich in B12 and folates

36. When is palliative care helpful to patients?

a. At any stage of cancer
b. At the end stage of cancer
c. At the onset of a cancer diagnosis
d. During transition from the hospital to hospice care

37. A patient underwent a biopsy of a lesion suspicious for melanoma. While waiting for the results, the nurse receives a call from the patient with complaints of nausea, vomiting, and fatigue for the past two days. The nurse anticipates which additional testing will be ordered based on symptoms and history?

a. Abdominal ultrasound
b. MRI of the brain
c. Abdominal CT
d. Head CT

38. Where should nurses assess for pallor in a patient with dark skin who is suspected to be anemic?
   a. Forearms
   b. Cheeks
   c. Conjunctiva
   d. Scalp

39. Elias is a 58-year-old lung cancer patient. Every morning, he wakes up with a swollen and puffy face. The swelling gradually decreases over the course of the day. In addition, he takes a prescription diuretic on some days, which helps the swelling subside faster. What condition is Elias showing symptoms of?
   a. Alcoholism
   b. Superior vena cava syndrome
   c. Early onset Alzheimer's disease
   d. Cauda equina syndrome

40. A nurse is performing pre-treatment education for a patient receiving radiation for oral cancer. Which of the following interventions should the nurse recommend to the patient?
   a. Regular laboratory tests to monitor for anemia
   b. Increase in dietary fiber to reduce risk of diarrhea
   c. Application of lotion to the radiation field prior to treatment
   d. A dental evaluation prior to starting treatment

41. Which of the following interventions would be least effective for managing and preventing caregiver burnout?
   a. Take regular short breaks.
   b. Coordinate respite care.
   c. Avoid neglecting personal care appointments.
   d. Make a to-do list to increase productivity.

42. A patient experiencing itching related to an allergic reaction likely has the substance histamine being secreted by which type of white blood cell?
   a. Lymphocytes
   b. Basophils
   c. Neutrophils
   d. Monocytes

43. The nurse is preparing to assess a patient's height and weight before their first chemotherapy treatment. This patient wears a turban. Which statement made by the nurse best demonstrates culturally congruent and safe nursing care?
   a. "You will be required to remove your scarf in order for me to provide your care."
   b. "I know your turban is an important part of your religious practice. You may leave it on."
   c. "We can submit a request to determine if you can continue wearing your turban."
   d. "Can we collaborate on a way to obtain an accurate height and weight that also honors your spiritual practice?"

44. What is the role of cytokines?
   a. Suppress the immune system
   b. Eliminate cancerous cells
   c. Increase the white blood cell count
   d. Decrease the red blood cell count

45. The nurse is providing care to a patient with a history of ovarian cancer. Which of the following tumor markers would most likely be found in this patient's laboratory history?
   a. CA 19-9
   b. CEA
   c. PSA
   d. CA-125

46. A male metastatic non-small cell lung cancer (NSCLC) patient is being seen for follow-up. The patient has an order for oxycodone 5mg every four hours as needed for cancer-related pain. He reports that he is taking the medication every time it is due during the day and feels it is somewhat helpful at managing his pain levels. He is not currently experiencing any side effects other than some intermittent difficulty sleeping at night. The nurse anticipates that the physician will most likely recommend which of the following?
   a. The physician will recommend the addition of a non-opioid analgesic.
   b. There will be no recommended changes to the patient's current opioid orders.
   c. The physician will recommend that the patient reduce the frequency of oxycodone usage.
   d. The physician will change the oxycodone order to a long-acting formulation.

47. A patient experiencing intermittent nausea during chemotherapy treatment is discussing their desire to try using peppermint oil during their treatment. Which application would be most appropriate for the nurse to suggest?
   a. Use an aromatherapy diffuser in the treatment area as needed.
   b. Apply oil to a cloth or napkin and place in a plastic bag for use as needed.
   c. Use drops of oil on the tongue or add drops to a glass of water as needed.
   d. Apply drops to the skin with or without a carrier lotion or oil as needed.

48. Which of the following may be responsible for increased sepsis rates in patients?
   a. Bacteria that have become resistant to antibiotics
   b. Poor personal hygiene
   c. Neglecting to regularly sanitize personal cellphones
   d. Grocery stores that have been built on superfund sites

49. A nurse is meeting with a 37-year-old female with newly diagnosed breast cancer prior to initiating chemotherapy. The nurse understands which of the following to be true about discussing fertility preservation?
   a. Most women over 35 years of age prefer to focus on initiating treatment instead of prioritizing future fertility.
   b. Pre-cancer fertility preservation counseling has little effect on the patient's quality of life post-treatment.
   c. Pre-treatment fertility counseling can decrease decisional regret post-treatment.
   d. Emergent treatment takes precedence over discussions of fertility.

50. Which of the following is a government-sponsored insurance program that covers all aspects of terminal care for patients over a certain age?
   a. Medicaid
   b. Medicare
   c. Lifecare
   d. Tricare

51. A nurse is counseling a patient who is beginning rucaparib for metastatic prostate cancer. The patient notes that he has already received several lines of chemotherapy and asks how this medication works. Which of the following best matches the mechanism of action for rucaparib?

a. Rucaparib inhibits the growth of new blood vessels by interfering with vascular endothelial growth factor.
b. Rucaparib interferes with cell division by interrupting the enzymes CDK4 and CDK6.
c. Rucaparib inhibits the ability of the PARP enzyme to repair DNA in the cell.
d. Rucaparib blocks a protein known as epidermal growth factor receptor, which is used for cell growth.

52. A 55-year-old male is undergoing an endoscopy to discover the source of his hematemesis. The gastroenterologist encounters an active, bleeding lesion. What procedure using the application of heat to seal the lesion will probably be used next?

a. Banding
b. Biopsy
c. Angioplasty
d. Cauterization

53. In the continuum of worsening illness, sepsis is systemic inflammatory response syndrome paired with what factor?

a. Organ dysfunction
b. Known source of infection
c. Hypotensive crisis
d. Lactic acidosis

54. According to the TNM model for tumor grading, which of the following definitions most closely describes a tumor classified as *TX*?

a. The primary tumor cannot be assessed.
b. The number of tumors cannot be determined.
c. It is unknown if the tumor is malignant or benign.
d. There is no evidence of a primary tumor.

55. What condition is treated through the medical procedure of pericardiocentesis?

a. Cardiac failure
b. Cardiac extravasation
c. Cardiac tamponade
d. Cardiac arrhythmia

56. To correct the hyponatremia associated with syndrome of inappropriate antidiuretic hormone, which of the following solutions is used?

a. Normal saline
b. Hypertonic saline
c. Hypotonic saline
d. Lactated ringer's solution

57. Which types of cancer have been shown to spread from a pregnant mother to her unborn fetus?
   a. Myeloma and lung
   b. Cervical and uterine
   c. Leukemia and melanoma
   d. Prostate and rectal

58. What are echocardiography and Doppler imaging generally used for?
   a. Combat carcinoid tumors
   b. Lower the risk of cardiovascular toxicity
   c. Monitor any damage to the heart
   d. Remove cancerous tumors affecting cardiovascular function

59. Common delayed effects of cancer treatments in pediatric patients include which of the following?
   a. Stunted bone length
   b. Hair loss
   c. Weight loss
   d. Chronic fatigue

60. A patient and her son have arrived for a follow-up visit to discuss a transition to hospice care. Which statement made by the patient's son would most closely align with the anger stage of anticipatory grief?
   a. "What types of services can the hospice team provide?"
   b. "Have we explored all of our potential treatment options for my mom?"
   c. "This is all just so overwhelming and stressful. I don't even know where to begin."
   d. "I am really not sure why we need to have this conversation now."

61. When is a colostomy bag used?
   a. When a breast cancer patient has a mastectomy on only one breast
   b. When a patient has severe nausea and vomiting from chemotherapy
   c. When a patient has severe bowel obstruction and cannot eliminate waste through the bowels
   d. When a patient is having a pessary device fitted

62. What should oncology nurses emphasize to patients in order to help prepare them ahead of chemotherapy?
   a. The need to stop receiving any further vaccinations
   b. The importance of not taking any flu shots
   c. The importance of proper hygiene and regular handwashing
   d. The need for family members and caregivers to toilet the patient

63. The nurse is caring for an incontinent patient who is currently receiving chemotherapy treatment every two weeks. The nurse knows that additional measures need to be taken to prevent exposure to contaminated body fluids for a minimum of how long after the last treatment?
   a. One day
   b. Two days
   c. Five days
   d. Seven days

64. TTP is a clotting disorder that is commonly treated with which of the following protocols?
   a. Pharmaceutical intervention only
   b. Localized Botox injections near the chest
   c. Stem cell injections
   d. Fresh or frozen plasma transfusion

65. When a high-intensity beam of light is used to remove affected tissue, what is this called?
   a. Biopsy
   b. Endoscopy
   c. Laparoscopy
   d. Laser surgery

66. The oncology nurse is providing an in-service program for the nursing students. Which of the following choices is appropriate to explain cellular differentiation?
   a. High-grade tumors are well differentiated.
   b. Aggressive tumors are usually moderately differentiated.
   c. Common cancer therapies will alter the differentiation of the cancer cells.
   d. Well-differentiated cells tend to grow more slowly.

67. Extreme fatigue, delirium, and loss of bowel and bladder control are some of the patterns of symptoms associated with what type or stage of cancer?
   a. Acute onset of cancer
   b. Chronic or recurring cancer
   c. Late stages of cancer
   d. Rare forms of cancer

68. What type of surgical procedure attempts to remove an entire tumor, along with some of the surrounding tissue known as the margin?
   a. Staging surgery
   b. Curative surgery (or primary surgery)
   c. Debulking surgery
   d. Laparoscopy

69. What is the fatality rate in patients diagnosed with DIC?
   a. Up to 10%
   b. Up to 25%
   c. Up to 50%
   d. Up to 75%

70. A nurse is administering FOLFIRI to a patient being treated for colon cancer. The nurse explains that one of the pre-medications is given to prevent acute onset diarrhea. Which medication is being referred to?
   a. Octreotide
   b. Loperamide
   c. Dexamethasone
   d. Atropine

71. The nurse is caring for a patient with increased intracranial pressure (ICP). Which of the following interventions would the nurse expect for the treatment of this patient?
   a. Burr holes
   b. 0.45% normal saline
   c. HOB at less than 30 degrees
   d. Mechanical hypoventilation

72. A nurse is providing education to a patient starting FOLFOX therapy. What education is important to include for management of integumentary symptoms?
   a. You may notice inflammation around your nail bed and should monitor this for infection.
   b. An acneiform rash is common. Therefore, you should use lotions liberally.
   c. You will likely lose all of your hair with this regimen. You may want to shave it, as losing it in clumps can be distressing.
   d. FOLFOX may make your skin sensitive to the sun. You should take care to thoroughly cover your skin when going out on sunny days.

73. A patient is currently receiving an infusion of etoposide. During a conversation with the patient, the nurse notices that the patient intermittently scratches around the IV site. When the nurse assesses the patient's IV site, they note that the area is slightly warm, and the skin appears pink. The nurse recognizes that this patient is most likely experiencing what type of skin reaction?
   a. Phlebitis
   b. Extravasation
   c. Flare
   d. Infection

74. A nurse is caring for a 44-year-old woman with breast cancer who has received 4 cycles of paclitaxel chemotherapy. The patient notes that she has noticed tingling in her hands and feet beginning with her last cycle. Which of the following interventions should be discussed with the patient?
   a. Vitamin E supplements to prevent further neuropathy
   b. Application of a lidocaine cream to decrease discomfort
   c. Close inspection of hands and feet for burns, cuts, and abrasions
   d. Rest and avoidance of unnecessary walking

75. Malignant cells are capable of altering the extracellular environment to promote growth. Which of the following processes is altered due to the malignant cell's ability to produce growth factors regardless of hormone levels?
   a. Initiation
   b. Density inhibition
   c. Angiogenesis
   d. Promotion

76. The nurse is performing intravesical instillation of *bacillus Calmette-Guerin* (BCG) in a patient with bladder cancer. The nurse knows that this treatment was originally developed as a vaccine to prevent which disease?
   a. Botulism
   b. Tuberculosis
   c. Smallpox
   d. Mad cow disease

77. What does a 65 percent positive predictive value mean?
    a. 65 percent of the individuals who test positive will have the disease.
    b. 65 percent of the individuals who test positive will not have the disease.
    c. Individuals who test positive have a 65 percent probability of having the disease.
    d. Individuals who test positive have the disease.

78. What are some ways that aspirin is beneficial to the human body?
    a. Helps patients to cope with stresses and anxieties of a cancer diagnosis
    b. Lowers the risk (and possibly prevents the development) of certain cancers
    c. Combats the HPV virus
    d. Alleviates extreme pain and discomfort

79. When an organ or gland is removed that doesn't yet show signs of cancer but may eventually become cancerous due to mutated alleles known to cause cancer, what surgical procedure is being employed?
    a. Diagnostic surgery
    b. Prophylactic surgery
    c. Radiofrequency ablation
    d. Mohs microscopic surgery

80. Which of the following is an independent, non-profit accrediting agency that focuses specifically on setting standards for and evaluating quality in various healthcare settings?
    a. The Oncology Nurses Society
    b. The Joint Commission
    c. The Commission on Cancer
    d. The American College of Surgeons

81. Sierra works in a manufacturing plant on the assembly line, a job that requires a moderate amount of movement from her upper body. She has recently transitioned into survivorship after experiencing breast cancer and a mastectomy. She is very excited to return to work and her specific job responsibilities, but still feels some tenderness and tightness across her chest, in her armpit area, and down one arm. Which of the following would assist in Sierra's transition back to work?
    a. A blood thinning prescription medication
    b. A new role at her place of employment
    c. Occupational therapy three times a week
    d. Night shift work, since less people are around

82. An elderly patient is receiving treatment in the infusion center and is accompanied by her daughter, who is the patient's fulltime caregiver. Just before leaving the unit to get lunch, the patient's daughter can be heard telling the patient, "Mom, you cannot get up on your own. You absolutely must call for the nurse if you need to use the bathroom." The nurse enters the patient's room to find her attempting to get up. The patient becomes frustrated and exclaims, "This is ridiculous! I am an adult, and I can do things on my own!" Which of the following statements by the nurse would be most appropriate?
    a. "It is very unsafe for you to get up on your own."
    b. "I know you are frustrated but you need to listen to your daughter."
    c. "Please lower your voice. I can assist you to the bathroom."
    d. "I can only imagine how difficult it has been with these changes. Is it OK if I walk with you?"

83. What is meant by neutropenic sepsis?
   a. A life-threatening complication during chemotherapy
   b. A life-threatening complication during radiation therapy
   c. Nerve and muscle numbness
   d. Persistent bruising

84. A 78-year-old male patient with squamous cell carcinoma of the head and neck is following up one year after completing treatment with bleomycin. Which of the following is the most critical follow-up assessment to perform related to this patient's chemotherapy treatment history?
   a. Thyroid examination
   b. Complete blood count
   c. Lung function test
   d. Dental examination

85. A patient with breast cancer is being started on trastuzumab. The nurse understands that which of the following needs to be completed before the patient can start therapy?
   a. Pulmonary function testing
   b. Molecular testing to ensure that the tumor is HER2 positive
   c. Baseline audiology exam
   d. Molecular testing to ensure that the tumor expresses PD-L1

86. Which statement is consistent with the epidemiology of breast cancer in the United States?
   a. BRCA 1 and BRCA 2 account for 30 to 40% of the incidence of breast cancer in women.
   b. All inherited breast cancers are related to mutations of the BRCA 1 and BRCA 2 genes.
   c. Breast cancer is the leading cause of death in women.
   d. Cowden syndrome is associated with an increased risk of inherited breast cancer.

87. A nurse is preparing to administer gemcitabine and cisplatin to a patient undergoing treatment for bladder cancer. Upon assessment, the patient notes that they have been more nauseated this cycle and have been unable to drink as much as they usually do. The nurse reviews the labs and finds the creatinine notable at 2.3. What can the nurse expect the plan of care to be for this patient?
   a. Provide the patient with IV antiemetics and proceed with chemotherapy.
   b. Proceed with chemotherapy as ordered.
   c. Hold gemcitabine and cisplatin today and proceed with IV hydration.
   d. Provide counseling to the patient on home antiemetic schedule and continue with gemcitabine but hold cisplatin.

88. The oncology nurse is participating in a shared decision-making model in all of the following examples EXCEPT:
   a. Discussing the side effects a patient is experiencing in treatment with the attending physician
   b. Reinforcing information about different treatment options with the patient after a visit with the physician
   c. Requesting referral to occupational therapy for a patient who is having difficulty managing ADLs after surgery
   d. Performing a chart review to determine if a patient has received the necessary education prior to treatment

89. A patient arrives for his first chemotherapy appointment and is given a diluted amount of the standard dosage. The nurse explains that the medical team will gradually increase the dose that the patient receives over the course of two to six weeks. Within a couple of months, the patient will receive a standard dosage for his body weight and cancer diagnosis. What is this practice called?
    a. Chemo break-in
    b. Compounding
    c. Desensitization protocol
    d. Radiation

90. A 25-year-old male is recommended bleomycin, etoposide, and cisplatin for treatment of testicular cancer. The patient notes that he has a history of smoking marijuana three times weekly for the past two years. The nurse should recommend which testing be completed prior to initiating therapy?
    a. Chest X-ray
    b. Pulmonary function test
    c. CT of chest
    d. Bronchoscopy

91. What surgical procedure uses liquid nitrogen to freeze and kill abnormal or cancerous cells?
    a. Cryosurgery
    b. Mohs surgery
    c. Laparoscopy
    d. Debulking surgery

92. A nurse is providing education to a patient prior to beginning chemotherapy in preparation for a bone marrow transplant. Which statement by the patient indicates understanding of the information?
    a. "My immune system will be compromised, but it is okay to see my young nieces and nephews because they are vaccinated."
    b. "My immune system will have trouble fighting infections, so I should avoid going to the ER and exposing myself to ill people."
    c. "My immune system won't be able to fight infections, so I should encourage friends and family to send fresh flowers instead of visiting."
    d. "I will be severely immunocompromised; therefore, I need to make sure I cook my food thoroughly and eat only fruits and vegetables that I can wash thoroughly."

93. A nurse is caring for a patient at the end of life who is reporting periods of high levels of pain throughout the day despite long-acting opioids. Which medication does the nurse anticipate orders for?
    a. Oxycodone 5 mg Q4 hours
    b. Gabapentin 200 QHS
    c. Fentanyl 25 mcg/hr transdermal patch Q72 hours
    d. Dexamethasone 8 mg daily

94. A 72-year-old male with prostate cancer has been receiving androgen deprivation therapy (ADT) for two years. His most recent DEXA scan showed osteoporosis. Which medication can the nurse expect to see ordered for this patient?
    a. Calcium infusion
    b. Sipuleucel-T
    c. G-CSF
    d. Bisphosphonates

95. A patient with lung cancer would be less likely to experience metastasis at which anatomical location?
  a. Intestines
  b. Bone
  c. Liver
  d. Brain

96. A nurse is caring for a patient after a double mastectomy. The patient notes that her partner will be the primary caregiver at home. The nurse should offer the following support options EXCEPT:
  a. Written instructions of the medication schedule
  b. Involvement in physical and occupational therapy sessions
  c. A list of bereavement resources in the community
  d. A referral to social work to review leave options

97. A female patient with lymphoma is being evaluated after she woke up with pain and swelling of the left lower leg. The nurse assesses the patient and finds that the posterior upper calf area has localized redness and is warm to the touch. The patient describes the pain as achy and cramping. Which intervention does the nurse anticipate next for this patient?
  a. Initiation of antibiotic therapy
  b. Initiation of anticoagulant therapy
  c. Diagnostic imaging
  d. Tissue culture

98. Which of the following practices is a non-pharmacologic, alternative form of therapy that has been shown to have statistically significant positive outcomes in cancer patients?
  a. Ayurvedic herb tinctures
  b. Vipassana meditation
  c. Rolfing
  d. Acupuncture

99. What surgical procedure removes all of the suspicious tissue during diagnostic surgery?
  a. Incisional biopsy
  b. Excisional biopsy
  c. Mastectomy
  d. Laparotomy

100. A patient is receiving their seventh dose of carboplatin and calls the nurse into the room to complain of flushing, tachycardia, and shortness of breath. The nurse understands that this reaction is unlikely to resolve without the use of which medication?
  a. Diphenhydramine
  b. Albuterol
  c. Epinephrine
  d. Dexamethasone

101. What is meant by symptom management?
  a. Coordinating care with the primary physician
  b. Collaborating with home caregivers
  c. The assessment of how well a patient reacts to treatment
  d. The prevention or treatment of side effects

102. What are targeted therapies?
  a. The use of living substances to help fight against cancer
  b. A class of drugs that work to prevent cancer from growing or spreading
  c. An endocrinological therapy
  d. An adoptive cellular therapy

103. A nurse is visiting with a patient who reports a metallic taste now that he has started chemotherapy and has not been eating as much because of it. The nurse should recommend which non-pharmacologic intervention to manage the taste changes?
  a. Avoid spices to prevent drying out of food.
  b. Use mouthwashes such as Listerine frequently to alter the taste in mouth.
  c. Eat candies such as lemon drops or chew gum prior to meals.
  d. Avoid foods with strong aromas.

104. A nurse is caring for a patient who has been ordered to have germline genetic testing. Which of the following supports patient autonomy?
  a. Providing the patient with written information about the testing after collecting the sample
  b. Scheduling an education session with the patient to ensure that they understand the risks and benefits surrounding genetic testing
  c. Providing the patient with the portal information to review the results and encouraging research prior to discussing the results with the provider
  d. Reviewing the notes from the patient's last visit and determining if the rationale for the test was shared by the provider during that visit

105. How is pain most routinely managed in palliative care settings?
  a. Breathing exercises
  b. Barbiturates
  c. Homeopathic medicines
  d. Opioids

106. What is biotherapy?
  a. A breakthrough approach to radiation therapy
  b. Chemotherapy treatment administered intravenously
  c. The use of living substances to help fight against cancer
  d. Chemotherapy treatment given orally

107. A patient with HER2-positive breast cancer is returning for follow-up six months after completing courses of chemotherapy, biologic therapy, and radiation therapy. Which of the following diagnostic tests would be most crucial to monitor this patient for one of the potential delayed-onset side effects of this combination of treatments?
  a. Chest X-ray
  b. Electrocardiogram
  c. Multigated acquisition scan
  d. Magnetic resonance imaging

108. A nurse is preparing to administer doxorubicin. Which medication should they ensure is ordered to be given prior to the chemotherapy dose?

a. Mesna
b. Dexrazoxane
c. Atropine
d. Dexamethasone

109. What is meant by Mohs microscopic surgery?

a. The removal of one layer of tissue at a time, examining the tissue under a microscope, and continuing in this fashion until the cells in a particular layer appear healthy
b. A small incision that is made in order to detect and remove abnormal cells
c. The freezing and destroying of cancer cells
d. A minimally-invasive procedure using a narrow and flexible tube

110. The nurse is performing a pre-treatment assessment of a patient with metastatic squamous cell carcinoma of the neck who is returning for radiation therapy. The patient complains of moderate pain (4/10) and reports that they can drink liquids and eat soft, bland foods. The nurse notes that the oral mucosa is red with several white patches to the buccal region and the tongue. What grade would the nurse document the patient's mucositis?

a. I
b. II
c. III
d. IV

111. If a patient bleeds for longer than normal and bruises easily, what might the patient's body be doing?

a. Producing higher levels of platelets
b. Producing lower levels of platelets
c. Producing lower levels of red blood cells
d. Producing higher levels of white blood cells

112. A patient is being seen for the treatment of breast cancer. Which of the following is considered a positive prognostic factor?

a. The tumor is 6 centimeters.
b. The cancer is node-positive.
c. The tumor is hormone receptor-negative.
d. The cancer cells are low grade.

113. A nurse is taking care of a patient receiving stereotactic body radiation therapy (SBRT) for prostate cancer. The patient asks the nurse to explain how this type of radiation differs from others. Which of the following is the best response by the nurse?

a. "This type of radiation uses multiple beams of radiation while accounting for tumor motion. This limits impact to surrounding tissues."
b. "This type of radiation uses X-rays to treat the tumor cells. Surrounding tissues are often impacted by the dose."
c. "This treatment uses the implantation of radioactive material near the tumor. The surrounding tissue can often be spared from damage."
d. "This type of radiation uses positively charged particles to target the tumor. Surrounding tissues see less damage because they can be stopped at certain depths."

114. Ashlee lost her mother to cancer one month ago. Even though Ashlee was told her mother had a terminal prognosis, spoke with her mother about it, and planned and attended the memorial services, she finds that she regularly tries to pick up the phone to call her mom and talks to her husband about her mother in the present tense. Which stage of grief does Ashlee appear to be in?

a. Denial
b. Anger
c. Acceptance
d. Habit

115. Which of the following drug classes can assist in preventing pain and fractures related to bone cancer?

a. Steroids
b. Antidepressants
c. Bisphosphonates
d. Anticonvulsants

116. What is meant by debulking surgery?

a. Removal of as much of a tumor as is medically possible
b. Entire removal of a tumor and surrounding tissues
c. Removal of an organ or gland
d. Removal of precancerous tissue

117. Which of the following may be a viable treatment option in the future to combat the influence that cancer and its treatments have on a patient's cognitive abilities?

a. A pescatarian diet
b. Reimbursing hospice services at an earlier stage of the cancer continuum
c. Audiobooks
d. Interventions typically administered to Alzheimer's patients

118. What is the primary difference between recurring malignancies and secondary malignancies?
a. Recurring malignancies refer to cancers that are genetically predisposed in family members; secondary malignancies refer to cancers that result from poor lifestyle habits.
b. Recurring malignancies occur in pediatric patients; secondary malignancies occur later in life.
c. Recurring malignancies refer to cancer that returns after treatment is complete and cancer has been undetectable; secondary malignancies occur as a result of treatment for another cancer.
d. Recurring malignancies refer to cancers above the torso, as these are more common; secondary malignancies refer to cancers below the torso, as these are more rare.

119. The oncology nurse in the breast center is counseling a patient who has received an abnormal mammogram report. Which of the following statements is consistent with a BI-RADS 0 result?
a. Continued monitoring with diagnostic mammograms of the affected breast every six months is recommended for two years.
b. No abnormalities were detected.
c. Abnormalities that were identified are benign.
d. Additional testing with diagnostic mammography and ultrasonography is required to assess the findings of the screening exam.

120. What is the expected prognosis for cancer patients who show symptoms of superior vena cava syndrome?
a. Likely to pass away in 24 to 48 hours
b. Likely to pass away in the next three years
c. Likely to pass away in the next six weeks
d. Likely to make a full recovery from their cancer

121. A 32-year-old patient with lymphoma is currently receiving chemotherapy treatment and is suspected of having tumor lysis syndrome. Which of the following lab values would support this diagnosis?
a. Calcium of 10.2 mg/dL
b. Potassium of 6.3 mEq/L
c. Phosphorus of 1.3 mg/dL
d. Uric acid of 1.5 mg/dL

122. When caring for affected skin in patients with GvHD, what should the nurse emphasize?
a. Avoid hydrating the skin, as this will lead to further damage.
b. Avoid application of any SPF, which acts as an irritant.
c. Hydrate and apply topical steroids and oil-based creams.
d. Cover all affected areas to lower the risk of infection.

123. When surgeons attempt to ascertain the size of a tumor or if a cancer has spread, what type of surgical procedure is being used?
a. Incisional biopsy
b. Diagnostic surgery
c. Staging surgery
d. Debulking surgery

124. A patient recently diagnosed with cancer asks the nurse to explain her disease. The nurse explains that her cancer interferes with the production of important proteins that are needed for the immune system. Which of the following types of cancer is consistent with this statement?

a. The cancer is a carcinoma.
b. The cancer is a myeloma.
c. The cancer is Hodgkin lymphoma.
d. The cancer is granulocytic leukemia.

125. As the nurse prepares to administer a patient's 5-fluorouracil bolus, they bring the patient a cup of ice chips. This intervention is performed to minimize the risk for which potential side effect?

a. Mucositis
b. Nausea
c. Taste changes
d. Neuropathy

126. Which of the following refers to any inflammation of tissues in and of the lung?

a. Pleural neuroma
b. Pneumonitis
c. Lung cancer
d. Emphysema

127. Which of the following is NOT one of the required patient education elements according to the American Society of Clinical Oncology's (ASCO) *Quality Oncology Practice Initiatives* (QOPI)?

a. Potential long-term side effects of ordered treatments
b. Safe handling of body fluids
c. Chemotherapy administration guidelines
d. Instructions for scheduling or rescheduling appointments

128. Which of the following would be suggested to minimize nose bleeds in cancer patients?

a. Get plenty of sleep.
b. Eliminate spinach from the diet.
c. Stop taking aspirin.
d. Use a dehumidifier.

129. A nurse provides care for a patient with colorectal cancer who is one-day post-op from a surgical colectomy with colostomy placement. Which of the following statements made by the patient regarding their new colostomy is most concerning to the nurse?

a. "I have not had any output yet."
b. "My stoma is very swollen."
c. "The stoma is kind of purple near the skin."
d. "My stomach is still tender."

130. A nurse is providing care to a patient post-endoscopic retrograde cholangiopancreatography (ERCP). Which priority action will the nurse perform to prevent aspiration?

a. Assess the gag reflex before feeding
b. Position the head of the bed to at least 30 degrees
c. Set up suction in the room post-procedure
d. Encourage coughing and deep breathing every hour

131. When would a fine-needle aspiration be appropriate?

a. To effectively treat a patient with cancer
b. To collect cells for a pathologist who will either confirm or rule out the presence of cancer
c. To prevent cells from spreading
d. To effectively remove a tumor

132. A nurse is caring for a patient who is struggling with making a treatment decision. The patient tells the nurse that they have been offered an IV therapy that is more aggressive but requires travel to the clinic on a weekly basis. The patient prefers a less aggressive oral medication that requires less travel to the clinic. By advocating for the patient's choice of the oral medication to the team, the nurse is practicing which leadership competency?

a. Professionalism
b. Communication and relationship management
c. Knowledge of the healthcare environment
d. Business skills and principles

133. The nurse is caring for a 32-year-old female patient with a history of breast cancer. The patient has completed four cycles of doxorubicin and cyclophosphamide, and she is currently receiving her seventh dose of paclitaxel and trastuzumab. The patient asks if her side effects will go away after she completes treatment. Which of the patient's reported symptoms has the greatest potential to become a chronic side effect of this regimen?

a. Numbness of the feet
b. Loss of hair
c. Nausea and vomiting
d. Dark nailbeds

134. In patients diagnosed with pancytopenia, which procedure is the best option for accurately determining the underlying cause?

a. A PCR test
b. A bone marrow biopsy
c. An amniocentesis
d. A CBC panel

135. Which of the following cancers is highly correlated with syndrome of inappropriate antidiuretic hormone secretion (SIADH)?

a. Kidney cancer
b. Small cell lung cancer
c. Bladder cancer
d. Pineal cancer

136. A patient has received general anesthesia for a surgical procedure. After surgery is initiated, the patient develops malignant hyperthermia. Which clinical value is consistent with this complication?

a. Heart rate of 54 beats/min
b. Temperature of 38.2 °C (100.7 °F)
c. Potassium level of 3.2 mEq/L
d. CO_2 level of 47 mmHg

137. What is required if a patient is experiencing opioid-induced respiratory depression?
   a. Weekly follow-ups to monitor the condition
   b. Antidepressant medication to lessen the severity of depressive symptoms
   c. A reevaluation of prescribed medications and treatments
   d. Immediate medication attention

138. A patient has arrived at an outpatient oncology clinic for their first visit after being diagnosed with cervical cancer. The patient visually appears to be male, and the nurse reads on the patient's chart that their gender is listed as male, while the sex assigned at birth is listed as female. Which of the following questions asked by the nurse would be the least helpful in establishing a trusting relationship with this patient?
   a. "Can you tell me what brings you in today?"
   b. "Have you completed gender reassignment surgery?"
   c. "What is your preferred name?"
   d. "What cultural or spiritual considerations should we know about?"

139. Irritability, weight fluctuations, sleep disruptions, and crying spells are most likely to be experienced by someone who is going through what process?
   a. Chemical-induced delusion
   b. Bereavement
   c. Adopting a plant-based diet
   d. Intravenous opioid titration

140. Which of the following is not a usual drug of choice when providing analgesia to the mechanically ventilated patient?
   a. Morphine
   b. Dopamine
   c. Fentanyl
   d. Propofol

141. Which of the following pharmaceuticals is commonly prescribed to combat nausea from chemotherapy?
   a. Ondansetron
   b. Amoxicillin
   c. Esomeprazole
   d. Hydrocodone

142. Which of the following statements made by a patient undergoing treatment for ovarian cancer indicates a possible need for additional teaching?
   a. "I stopped my morning walks so I wouldn't be so tired."
   b. "I have been eating with plastic utensils."
   c. "I have been trying to eat a small amount of food every hour or so."
   d. "My skin has been drier, so I have been using lotion in the morning and at night."

143. What is a pathological laparotomy?
  a. Complete removal of an organ or gland
  b. A procedure that allows the surgeon to look for evidence of cancer and remove samples as needed for further examination
  b. Removal of a tumor and surrounding tissue
  d. Partial removal of a tumor

144. Since cells are able to repair mutations, how are the mutations passed on to new cells as inheritable defects?
  a. The mutations suppress the cell's ability to block tumor formation.
  b. Multiple mutations exceed the cellular repair capabilities.
  c. If the cell divides before the DNA repairs are complete, the damage is permanent and will be inherited.
  d. The mutations decrease the rate of cellular proliferation.

145. The nurse is assisting a colleague with a patient experiencing possible extravasation of intravenous vincristine. The nurse has stopped the infusion and attempted aspiration of the peripheral IV. The physician has also been notified. Which of the following interventions can the nurse perform to assist the colleague in this situation?
  a. Place the affected arm below the level of the patient's heart.
  b. Apply a tourniquet above the site.
  c. Administer sodium thiosulfate at the site.
  d. Apply a warm compress to the site.

146. A nurse is preparing a patient for an allogeneic transplant. Which of the following statements indicates patient understanding of the information?
  a. "I will have cells collected after several rounds of chemotherapy."
  b. "My brother is guaranteed to be the best match since we have the same parents."
  c. "After the transplant, I won't need to be immunosuppressed."
  d. "I will undergo testing to ensure an HLA-compatible donor."

147. Which form of disseminated intravascular coagulation (DIC) are cancer patients most likely to experience?
  a. Acute
  b. Chronic
  c. Fatal
  d. Mild

148. Which of the following common supplements would be least concerning for use with a patient experiencing thrombocytopenia?
  a. Chamomile
  b. Ginseng
  c. Melatonin
  d. Ginger

149. Melvin lives in a small, rural town with less than 6,000 people. He was recently diagnosed with kidney cancer and has to travel two hours away into the closest metropolitan area to receive care. Melvin is exhausted by the travel and feels very alone. He does not know anyone in his town who has experienced cancer, and he only gets a chance to express his feelings when he sees his nursing team. How can Melvin most easily alleviate his distress?

a. Ask his insurance company to pay for long-term overnight visits at his metropolitan hospital.
b. Try to get more sleep.
c. Join a closed Facebook group consisting of kidney cancer patients and survivors.
d. Move to the metropolitan area so he can meet more people and not have to travel so far.

150. Ben is an avid golfer, cyclist, and runner. One day, he feels some lower back pain and an ache in his left hip. The next morning, he feels some tingling down the length of his left leg. He rests, applies ice, performs gentle stretching exercises, and takes a break from his activities for a week. While golfing the next weekend, his lower body suddenly goes numb, and he accidentally urinates in his pants. What condition is Ben showing symptoms of?

a. Trigeminal neuralgia
b. Aging
c. Meningitis
d. Cauda equina syndrome

151. Paula has a routine cervical exam which shows the presence of abnormal cells on her cervix. A biopsy shows that she has stage one cervical cancer. Paula has surgery to remove all of the cancerous cells, and her medical team feels she has a very good prognosis due to early detection. However, why will Paula need to continue to be monitored with follow-up visits?

a. She appears to have a genetic predisposition to reproductive cancers.
b. She is of child-bearing age and hopes to become pregnant.
c. Cancerous cells can spread before becoming detectable.
d. She is nearing menopause.

152. Which of the following foods is associated with the development of cancerous conditions?

a. Aged cheese
b. Red wine
c. Oxalate-containing vegetables
d. Bacon

153. Although cancer survivors have found themselves free of their disease, which of the following distressing experiences are they most likely to experience compared to other demographics?

a. Debt or bankrupt
b. Estrangement from family
c. Relocation
d. Marriage

154. Which of the following patients is most likely to be recommended for prophylactic gastrostomy tube placement?

a. A female patient with stage IIIB breast cancer
b. A male patient with stage III squamous cell carcinoma of the larynx
c. A male patient with stage IB non-small cell lung cancer
d. A female patient with stage IIC colorectal cancer

155. A manager of an inpatient oncology unit is implementing a program for staff that focuses on cultivating optimism, purpose, spirituality, social connection, and self-care strategies. Which of the following is most likely to be the unit manager's primary goal for the development of this program?
   a. Improving patient satisfaction
   b. Reducing medication error rates
   c. Maintaining standards of practice
   d. Increasing staff resilience

156. Which procedure is commonly used to both treat and relieve intracranial pressure?
   a. Meditation
   b. Lumbar puncture
   c. Trigger point therapy under the occipital ridge
   d. Desensitization protocol

157. A 23-year-old male patient arrives to the infusion center for treatment for testicular cancer. As the nurse is preparing to place the patient's intravenous catheter, the patient asks for an emesis basin and states, "Every time I get my IV, I feel sick to my stomach." The nurse knows that the patient may benefit most from premedication with which of the following medication classes?
   a. Benzodiazepine
   b. Proton pump inhibitor
   c. Selective 5-HT3 receptor antagonist
   d. Antihistamine

158. A nurse provides care for a 50-year-old patient with metastatic colorectal cancer. During a conversation, the patient states, "I'm not sure how much longer I have left. I sometimes wonder if I have had a chance to do enough good in my life." Regarding the patient's statement, which of the following is most indicated for this patient?
   a. Notify the physician.
   b. Request referral to psychiatry.
   c. Request chaplain services.
   d. Request referral to palliative care.

159. The nurse is assisting with the admission of a patient with ovarian cancer. The patient is very tearful and appears emotionally distraught. When asked if she has had thoughts of harming herself, the patient responds that she has been saving up her pain medications in plans of taking them to go to sleep forever. Which of the following is the most appropriate response by the nurse?
   a. "I am concerned about what you have shared, and I think it would be a good idea to speak with someone about this."
   b. "I am going to have to leave to contact your doctor about how you're feeling."
   c. "You can't let life get you down. Don't give up."
   d. "I am so sorry that you're dealing with these feelings."

160. What are some of the areas that should be captured in the assessment section of a patient's medical care plan?
   a. Current symptoms and pain levels
   b. Confirmation of financial clearance
   c. Role of caregivers and logistics of care coordination
   d. Communication and collaboration with referring physician's office

161. What is meant by palliative surgery?
    a. Surgery that alleviates as much pain and discomfort as possible for patients with advanced forms of cancer in order to improve their quality of life
    b. A term used interchangeably with curative surgery
    c. Minimally-invasive surgery to examine suspicious tissue
    d. Highly-invasive surgery that may negatively impact a patient's physical appearance and/or physical function

162. Which of the following is an example of a situation where a verbal order should never be accepted?
    a. The patient's chemotherapy dose requires recalculation due to a weight change.
    b. The patient's chemotherapy is being held due to neutropenia.
    c. Additional orders for premedication are being added to the patient's treatment plan.
    d. Additional hydration is being added to the patient's treatment today.

163. Cancer cells are capable of blocking the function of the immune system. Which of the following choices is consistent with this statement?
    a. Cell surface proteins are inactivated by antibodies.
    b. The release of immune cell suppressants by adjacent cells is triggered.
    c. Angiogenesis is initiated.
    d. Cellular contact inhibition is increased.

164. Which of the following treatments would typically be discontinued after an oncology patient transitions to hospice care?
    a. Transfusion of two units of packed red blood cells to improve shortness of breath and fatigue
    b. Radiation therapy to assist with pain management for a lung cancer patient
    c. Administration of intravenous fluids to a patient who is having difficulty with oral intake
    d. Treatment with bevacizumab to control glioblastoma growth

165. The nurse provides care for a patient with bladder cancer. Which of the following is the most common cause for this type of malignancy?
    a. History of cigarette smoking
    b. History of obesity
    c. History of chronic urinary tract infections
    d. History of exposure to certain environmental chemicals

Answer Explanations #1

1. B. Macrophages are part of innate immunity and recognize, ingest, and kill microbes; clear out debris and dead cells; and stimulate other cells of the immune system. Choice *A* refers to cytokines, Choice *C* describes the role of T-cells, and Choice *D* refers to B-cells.

2. C: Survivorship refers to the period when a patient has finished cancer treatment and cancerous cells are undetectable until the time of patient death, regardless of the cause of death. This specific time period is called survivorship because the patient is said to have "survived" the diagnosis, but now must make a number of personal and lifestyle adjustments that will dictate their quality of life for the rest of their lifespan.

3. C: Testicular cancer can be treated with an autologous stem cell transplant if there is recurrence after initial chemotherapy treatment. Other solid tumors include neuroblastoma, Ewing sarcoma, hepatoblastoma, and osteosarcoma. Choices *A, B,* and *D* are incorrect.

4. B: Inflammatory reactions in all body tissues release carcinogenic substances that can initiate carcinogenesis and damage DNA. Inflammatory diseases are treated with non-steroidal anti-inflammatory agents, which have an anti-tumor effect, making Choice *A* incorrect. Chronic inflammation does not slow the process; instead, it is associated with acceleration of the process of initiation, making Choice *C* incorrect. There is no evidence that inflammation in any specific system has a greater effect on the development of cancer, making Choice *D* incorrect.

5. C: The best way to evaluate if an oncology practice is meeting the requirements of their current patient education program would be to review the current standards of practice, such as the *Chemotherapy and Immunotherapy Guidelines and Recommendations for Practice*, written by the Oncology Nursing Society in 2018. Choice *A* is not the best choice because patient satisfaction surveys would be best suited for identifying ways to improve patient experience, as opposed to compliance with current requirements. Choice *B* is not the best choice, as staff polling would be better for identifying adherence to the process rather than identifying whether the program is meeting guidelines. Lastly, Choice *D* is not the best choice because discussion with community stakeholders would be better suited for identifying needs and concerns within the community, rather than evaluating adherence to requirements.

6. A: Radiofrequency ablation involves the use of heat created by radio waves to destroy cancer cells. A tube is inserted through the skin into the tumor, and an electrical current then heats the cancer cells to extremely high temperatures in order to terminate them. Choice *B* refers to laser surgery, which employs a high-intensity beam of light to remove tissue. Choice *C* describes cryosurgery, in which liquid nitrogen is applied to cause the cells to freeze and die. Choice *D* refers to preventative surgery, in which precancerous cells are removed from the body.

7. A: Choice *A* is the correct answer because patients at risk for lymphedema are recommended to remain active and strength train. This improves circulation, and it also assists the patient to maintain control of their weight. Choices *B, C,* and *D* would not be the correct answer because these items would be included in patient education related to preventing lymphedema.

8. C: Absolute neutrophil count (ANC) is calculated by taking the total number of white blood cells (WBC) per microliter and multiplying that by the percentage of neutrophils as a decimal. In this example, 4.5

thousand cells/microliter is converted to 4500 cells/microliter. Then, 4500 cells/microliter x 0.15 (15%) = 675 cells/microliter. This ANC would be below the physician's parameters of an ANC of above 1000 cells/microliter, and this patient's treatment would be held. Choices *A, B,* and *D* are not the correct answer choices.

9. B: The most appropriate next step for the nurse to take is to clarify the orders with the research nurse. Research protocols may differ from monographs, and the nurse may be administering the patient's medications using different guidelines than is typically advised. However, the nurse should immediately seek to clarify the orders if there are any concerns or questions. Choice *A* is not the most appropriate answer because the nurse is unsure of the orders and should clarify before administering the treatment. Choice *C* is incorrect because the nurse should follow the appropriate research protocol for this patient after confirming the orders are correct. Lastly, Choice *D* is incorrect because it would not be appropriate to make treatment decisions based on the administration technique of a previous caregiver.

10. A: Chemotherapy treatment refers to the administration of one or a combination of medications that work to fight cancer. The medications work to stop or slow down the growth of cancer cells. Choice *B* is incorrect since chemotherapy is not a surgical procedure. Choice *C* is another name for a CT scan. Choice *D* refers to a form of radiation therapy used to treat patients with prostate cancer.

11. A: Hodgkin's lymphoma patients normally have positive prognoses for this specific cancer, but are also screened at higher rates due to the high correlation that Hodgkin's lymphoma has with secondary malignancies. Most patients are told to expect another malignancy at some point during their survivorship; these can be far more serious than the initial Hodgkin's diagnosis.

12. A: Spinal cord compression occurs when there is an impact to the spinal cord or cauda equina by the tumor, resulting in direct pressure, vertebral collapse, or both. Patients with breast, lung, prostate, renal, and melanoma are at high risk due to the affinity of the tumor to metastasize to the bone. Patients with metastatic disease at presentation are at higher risk than those with localized disease. Choice *A* is at highest risk due to having breast cancer that is widely metastatic. Choice *B* is low risk, as the patient has a locally advanced colon cancer. Choice *C* is incorrect, as the patient has localized bladder cancer. Choice *D* is incorrect, as the patient has a locally advanced prostate cancer.

13. C: Although a diet high in fat and calories is not considered a particular healthy regime, it is important for patients undergoing chemotherapy and radiation to maintain their current body weight and lessen the risk of too much weight loss. Choices *A* and *B* are not recommended as patients may lose too much weight, which can further complicate their ability to fight the disease. Choice *D* is incorrect; although fiber is known to be an excellent cancer fighter, a diet high in fat and calories is more important.

14. A: Acupuncture would be contraindicated for a patient who is neutropenic, as this procedure requires the placement of small needles to certain points on the body. This places the neutropenic patient at risk for potential infection. Choices *B*, *C*, and *D* are all examples of non-pharmacological comfort measures which would typically be considered safe for a neutropenic patient.

15. A: In the autosomal dominant pattern of inheritance, the child inherits the mutated gene from one parent, and both the child and the parent will manifest the disease. In the autosomal recessive pattern, the child must inherit the gene from both parents, and the parents may or may not manifest an increased cancer risk.

16. D: Choice *D* is correct because the suffixes of *-omab* and *-opab* designate that the antibody is derived from mice. Choice *A* is incorrect, as the suffixes *-umab* and *-upab* designate a human-derived antibody. Choice *B* is incorrect because *-amab* or *-apab* are designations associated with antibodies derived from rats. Choice *C* is also incorrect because monoclonal antibodies of a primate origin are associated with the suffixes *-imab* and *-ipab*.

17. A: Beck's triad of muffled heart sounds, distended neck veins, and hypotension are cardinal signs of cardiac tamponade. Chest pain and back pain are the most common presenting symptoms with an AAA. Heart function, breathing, and consciousness are not evident in cardiopulmonary arrest. Cardiogenic shock includes ashen, cyanotic, or mottled extremities; distant heart sounds; and rapid and faint peripheral pulses.

18. D: Implanted port needles and dressings should be replaced at least every seven days or more often as required (e.g., due to compromised dressing, signs of infection, leaking, etc.). Choices *A, B,* and *C* are not the correct answer because current evidence supports that needles and dressings may safely remain for up to seven days without increased risk for infection.

19. A: Choice *A* is the correct answer, as an allogeneic stem cell transplant is received by a related or unrelated donor and carries the highest risk of graft versus host disease (GvHD). Choice *B* is not correct as this procedure reduces the amount of donor T-cells received, which decreases the risk of GvHD in the recipient. Choice *C* is incorrect as cord blood transplant is obtained by collecting blood samples from healthy newborn umbilical cords and placentas, which carries a lower risk for development of GvHD. Lastly, Choice *D* is incorrect because the term *autologous stem cell transplant* refers to when the donor and the recipient are the same person, which also carries a much lower risk of development of GvHD.

20. B: Acute lymphoblastic leukemia is the most common class of leukemia diagnosed in children. This form is rare in adults. Choices *A* and C are incorrect because chronic lymphocytic leukemia and chronic myelogenous leukemia are primarily seen in adults. Choice *D*, acute myelogenous leukemia, is the second most common form of pediatric leukemia but is one of the most commonly diagnosed leukemias in adults.

21. C: Cushing's triad of manifestations are late signs of increased ICP. Choice *C* is an example of widening pulse pressure: Normal pulse pressure is 40 to 60 mmHg, while the pulse pressure in Choice *C* is 130 mmHg, and thus is the correct choice. Choices *A, B,* and *D* are all early signs of increased ICP and, therefore, are incorrect.

22. D: Choice *D* is a likely imbalance that presents in a patient with acute renal failure and will require diligent management. Choices *A*, *B*, and *C* are unlikely as the patient is at risk for a decreased GFR, increased BUN, and decreased calcium level. Acute renal failure involves poor filtering ability and a buildup of waste in the blood.

23. B: Opiates are a mainstay in the medical profession when patients are experiencing severe, debilitating pain and discomfort. Great care must be taken when prescribing and administering opiates as they can cause opioid-induced respiratory depression—a potentially life-threatening side effect. Choice *A* is incorrect since HPV infections are best fought with antibiotics. Choice *C* is incorrect since antidepressants and antianxiety medications would be prescribed for patients with acute anxiety and/or depression. Choice *D* is incorrect since opiates are used to help patients who are in severe pain and are not used as a prevention in developing any kind of illness.

24. A: Breast cancer, lung cancer, and myeloma are most commonly correlated with hypercalcemia. This can be indicative that the cancer has spread to the bones, causing osteoclasts to work excessively. Osteoclasts break down the bones; when cancer spreads to the bones, the osteoclasts break the bones down faster than osteoblasts can build them.

25. D: Sepsis specifically refers to infectious agents in the blood, while SIRS refers to any kind of inflammation. Sepsis can be a type of SIRS if it causes inflammation. However, SIRS is not considered equivalent to sepsis on its own since it can result from infectious or non-infectious agents.

26. B: Value stream mapping is an analytic tool that examines a specific workflow. It breaks the workflow down into steps and examines each step for the value it adds. Often, this process indicates that some steps are wasteful and unnecessary for the procedure. Thus, the procedure can be reworked for efficiency. Gap analyses identify holes in a procedure that need steps or a new procedure added. PDCA cycles examine a test of change. Step charts are not a process improvement tool.

27. B: The Americans with Disabilities (ADA) Act provides certain rights and protections to individuals with qualifying disabilities to ensure they have equal opportunities in many areas, including employment. Employers with fifteen or greater employees are obligated to provide reasonable accommodation as long as employees can perform the essential functions of their position. For the patient in the example, permanent neuropathy may be considered an ADA-qualifying disability because it impacts daily activities. A reasonable accommodation may be to provide seating to the patient while she performs her duties as cashier. Choice *A* is not the correct answer because the Family and Medical Leave (FMLA) Act is a law that provides the ability for eligible employees to take up to 12 weeks per year of qualifying medical or family leave from their place of employment without risk of losing their job. Choice *C* is incorrect because the Fair Labor Standards Act (FLSA) provides certain rights with respect to minimum wage, overtime pay, and child labor. Choice *D* is incorrect because the Occupational Safety and Health Act (OSHA) provides standards and regulations that employers must follow to safely operate their business.

28. B: Choice *B* is the most appropriate response by the nurse because it includes empathy and seeks to determine whether the patient has discussed this with another professional. The patient's statements could indicate they are experiencing depression, which is a very common experience amongst cancer patients. Choices *A* and *C* are not the most appropriate responses since these statements do not empathize or validate the patient's statement. Choice *D* is not the most appropriate response because responding with "I know how you feel," or responding with personal experiences would not be the most professional, therapeutic, or validating statement to make.

29. A: Laparoscopy is a special type of surgery that employs the use of a narrow, lighted tube inserted into the abdomen through an incision. Laparoscopies are often used to detect cysts, fibroids, infection, or adhesions. Choice *B* involves the removal of affected tissues by employing a high-intensity beam of light. Choice *C* also employs the use of a narrow and flexible tube, which is inserted into the patient's mouth, rectum, or vagina, rather than their abdomen. If abnormal tissue is discovered, the surgeon may opt to remove some or all of this tissue for further examination. Choice *D* refers to the removal of tissue that will be examined more closely under a microscope. Although several tests exist that help to determine if cancer is present, a biopsy will make a definite diagnosis or definitively rule it out.

30. D: In this case, the patient is blatantly ignoring Doug's attempts to provide patient education. Often, cancer patients who are overwhelmed with their health situation are not cooperative in discussing their treatment options and what to expect. Some simply do not want to know any more than they have to.

In these cases, speaking with a close family member (such as a spouse) or caregiver can ensure that adequate patient education is still disseminated to someone who can benefit the patient with it. However, staff must make sure they are speaking with authorized family members or caregivers to ensure they are not violating any privacy laws.

31. A: The patient's history and presenting symptoms are most consistent with nivolumab-related pneumonitis. Programmed cell death protein-1 inhibitors (PD-1), such as nivolumab, have been shown to carry a risk for potentially life-threatening immune-related adverse events (irAEs) that include pneumonitis. The condition often presents with varying severity of cough, shortness of breath, and chest pain and can begin anytime in the first year of treatment with nivolumab. History of radiation therapy to the chest also increases the risk for pneumonitis development. Choice *B* is not the best answer because this irAE can present with chest pain and shortness of breath, but it also tends to be accompanied by arrhythmias, swelling, and fatigue. Choice *C* is not the best answer because cancer progression is not a treatment-related complication. Choice *D* is also not the best answer choice because the patient is afebrile, and there are no additional indicators to suggest that the patient is experiencing low white blood cell count.

32. D: Radiation therapy can result in damage to tissue and blood vessels. Choices *A* and *B* are incorrect since there is no evidence to suggest that radiation therapy causes an overstimulation of the body's blood supply or impairs the body's ability to produce protein. Choice *C* is incorrect since chemotherapy treatment often leads to damaged hair follicles.

33. C: Neutrophils are the most numerous of the white blood cells, which is the reason why the general term leukopenia is often used interchangeably with the slightly more specific term neutropenia. Monocytopenia and lymphocytopenia both refer to lower than normal levels of two other types of white blood cells. Thrombocytopenia is unrelated to the white blood cells, but rather refers to a lowered platelet count, a different component of the blood.

34. D: An early sign of respiratory distress is agitation, along with confusion and oxygen hunger. Later signs of respiratory distress occur when the patient has become fatigued because of the respiratory effort they have put forth. These signs include decreased respiratory rate, unconsciousness, and cyanosis.

35. D: For patients experiencing low platelet count, or thrombocytopenia, it is important to stress the importance of consuming foods rich in B12 and folates. Some other interventions include lowering alcohol consumption, limiting sugary drinks, and stopping the use of ibuprofen, which are known to thin the blood. Choice *A* is used to stimulate the production of red blood cells, while Choice *B* is important for those with low white blood cell counts. Choice *C*, limiting iron-rich foods, is incorrect since this would further deplete the body of necessary platelets.

36. A: Palliative care, also known as comfort care, symptom management, and supportive care, refers to the special care of patients that helps them to manage the physical, social, and emotional challenges they face at any stage of cancer. Palliative care may involve teaching breathing exercises and relaxation techniques, proper diet, an exercise regime, or many other approaches. While palliative care can take place during the options mentioned in Choices *B*, *C*, and *D*, palliative care is not exclusive to these stages.

37. B: Melanoma has a 20 percent risk of metastasis to the brain and CNS. Symptoms of a brain tumor include fatigue, weakness, nausea, vomiting, headaches, vision changes, and confusion. The nurse can expect orders for an MRI of the brain, as an MRI is preferred for visualizing brain and spine lesions. A CT is better used for evaluating bony metastasis or to evaluate for stroke, making Choice *D* incorrect. While an abdominal CT may be indicated as part of initial staging, it would not evaluate for brain metastasis, so Choice *C* is incorrect. An abdominal ultrasound is used to evaluate the gallbladder, pancreas, bile ducts, and spleen. The patient's symptoms would not immediately call for this evaluation, making Choice *A* incorrect.

38. C: A person with dark skin tones who is suspected to be anemic will show pallor in the conjunctiva of the eyes, along with the palms of the hands, bottoms of feet, buccal mucosa, and lips. Forearms, scalp, and cheeks will not show pallor, per se, but may show a gray, ashy hue if they are truly anemic.

39: B: Facial swelling that decreases throughout the day is indicative of superior vena cava syndrome. It is common in lung cancer patients due to the proximity of masses near the superior vena cava and is often treated with diuretics that promote increased circulation through the vein.

40. D: Radiation to the oral cavity puts patients at risk for xerostomia, tooth decay, and permanent taste changes. Patients should be seen by their dentist prior to starting treatment to assess for any dental work that should take place before radiation. Choice *A* is incorrect, as risk for anemia is low with radiation to the oral cavity. Choice *B* is incorrect, as diarrhea is more often seen when the lower GI tract is in the radiation field. Lotions and ointments applied shortly before radiation treatment can intensify the effects of the radiation, making Choice *C* incorrect.

41. D: The least helpful intervention to prevent caregiver burnout would be to make a to-do list with the intent to increase productivity. A better intervention would be to make a to-do list and try to delegate some tasks to other family or friends. Choices *A*, *B*, and *C* are not the correct answer because these answers represent helpful strategies to prevent and manage caregiver burnout.

42. B: Basophils are the white blood cells that secrete histamine, the substance that causes itching in allergic reactions. Lymphocytes are responsible for antibody creation. Neutrophils take out bacterial and fungal organisms and are quite numerous. Monocytes assist in breaking down bacterial organisms.

43. D: The statement that promotes culturally competent and safe nursing care is Choice *D*, which addresses the need for accurate height and weight measurement while also respecting the patient's cultural practices. Choice *A* is incorrect because this statement addresses safe care but does not address cultural significance to the patient. Choice *B* is incorrect because this statement addresses the cultural significance of the turban but does not address the need for accurate height and weight measurement in providing safe nursing care. Choice *C* is incorrect because this statement does not address the conflict at the time of the incident; instead, it suggests that the patient should submit a request to another party to approve or deny the patient's cultural practice.

44. B: Cytokines are responsible for enhancing communication between cells that work to signal effective immune responses and stimulate the movement of cells to fight disease. Choices *A*, *C*, and *D* are incorrect since cytokines do not suppress the immune system, increase a patient's white blood cell count, or decrease a patient's red blood cell count.

45. D: Cancer antigen 125 (CA-125) is the correct answer, as this tumor marker is most associated with ovarian and uterine cancers. Choice *A* is incorrect because cancer antigen 19-9 (CA 19-9) is most associated with colon and pancreatic cancers. Carcinoembryonic antigen (CEA), Choice *B*, is incorrect because this tumor marker is most associated with colon and breast cancers. Lastly, prostate-specific antigen (PSA), Choice *C*, is incorrect because this is most associated with prostate cancers.

46. D: The nurse anticipates that the physician will change the current as-needed (PRN) oxycodone order to a long-acting formulation. One of the major reasons for this is that the patient is currently using the medication around the clock during the day with moderate efficacy; this indicates that the patient's pain level is greater than the as-needed basis of the original oxycodone order. Therefore, the current order is no longer appropriate for this patient. Additionally, the long-acting formulation will provide more consistent pain relief throughout the day and night and may also improve the patient's intermittent insomnia. Furthermore, reducing the number of daily pills can be helpful for cancer patients who experience gastrointestinal side effects, such as anorexia, nausea, and vomiting. Choice *A* is not the most likely recommendation, as the patient is currently having moderate pain relief and no reported adverse effects. Choice *B* is not the most likely answer since the patient is utilizing the PRN medication around the clock, which means that a PRN order may not be the most appropriate choice for this patient. Choice *C* is not likely to be recommended by the physician since the patient is having moderate analgesia with no side effects at the current frequency of dosing.

47. B: Choice *B* is the safest and most appropriate choice for the nurse to suggest regarding use of aromatherapy in the chemotherapy treatment area. Applying drops to a cloth, napkin, or cotton ball and placing them in a plastic bag allows the patient to have control over use of the product while containing the strong scent. Choice *A* would not be the most appropriate choice, as diffusers can disperse the aromatherapy beyond the immediate location. Peppermint has a strong smell and could have an adverse effect (e.g., headache, nausea, or breathing difficulties) on patients, caregivers, or healthcare providers. Removing the odor from the area would be challenging if an adverse event occurred. Choice *C* is incorrect because the nurse should not advise the patient to consume essential oils orally. Choice *D* is incorrect because the nurse would not recommend topical use of essential oils, as some individuals could experience irritation or allergic reactions. It would be challenging to remove the product quickly from the skin if this were to occur.

48. A: Antibiotic-resistant strains of bacteria easily cause unmitigated infection in patients, which can then turn into sepsis. Antibiotic-resistant strains of bacteria have become more common due to over-prescription and improper consumption of antibiotics. While Choices *B*, *C*, and *D* may expose people to bacteria, these events are not commonly linked with developing sepsis.

49. C: It is important to provide counseling on fertility preservation before the start of treatment, as it has a significant impact on quality of life during survivorship. The ability of a patient to have their own children is a central aspect of survivorship for all patients regardless of age, making Choice *A* incorrect. Fertility preservation counseling increases post-treatment quality of life by decreasing stress, depressive symptoms, and decisional regret, making Choice *B* incorrect. Oncofertility discussion is the standard of care and is recognized by ASCO even when emergent treatment is needed, making Choice *D* incorrect.

50. B: Medicare is a single-payer, social benefit that pays for most healthcare needs for patients over 65 years of age. There are limited stipulations on the type of care provided through Medicare.

51. C: Rucaparib is a PARP inhibitor and interferes with the PARP enzyme's ability to repair DNA in the cell, leading to cell death. Choice *A* refers to a VEGF inhibitor, such as pazopanib. Choice *B* refers to CDK4 and CDK6 inhibitors, such as abemaciclib. Choice *D* refers to an EGFR inhibitor, such as erlotinib.

52. D: The gastroenterologist will likely use cauterization, an application of heat, to seal the bleeding lesion. Banding is a procedure used to help stop bleeding in esophageal varices. Biopsy is where tissues are removed for histological analysis. Angioplasty is performed in cardiac catheterizations and involves balloon inflation and stent placement to open up occluded blood vessels.

53. B: Systemic inflammatory response syndrome (SIRS) paired with a known source of infection is called sepsis. Organ dysfunction is part of severe sepsis and lactic acidosis is a hypoperfusion abnormality that presents when severe sepsis has advanced to septic shock.

54. A: The *T* in TNM refers to the size of the primary tumor. A tumor graded as *TX* indicates that there is a primary tumor that cannot be assessed, making Choice *A* correct. Choice *D* is incorrect because no evidence of a primary tumor would be graded as *T0*. Choices *B* and *C* are incorrect because these criteria are not part of the TNM model of tumor grading.

55. C: Pericardiocentesis is used to treat cardiac tamponade, in which the pericardium has an open wound or hole through which fluid can fill the space. Pericardiocentesis is the procedure of drawing out fluid from this space using a syringe. This procedure relieves pressure on the ventricles of the heart and allows blood circulation to stay relatively stable.

56. B: Hypertonic saline, in which the sodium is more concentrated, is often used to correct the dilutional hyponatremia of SIADH. Normal saline has a 0.9% concentration of sodium, which is the same as circulating blood and thus will not be helpful in correcting hyponatremia. Hypotonic saline, in which there is less than 0.9% concentration of sodium, will also not be helpful in restoring normal sodium levels to the blood. Lactated ringer's solution is not a fluid used for the purpose of restoring normal sodium levels.

57. C: These two cancers have been shown to cross through the placenta, and the fetus may develop the same cancer as the mother. It is believed the cells of leukemia and melanoma can cross the placental barrier, perhaps due to the immune support that mothers provide the fetus. However, this is a speculative conclusion, and further research is required.

58. C: Echocardiography and Doppler imaging are noninvasive procedures commonly used to monitor any damage to the heart caused by chemotherapy treatment, making Choice *C* correct. 2D and 3D strain and torsion analysis, as well as 3D measures of cardiac size, are also used to detect possible heart damage. Choices *A*, *B*, and *D* are all incorrect, as echocardiography and Doppler imaging are monitoring techniques. They are not classified as surgical procedures.

59. A: Stunted bone growth is a commonly seen delayed side effect in pediatric patients. This is often the result of disrupted endocrine functioning, including disruption of hormones that control growth and epiphyseal fusion after puberty. The other effects listed may be seen during the treatment period, but usually not once the treatment ends.

60. C: Choice *C* is correct since being overwhelmed, feeling stress, and experiencing frustration can all indicate that an individual is experiencing the anger stage of anticipatory grief. Choice *A* is not correct because the son is asking questions about hospice services, which would indicate that they have reached the acceptance stage of anticipatory grief. Choice *B* is incorrect since this statement more closely aligns with the bargaining phase, in which the son is seeking to find ways to avoid a transition to hospice care. Choice *D* is incorrect because the patient's son is wondering why a hospice discussion is occurring at all, which would indicate he is in the denial stage of anticipatory grief.

61. C: Patients who cannot eliminate waste are given a colostomy bag, or a pouch that is placed over a hole made through the abdomen for the sole purpose of waste collection. All waste goes directly into the bag rather than through obstructed bowels. Colostomy bags are not used for the conditions listed in Choices *A*, *B*, and *D*.

62. C: Proper hygiene and handwashing, Choice *C*, are important practices for chemotherapy patients in order to prevent infection. Choices *A* and *B* are incorrect. In fact, patients are encouraged to have their vaccinations up to date and receive a flu shot. Choice *D* is incorrect since exposure to chemotherapy medications through bodily fluids can be harmful to caregivers. Patients are advised to properly clean the toilet after use and to flush twice to help protect family members and caregivers.

63. B: Most hazardous drugs are excreted by the body within forty-eight hours from the last treatment. This is the minimum amount of time that caregivers and patients should use enhanced precautions when handling body fluids. Choices *A*, *C*, and *D* are incorrect since the minimum is forty-eight hours. However, it is important to note that some hazardous drugs do have the potential to be excreted for longer periods of time (up to seven days).

64. D: Thrombotic thrombocytopenia purpura (TTP) is treated with plasma infusions until clotting stabilizes, at which point transfusions are stopped. This can take days or weeks. While pharmaceuticals may be used to aid this process, all TTP patients will receive plasma transfusions, making Choice *A* incorrect. Choices *B* and *C* are not applicable treatments.

65. D: Laser surgery involves the use of a laser beam in order to remove diseased tissue and treat blood vessels that are bleeding. Choice *A* refers to a medical procedure that removes a small piece of tissue or a sample of cells for further examination by a pathologist. Choice *B* refers to a surgical procedure in which an endoscope is inserted into an opening in the body, such as the mouth. This allows the physician to take a closer look at the body's tissues. Choice *C* refers to the insertion of a thin, lighted tube (called a laparoscope) into the abdomen in order to detect any organ abnormalities.

66. D: The more similar the malignant cells are to the original cells (well differentiated), the more likely that the resulting tumor will grow and metastasize more slowly than a poorly differentiated cell. High-grade and aggressive tumors are considered the most lethal and are most often poorly differentiated, making Choices *A* and *B* incorrect. Cancer therapies are focused on the destruction of the cell, rather structural changes, making Choice *C* incorrect.

67. C: In the late stages of cancer, some patients will experience extreme fatigue, delirium, and complete loss of bowl and bladder control. Symptoms of acute onset of cancer (Choice *A*) as well as chronic or recurring cancer (Choice *B*) have completely different symptoms, although bowel and bladder problems and fatigue may also be present. Rare forms of cancer (Choice *D*) can have many varying symptoms.

68. B: Curative surgery, or primary surgery, refers to the removal of an entire tumor and some of the surrounding tissue to lessen the chances of cancer recurrence. If lymph nodes are adjacent to the tumor, they may also be removed. Choice *A*, staging surgery, is used to determine the stage of cancer and whether or not the cancer has spread. Choice *C*, debulking surgery, refers to the removal of as much of the cancerous tumor as is medically safe. Choice *D*, laparoscopy, is a minimally invasive procedure in which a thin, lighted tube is inserted into the abdomen to detect any abnormalities, such as cysts or fibroids.

69. C: Up to 50% of patients who are diagnosed with DIC (disseminated intravascular coagulation) will pass away, even with treatment.

70. D: Atropine is given immediately prior to administration of irinotecan, which is part of the FOLFIRI regimen, to prevent acute cholinergic diarrhea. Choice *A*, octreotide, is used to treat diarrhea by increasing the gut transit time but is not used routinely for FOLFIRI. Choice *B*, loperamide, is a first-line medication used to treat chemotherapy diarrhea, but it is not use prophylactically. Choice *C*, dexamethasone, is used to treat colitis. Although it is often given as a pre-medication, it is used to prevent reactions, not diarrhea.

71. A: A patient with increased intracranial pressure (ICP) is at risk of seizure, coma, and death due to increased fluid in the brain, called hydrocephalus. Burr holes, or decompressive craniectomy, can be used to relieve this pressure and may done on these patients. They may also have ventricular drains placed to help remove fluid. Choice *B* is incorrect because 0.45% normal saline is hypotonic and could cause an increase of fluid and therefore pressure in the brain. Typically, 3% normal saline, which is hypertonic, or mannitol is used to help pull fluid off of the brain back into the vascular space to help reduce pressure. Choice *C* is incorrect because the head of the bed should be maintained at 30 degrees or higher to help promote fluid drainage from the brain. Choice *D* is incorrect because, although these patients often require mechanical ventilation, they should be hyperventilated because it can cause arterial vasoconstriction which would lower cerebral blood flow and decrease ICP.

72. D: FOLFOX can cause phototoxicity or an allergic response to sun-exposed areas, leading to edema and blistering. Patients should be advised to cover exposed skin with clothing, use sunscreen, and limit time outside when the sun is strongest. Choices *A* and *B* are side effects associate with EGFR inhibitors and taxanes, making them incorrect. Choice *C* is incorrect, as FOLFOX typically causes hair thinning but rarely results in full hair loss.

73. C: The itching, warmth, and redness of the IV site are most likely associated with a flare reaction, which is a localized sensitivity reaction. Choice *A* is incorrect because phlebitis would present with redness, swelling, and sensitivity of the proximal vein to the IV site and is associated with irritation to the vein. Choice *B* is incorrect because extravasation is a serious reaction to infiltration of a vesicant medication into the subcutaneous tissue and can result in severe tissue damage and tissue death. Etoposide is designated as an irritant, rather than a vesicant. Choice *D* is also not correct because infections of the IV site would be unlikely to develop at the time of infusion, and the site would be more likely to be painful than to have pruritus.

74. C: Patients with neuropathy often have limited sensation to their hands and feet, making them more prone to injury that can lead to infection. Patients should be counseled on regular examinations and care of hands and feet to prevent infection. Choices *A* and *B* are incorrect, as there is little data that exists to recommend routine vitamin E for the prevention of chemotherapy-induced peripheral neuropathy or lidocaine cream for the treatment of pain. For physical and emotional wellbeing, patients with neuropathy should continue to exercise as they are able, making Choice *D* incorrect. This may require a referral to physical therapy for an optimal program.

75. B: In order to initiate and sustain tumor growth, malignant cells are able to produce growth factors even when the cellular density level has been reached and the levels of growth hormones and growth factors associated with normal cell growth have diminished. This results in altered density inhibition, which is one of the cellular properties that maintains the normal structure of tissues so cells do not "crowd" one another. Angiogenesis, Choice *C*, is the process whereby malignant cells trigger the development of new blood vessels that supply nutrients to the developing tumor and also facilitate metastasis. The process is triggered when the new tumor reaches a density of one million cells. Initiation (Choice *A*) is the first step in the mutation of normal cells by carcinogens, while promotion (Choice *D*) is the second stage of that process.

76. B: *Bacillus Calmette-Guerin* (BCG) is a live vaccine originally developed to prevent tuberculosis. For this reason, patients with tuberculosis and those at risk for infection should not receive this treatment. Additionally, exposure through needle stick or accidental laceration can result in patient and/or healthcare provider infection. Therefore, extreme care must always be taken with handling and administering this product. Choices *A, C,* and *D* are incorrect because BCG is not associated with these diseases.

77. C: The positive predictive value is expressed as the probability that the individual has the disease when the screening test is positive. Sensitivity is expressed as the degree to which the test correctly identifies individuals who have the disease, while specificity is expressed as the degree to which the test correctly identifies individuals who do not have the disease.

78. B: Although aspirin has been used for years to prevent (or decrease the risk of) heart attack and stroke, research is now finding very promising evidence that it may also significantly reduce and possibly prevent certain types of cancer. The results have been most evident with colorectal cancer. Choice *A* refers to antidepressant and antianxiety medications. Choice *C* refers to the Gardasil vaccine, and Choice *D* refers to opioids.

79. B: When patients are found to carry mutated alleles that are known to cause cancer, prophylactic surgery may be an effective technique. This involves the complete removal of organs, such as prophylactic oophorectomy (removal of both ovaries) and mastectomy (removal of one or both breasts). Choice *A*, diagnostic surgery, refers to surgery performed to diagnose or locate the presence of cancer. Choice *C*, radiofrequency ablation, involves the use of electrical energy and heat to kill cancer cells. Choice *D*, Mohs microscopic surgery, involves the removal of one layer of skin at a time which is viewed under a microscope until the cells appear healthy. This is an effective technique for patients diagnosed with basal cell or squamous cell carcinoma.

80. B: The Joint Commission (TJC) is an independent agency that certifies various healthcare organizations (e.g., hospitals, clinics, pharmacies, etc.) according to stringent quality standards. TJS utilizes 250 auditing and compliance measures relating to patient satisfaction, handoff procedures, cleanliness, and documentation (among others) to ensure organizations that receive their accreditation are upholding the required quality of care.

81. C: Occupational therapy is a type of rehabilitation that supports individuals in returning to a specific type of movement, often for their occupation or routine activities. Sierra is excited to return to her specific job role, and an occupational therapist can provide emotional and mental support, along with physical exercises to strengthen specific areas and build range of motion, that can help her on the job. Blood thinners, Choice *A*, are not necessary in this situation. Since Sierra wants to return to her original position, switching her to a new role or new shift (Choices *B* and *D*) are not the best options for her mental or emotional state; these are prohibitive to returning to "normalcy."

82. D: Choice *D* is the most appropriate response, as it successfully de-escalates the patient and maintains their safety in a non-confrontational way. Choices *A* and *B* are not the most appropriate responses, as they do not address the patient's frustration and would likely result in increased patient frustration. Choice *C* is not an appropriate response because it could potentially escalate the patient's emotional state to ask them to calm themselves.

83. A: Neutropenic sepsis, a life-threatening complication of chemotherapy, presents with fever, diarrhea, and breathlessness for which immediate medical attention is required. Choice *B* is incorrect, as neutropenic sepsis is not a side effect of radiation therapy. Choice *C* is incorrect since nerve or muscle numbness is not associated with neutropenic sepsis. Choice *D* is incorrect since bruising is also not associated with neutropenic sepsis.

84. C: Lung function testing is important in this scenario because bleomycin is most significantly associated with a risk for severe pulmonary toxicity in the form of pneumonitis and pulmonary fibrosis. Choice *A* is incorrect because thyroid examination addresses the patient's risk for thyroid injury following *radiation therapy*, not the patient's chemotherapy treatment. Choice *B* is not the most appropriate answer choice because a complete blood count does not provide the most pertinent information about the patient's lung function. Choice *D* is not correct because dental issues are not the most significant potential side effect of bleomycin.

85. B: Trastuzumab is a biotherapy approved for use in breast cancer for patients whose tumor over expresses HER2 (human epidermal growth factor receptor 2). Pulmonary function and baseline audiology exams are not required prior to starting treatment, making Choices *A* and *C* incorrect. PD-L1 is targeted by agents such as pembrolizumab; therefore, molecular testing for this purpose is not needed for trastuzumab therapy, making Choice *D* incorrect.

86. D: Cowden syndrome is the result of the mutation of gene PTEN, which produces a protein that suppresses tumor growth, and is associated with an increased risk of breast, thyroid and endometrial cancer. BRCA 1 and BRCA 2 are estimated to cause 5 to 10 percent of the incidence of inherited breast cancer, making Choices *A* and *B* incorrect. As noted, alterations in multiple genes are associated with the incidence of inherited breast cancer. The leading cause of death in women is cardiovascular disease, making Choice *C* incorrect. Breast cancer is the most frequently diagnosed cancerous condition in women; however, lung cancer is the leading cause of cancer death in both men and women.

87. C: Because cisplatin is a nephrotoxic chemotherapy, it should not be administered if the patient's creatinine levels are abnormal; however, hydration should follow to provide intervention. While the patient should be counseled on encouraging adequate hydration at home and controlling nausea and vomiting with antiemetics, Choices *A, B,* and *D* are incorrect, as all chemotherapy should be held.

88. D: A shared decision-making model is the process in which health professionals and patients work together to select tests and treatments and manage side effects based on clinical evidence as well as the patient's preferences. Choice *D* does not consider any discussion with the patient to determine if they feel the education thus far has been sufficient and, therefore, does not represent shared decision making. Choices *A, B,* and *C* show examples of shared decision making.

89. C: The desensitization protocol is used to minimize patient reaction to chemotherapy, which is an aggressive agent to a patient's body. By gradually exposing the patient to chemotherapy medications, the body is able to better recognize and adapt to its presence. Without this progressive dosing schedule, patients may experience severe allergic reactions to the medications, especially if their immune system is already relatively weak. Choices *A, B,* and *D* do not represent this process.

90. B: A baseline pulmonary function test (PFT) should be performed in order to evaluate whether any changes to lung function occur during treatment, as bleomycin is associated with several lung alterations. A chest X-ray, CT of the chest, or bronchoscopy are unnecessary for this function; thus, Choices *A, C,* and *D* are incorrect.

91. A: Cryosurgery (cryotherapy) employs the use of liquid nitrogen with the intent of destroying abnormal tissue. This surgery is primarily used to treat external tumors which may be found on the skin. Liquid nitrogen is placed on a cotton swab or in a spraying device and is then directly applied to the cancer cells. Choice *B* involves the removal one layer of tissue at a time. Choice *C* is a minimally-invasive procedure and only requires a small incision to more closely examine the body's tissues. Choice *D* refers to removing as much of the tumor as possible when it is impossible to remove the entire tumor.

92. D: Chemotherapy regimens, especially those used to prepare for transplant, are immunosuppressive, and patients need to be counselled on avoiding infection. An effective way to prevent infection is to cook food, such as meat and fish, thoroughly. Fresh fruits and vegetables are okay to eat if they can be thoroughly washed. Choice *A* is incorrect, as young children are prone to transmitting pathogens, and contact should be limited unless they are asymptomatic, regardless of vaccination status. Choice *B* is incorrect, as patients should be seen in the ER in emergent situations despite concern for other illness. Choice *C* is incorrect because fresh flowers should be avoided due to the possibility for pathogens in the stagnant water.

93. A: The patient is experiencing breakthrough pain, so the addition of a short-acting opioid, such as oxycodone, will likely be added into the patient's pain regimen. Gabapentin is often prescribed for neuropathic pain but will not address breakthrough pain, so Choice *B* is incorrect. Fentanyl is a strong pain medication and, depending on formulation, can be used for breakthrough pain. However, a transdermal patch is meant to be long acting, making Choice *C* incorrect. Dexamethasone is prescribed for many different indications at the end of life and can be useful for pain caused by inflammation. However, it is not meant to treat breakthrough pain and is intended to be used for short durations of time, so Choice *D* is incorrect.

94. D: Bisphosphonates, such as zoledronic acid or denosumab, are used to reduce bone loss and the risk of spine and hip fractures. Bone loss is a common side effect with hormonal therapies, such as ADT. Calcium infusions are not indicated to increase bone density, so Choice *A* is incorrect. Sipuleucel-T is a type of cancer vaccine used to treat prostate cancer, so Choice *B* is incorrect. G-CSF is used to boost the production of white blood cells and is generally used in conjunction with chemotherapy, so Choice *C* is incorrect.

95. A: Although lung cancer can spread to the intestines, this location has a lower chance for metastasis than the other answer choices. Choices *B, C,* and *D* are incorrect because these represent some of the most common sites for metastasis of lung cancers.

96. C: For a patient who received a double mastectomy, bereavement services are unlikely to be needed. The nurse should perform an assessment for caregiver needs. After surgery, this can include written instructions on pain medication schedules, education by physical and occupational therapy to make caregiving less strenuous, and a discussion with a social worker or vocational therapist to review work leave options for the recovery period. Therefore, Choices *A, B,* and *D* are incorrect answers.

97. C: The nurse would anticipate the next intervention for this patient to be diagnostic imaging (e.g., ultrasound, CT, MRI) to confirm or rule out deep vein thrombosis (DVT), which often presents with acute unilateral swelling, cramping pain, and redness of the affected extremity. Cancer alone places patients at increased risk for blood clots. Additionally, lymphoma is one form of cancer that carries additional clotting risk. Choice *A* is not the most appropriate next intervention, since initiation of antibiotic therapy for suspected cellulitis infection would be more likely to happen after thromboembolism is ruled out. Choice *B* is not the most appropriate next intervention because initiation of anticoagulant therapy would occur following confirmation of thromboembolism via diagnostic imaging. Choice *D* is also wrong because a tissue culture to assess for infection or other differential diagnosis would be considered less critical than diagnostic confirmation of DVT, which could mobilize, lead to pulmonary embolism (PE), and quickly become life-threatening.

98. D: Acupuncture, a Chinese technique in which micro-needles are inserted into specific pathways of energy in the body, has been shown in controlled research studies to have positive effects in cancer patients specifically. While Ayurvedic techniques (therapeutic, tailored techniques from ancient Indian sciences), Vipassana meditation (a Buddhist tradition of silence that encourages deep introspection), and Rolfing (a method of fascial realignment) can all be therapeutic, they have not yet been studied in a randomized and controlled manner.

99. B: An excisional biopsy refers to the entire removal of a tumor, including some normal tissue around it (margin). Choice *A* refers to the partial removal of a tumor. Choice *C* refers to the removal of one or both breasts, while Choice *D* refers to a surgical incision of the abdomen.

100. C: Anaphylaxis is an acute, potentially fatal, reaction that involves prior sensitization to an allergen with later re-exposure. Although other drugs such as diphenhydramine, albuterol, and dexamethasone can be given to lessen effects, administration of epinephrine is needed to stop the reaction.

101. D: Symptom management aims to prevent the onset of side effects that a patient faces following radiation, chemotherapy treatment, or any surgical procedure. In the event that side effects do occur, symptom management aims to minimize the severity, pain, and discomfort of those side effects. Choices *A*, *B*, and *C* are aspects of medical care but do not describe symptom management.

102. B: Targeted therapies work by targeting specific genes and/or proteins that are found within the cancer cells or within the cells linked to cancer growth. Targeted therapies are commonly used in conjunction with chemotherapy and other treatments. Choice *A* refers to biotherapy. Choice *C* refers to a type of therapy that works to slow down or stop the growth of cancer by adding, blocking, or removing certain hormones that may be responsible for the cancer. Choice *D* refers to a specific therapy that infuses cytotoxic T-cells into cancer patients in order to recognize, target, and kill cancerous cells.

103. C: Candies and gum can be used prior to meals and chemotherapy to reduce the metallic taste and change the taste of the mouth prior to eating. Experimentation with spices should be encouraged, making Choice *A* incorrect. Mouthwashes like Listerine contain alcohol, which can dry the mucous membranes and make taste changes more pronounced, so Choice *B* is incorrect. Aromas help to intensify the taste of foods, so foods with strong aromas should be encouraged, making Choice *D* incorrect.

104. B: Autonomy is the ethical principle that patients have the right to self-determination. Nurses play a vital role in ensuring that patients have accurate and timely information prior to making decisions. Patients should be provided with written information explaining the risks of discrimination if they share the results of the testing. This information should be provided prior to testing, not after, so Choice *A* is incorrect. While patients should have access to their results, having the results and performing their own research may result in false information and patient distress, making Choice *C* incorrect. The nurse should always verify with the patient that they understand the need for tests being ordered rather than relying on a visit note, making Choice *D* incorrect.

105. D: Opioids, provided orally or intravenously, are the most common method of managing pain in palliative and hospice care settings. They are often coupled with a laxative agent, as the dosing amounts needed for end-of-life patients can cause chronic constipation.

106. C: Biotherapy is the use of living substances that work to stimulate or suppress the immune system, attack specific cancer cells, and help the body fight cancer, infection, or other diseases. Choices *A*, *B* and *C* are incorrect since biotherapy is not a form of radiation or chemotherapy.

107. C: A multigated acquisition scan (MUGA scan), Choice *C*, is a non-invasive test used to visualize the function of the heart. This type of scan would be most indicated for a patient with breast cancer who has completed chemotherapy, biologic therapy, and radiation therapy. Common chemotherapy agents used for treatment of breast cancer, particularly anthracyclines, carry a significant risk of cardiotoxicity. Additionally, biologic treatment for HER2-positive breast cancer (e.g., trastuzumab) also has varying degrees of risk for cardiotoxicity, especially when used in combination with anthracyclines. Lastly, radiation therapy to the chest also adds risk for injury to the cardiac tissue. Choice *A* is not the most appropriate choice, as an X-ray would be better suited for identifying metastasis to the lungs or bones, not a delayed side effect of the patient's treatment. Choice *B* is not the most appropriate answer because an electrocardiogram (EKG) would only provide information about the electrical conduction of the heart and not the function of the cardiac muscle. Choice *D* is also not the most appropriate answer choice because magnetic resonance imaging (MRI) is a more precise means of identifying malignancy throughout the body and would be used to monitor for recurrence rather than a delayed side effect of the patient's treatment.

108. B: Dexrazoxane is a protectant given to prevent the cardiotoxicities of free radicals from anthracyclines, such as doxorubicin, daunorubicin, epirubicin, idarubicin, and mitoxantrone. Choice *A* is given with ifosfamide administration to protect the bladder. Choice *C* is given to prevent cholinergic diarrhea with irinotecan administration. Choice *D* is given prior to many chemotherapies to prevent hypersensitivity reactions.

109. A: Mohs microscopic surgery is regarded as the most effective procedure for treating basal cell and squamous cell carcinomas, which are the two most common types of skin cancer. The procedure involves the removal of one layer of tissue at a time, examining the tissue under a microscope, and continuing in this fashion until the cells in a particular layer appear healthy. Choice *B* refers to a biopsy, in which a small incision is made in order to better examine the body's tissues and organs. Choice *C* describes a procedure known as cryosurgery, in which the abnormal or cancerous cells are destroyed using liquid nitrogen. Choice *D* describes an endoscopy, in which a narrow and flexible tube is inserted into an opening in the body to more closely examine affected organs and tissues.

110. B: Oral mucositis that consists of erythema, pain, ulceration, and the ability to eat solid food would be considered grade II mucositis. Choice *A* is incorrect, as grade I mucositis consists of redness and irritation without the presence of ulcers. Choice *C* is incorrect because grade III mucositis consists of erythema, pain, ulceration, and the ability to consume liquids only. Lastly, Choice *D* is incorrect, as grade IV mucositis is reserved for patients who are unable to consume solids or liquids by mouth due to the ulceration and pain.

111. B: When a person is not producing enough platelets, the body has a more difficult time in clumping or clotting, which results in longer bleeding times and easy bruising. Choices *A*, *B*, and *C* do not refer to conditions which would cause increased bleeding times or bruising easily.

112. D: Low-grade cancer cells are malignant cells that look similar to healthy cells, which is a positive prognostic factor. Choice *A* is incorrect because tumors larger than 1 centimeter become associated with less favorable outcomes as they grow bigger. Choice *B* is incorrect because node-positive cancers have started spreading to surrounding lymph nodes and are associated with less favorable prognosis. Choice *C* is incorrect because hormone receptor-negative tumors have a less favorable initial prognosis than hormone receptor-positive tumors. However, hormone receptor-negative tumors do tend to have a lower recurrence rate than hormone receptor-positive tumors.

113. A: Stereotactic body radiation (SBRT) is a very precise type of radiation that is often used to treat spine, liver, pancreas, lung, prostate, and kidney lesions. Motion of the tumor is accounted for to precisely target the tumor, which limits the damage to surrounding tissues. While all these options can be used to treat prostate cancer, Choice *B* describes photon radiation, Choice *C* describes brachytherapy, and Choice *D* describes proton therapy.

114. A: Ashlee seems to be in denial about her mother's death. She continues to act as if she is still alive and present in Ashlee's regular life. This is typically seen in the first stage of grief, when a bereaved individual does not accept the loss. Anger comes later when the individual becomes upset about the loss, followed by acceptance in the final stage. Although it appears Ashlee may have some habits relating to her relationship with her mother, habit is not a stage of grief.

115. C: Choice *C* is the correct answer because bisphosphonates are a non-analgesic drug class and effective at preventing bone pain and fractures in patients with bone cancer. Bone cancer results in an overactivity of osteoclasts, the bone cells that facilitate the breakdown and remodeling of bone. Bisphosphonates are effective at inhibiting these overactive osteoclasts, thereby preventing bone thinning, weakness, fractures, and pain that can accompany this diagnosis. Choice *A* is incorrect because although steroids can be an effective non-opioid option for pain resulting from inflammation, they can also adversely impact how calcium and vitamin D are utilized by the bone. This can result in lower bone density, which could increase risk of fracture. Choice *B* is incorrect because although antidepressants have been shown to have a positive impact on cancer pain, they can also increase the risk of decreased bone mineral density and bone fracture. Choice *D* is also incorrect because anticonvulsants, such as gabapentin or pregabalin, can be effective in the management of neurological pain; however, there is evidence that these medications may cause increased bone loss and risk for bone fracture.

116. A: When it is determined too risky to remove the entire tumor, surgeons may opt to perform a debulking surgical procedure to remove as much of the tumor as is medically safe for the patient. Choice *B* refers to curative or primary surgery, in which the entire tumor and some of the surrounding tissue is removed. Choice *C* refers to prophylactic surgery, while Choice *D* refers to preventative surgery.

117. D: Cancer and its treatments appear to mimic rapid aging in patients, thus resulting in cognitive decline for a temporary or long-term period. Much of the future research in cancer treatment is focusing on anti-aging and Alzheimer's treatments, including medications, cognitive exercises, and certain protein chains used to treat cognitive decline in the same manner. The other options listed are not treatment options, but they could serve as general comfort measures in patients.

118. C: Recurring malignancies refer to the re-emergence of a cancer that had previously gone into remission. Recurring malignancies have the same appearance and behavioral mannerisms as the initial cancer that was detected. Secondary malignancies occur as a result of treating a primary malignancy. As radiation and chemotherapy are quite stressful and damaging to the body, these treatments can cause new cancers in the body at a later time. Secondary malignancies will look and behave differently from the primary cancer. Choices *A*, *B*, and *D* are not the correct definitions of recurring and secondary malignancies.

119. D: A BI-RADS 0 report means that abnormalities have been identified on the screening mammogram that require additional testing. A diagnostic mammogram uses additional views, often spot compression and magnification views, to assist in the diagnosis. If the abnormality is a tumor rather than a calcification, ultrasonography may also be used to establish the diagnosis. BI-RADS 1 indicates that no abnormalities were detected in either breast, making Choice *B* incorrect. BI-RADS 2 indicates that the identified abnormalities are benign, making Choice *C* incorrect. BI-RADS 3 means that the identified abnormalities are probably benign, however diagnostic mammograms of the affected breast every six months for two years is recommended, making Choice *A* incorrect. BI-RADS 4 indicates that the identified lesions are highly suspicious of malignancy. BI-RADS 5 indicates that the lesions are malignant; however, this result will be verified with a biopsy to confirm the diagnosis and assess the lesion.

120. B: Patients who show symptoms of superior vena cava syndrome are likely to pass away within three years, making Choice *B* correct. It is not due to the syndrome; rather, this syndrome primarily develops in patients with advanced stages of aggressive cancer. Therefore, the syndrome is correlated with a shortened lifespan.

121. B: Tumor lysis syndrome (TLS) is an oncologic emergency associated with the rapid breakdown of a very large number of cancer cells due to the administration of cytotoxic treatment. This results in a flooding of potassium, phosphate, and nucleic acid into the circulation and results in serious systemic complications, including cardiac and renal injury and/or failure. Lab findings associated with TLS include hyperkalemia, hyperphosphatemia, hypocalcemia, and hyperuricemia. Choice *B* is the correct answer because it would be expected that a patient experiencing TLS would have a potassium level of greater than 6.0 mEq/L (or an increase of 25 percent from baseline). Choice *A* would be incorrect because a patient experiencing TLS would be expected to have a calcium level of less than or equal to 7.0 mg/dL (or a decrease of 25 percent from baseline). Choice *C* is incorrect because an adult patient experiencing TLS would be expected to have a phosphorus level of greater than 4.5 mg/dL (or an increase of 25 percent from baseline). Choice *D* is incorrect because a patient experiencing TLS would be expected to have a uric acid level of greater than 7.0 mg/dL (or an increase of 25 percent from baseline).

122. C: The affected skin of patients diagnosed with GvHD can be very dry and damaged. Hydrating the skin is one of the most effective ways to lessen this damage and alleviate the pain and discomfort. Choice *A* would be highly inappropriate, as the skin is already very dry. Choice *B* is incorrect since SPF lotion will not irritate the skin and is necessary to apply if the patient goes outside. Choice *D* is not recommended unless there are open wounds that need to be protected.

123. C: Staging surgery allows the doctor to fully assess the extent of cancer and helps the medical team make decisions regarding effective treatments and therapies. Staging surgery also attempts to remove all of the visible disease. Choice *A* refers to the partial removal of a tumor. Choice *B* refers to surgery that attempts to diagnose and/or locate the presence of disease. Choice *D* refers to the surgical removal of as much of a tumor as is medically safe to remove.

124. B: Myeloma is a cancer of the plasma cells in the bone marrow, which are normally responsible for the production of the proteins that are used to develop antibodies. The cancer may present as a single tumor, or multiple growths may be present, which is identified as multiple myeloma. Granulocytic leukemia, Choice *D*, also arises in the bone marrow; however, the disease is associated with excessive production of immature white cells rather than proteins. Carcinoma, Choice *A*, is the most common form of cancer and most often originates in the skin, breast, lungs, and pancreas. Hodgkin Lymphoma, Choice *C*, is a cancer that affects the lymphatic system and the lymphoid organs.

125. A: The nurse provides the cup of ice chips for the patient to hold in their mouth during administration of the 5-fluorouracil bolus to prevent mucositis. The use of ice chips, a form of cryotherapy, causes vasoconstriction of the blood vessels in the mouth and reduces the exposure of oral mucosa to this mucotoxic drug. Choices *B* and *C* are incorrect because cryotherapy is not commonly associated with a reduction in nausea or taste changes. Choice *D* is incorrect because cryotherapy for use in preventing neuropathy occurs at the point of risk (e.g., hands or feet).

126. B: Pneumonitis is the term for lung tissue inflammation. Lung cancer (Choice *C*) and emphysema (Choice *D*) may lead to pneumonitis, but these two diagnoses are far more complicated than only tissue inflammation. Choice *A* is not a real condition.

127. C: Chemotherapy administration guidelines are not required to be addressed as an element of patient education prior to beginning treatment. Choices *A*, *B*, and *D* are all examples of items which are a requirement of patient education in accordance with the QOPI standards of care.

128. C: Aspirin thins the blood, which can cause nosebleeds, so Choice *C* is correct. Getting plenty of sleep would not be an appropriate suggestion to minimize nose bleeds, making Choice *A* incorrect. Spinach is a good source of B12 and folate, which helps to increase platelet count. It also provides vitamin K, which helps with clotting. Therefore, eliminating spinach from the diet would not be a wise choice, making Choice *B* incorrect. Choice *D* is incorrect because adding humidity to the air would be a better choice than dehumidifying the air.

129. C: Choice *C* is most concerning to the nurse, as a stoma with a purple color could be indicative of issues with blood flow or necrosis of the new stoma. Choice *A* is not correct because there may be no output from the stoma for two to four days after colostomy placement. Choice *B* is incorrect because it is expected that the stoma will be quite swollen for several days following surgery. Choice *D* is also incorrect because tenderness would be expected on post-op day one; however, the nurse would still perform a full assessment to ensure there are no additional concerns.

130. A: Choice *A* is correct because the gag reflex is often affected during moderate sedation and/or topical anesthesia used to perform an endoscopic procedure. Assessing the gag reflex before feeding ensures the patient can swallow adequately. Choice *B* is incorrect because, although positioning the head of the bed to at least 30 degrees facilitates the passage of oral secretions, this is not a priority action to prevent aspiration in a patient who underwent an endoscopic procedure. Choice *C* is incorrect because setting up suction is a safety precaution in case the patient's airway is compromised. However, this intervention does not specifically prevent aspiration. Choice *D* is incorrect because coughing and deep breathing promote removal of oral secretions, but this is a standard intervention for every patient receiving anesthesia.

131. B: Fine-needle aspirations are a specific type of biopsy involving the insertion of a thin needle into an area of tissue or body fluid that appears abnormal. This sample will be collected and sent to a pathologist to either confirm or rule out certain diagnoses. Choice *A* would refer to any number of procedures that are performed to treat cancer, rather than to confirm or rule out a diagnosis. Choice *C* refers to medical treatments and surgeries that attempt to prevent the spread of cancer. This does not involve fine-needle aspiration. Choice *D* refers to curative surgery, also known as primary surgery.

132. A: Competencies that define the necessary skills for oncology nurse leaders have been created by the Oncology Nurse Society (ONS) with the support of the American Organization for Nursing Leadership (AONL). These core competencies are professionalism; communications and relationship management; knowledge of the healthcare environment; and business skills and principles. Professionalism best supports this scenario, as it encompasses advocacy for patients and keeping their voice central in decision making. Choice *B* focuses on clear communication and fostering strong relationships across the care continuum. Choice *C* refers to the application of nursing practice at a higher level, influencing delivery systems, regulations, and economics. Choice *D* focuses on fiscal responsibility and human resource management required to support a healthcare system.

133. A: Of the answer choices, *numbness of the feet* is the side effect with the greatest potential for becoming a chronic side effect. Peripheral neuropathy is one of the dose-limiting potential side effects of treatment with taxane medications (e.g., paclitaxel). The presence of peripheral neuropathy can result in decreased dosing or discontinuation of this therapy completely. Choices *B, C,* and *D* are all examples of common side effects associated with this patient's chemotherapy regimen. However, these side effects carry a low risk of persisting after completion of treatment.

134. B: Pancytopenia refers to an abnormally low blood cell count. It can result from a variety of causes including, but not limited to, viral infections, complications of pregnancy, pharmaceutical drugs, autoimmune disorders, and congenital issues. A biopsy of the patient's bone marrow quickly eliminates many of the possible causes, saving time and unnecessary testing for the patient and allowing for more prompt care. Choice *A* is incorrect because a PCR test detects the presence of specific viral particles, which may or may not relate to the pancytopenia diagnosis. Choice *C* is incorrect because an amniocentesis is a procedure performed during pregnancy to detect specific congenital diseases in the fetus. It is generally not used to detect pancytopenia in the mother or the fetus. Choice *D* is incorrect because, although a complete blood count (CBC) panel is often the first indicator that a patient is experiencing pancytopenia, this test does not provide helpful information to determine the underlying cause.

135. B: Small cell lung cancer is the only option listed that has been shown to have a high correlation with syndrome of inappropriate antidiuretic hormone secretion (SIADH). This may be due to specific interactions that this type of cancer cell has with the endocrine system that negatively affects ADH production. It is thought that small cell lung cancer may cause the body to feel as if there is excessive ADH available when there is not. In turn, this leads to electrolyte imbalances and other symptoms of SIADH.

136. D: Choice *D* is correct because one of the primary manifestations of malignant hyperthermia is hypercarbia. A carbon dioxide level of 47 mmHg is above normal. The normal CO_2 level is 35-45 mmHg. Choice *A* is not correct because a heart rate of 54 beats/min is not expected with hyperthermia. Tachycardia, or increased heart rate, is expected. Choice *B* is not correct because a temperature of 38.2 °C (100.7 °F) is on the higher end of normal. Choice *C* is not correct because a potassium level of 3.2 mEq/L is not expected in malignant hyperthermia. Hyperkalemia, an elevated potassium level, is consistent with the complication.

137. D: Opioid drugs, such as morphine, greatly suppress a patient's level of pain; however, they can also greatly reduce a patient's respiratory function. When opioid-induced respiratory depression occurs, a patient's ability to breathe is greatly compromised in a life-threatening manner. Choice *A* would be highly unethical and may lead to a patient's untimely death. Choice *B* assumes that opioid-induced respiratory depression is referring to a depressive emotional state. Antidepressant medication would be a highly inappropriate treatment response. Although Choice *C* would likely occur, it would certainly follow an immediate medical intervention.

138. B: The *least* helpful question asked by the nurse would be about gender reassignment surgery because this question is invasive and can feel insensitive to a new patient. Additionally, this question would not be required or indicated during an initial intake with the nurse. The patient in this example is a transgender male (assigned female at birth) who has been diagnosed with cervical cancer. Choice *A* is incorrect because asking the reason for the visit is a required intake question and would be a neutral, open-ended item to ask. Choice *C* is incorrect because the name listed in their medical record may be different than their preferred name, which is very important in building a trusting relationship with the patient. Choice *D* is also incorrect because asking about cultural and spiritual considerations related to the provision of care is helpful in establishing trust with the patient. This open-ended question provides an opportunity for the patient to share their individual needs and enables the healthcare team to provide higher quality, culturally competent care for the patient.

139. B: These are all indicators of bereavement that may take place during the grieving process as a person adjusts to the loss. It is important to seek counseling intervention if these symptoms persist for longer than a few weeks, as it can turn into a major depressive episode and interfere with the person's daily life. Patients who are receiving medications and become delusional, are receiving opioid titration for pain, or are shifting to a plant-based diet typically do not experience these symptoms.

140. B: Dopamine is a commonly infused drug in a mechanically ventilated patient, but not for the purpose of analgesia. Rather, it is used to maintain a normal blood pressure in a hemodynamically unstable patient. The usual drugs of choice include morphine, fentanyl, and propofol. These three are commonly used to provide analgesia to a mechanically ventilated patient.

141. A: Ondansetron is an anti-nausea medication. Choices *B*, *C*, and *D* are used as an antibiotic, to treat GERD, and for pain relief.

142. A: Choice *A* is the correct answer because light activity (e.g., walking) has been shown to improve cancer-related fatigue. Choice *B* is incorrect because eating with plastic utensils can help with treatment-related taste changes. Choice *C* is incorrect because eating small, frequent meals is advised for patients having trouble with appetite. Choice *D* is also incorrect, as application of lotion can assist patients who experience dry skin from cancer treatment.

143. B: Pathological laparotomy refers to a procedure that allows the surgeon to look for evidence of cancer and remove samples as needed for further examination. They may also cause certain complications, including infection and the development of scar tissue, but surgeons who opt to perform a laparotomy believe that the benefits greatly outweigh the risks. Choice *A* refers to prophylactic surgery, Choice *C* refers to curative or primary surgery, and Choice *D* refers to debulking surgery.

144. C: If cells replicate before the damage to the cellular DNA is repaired, the defective DNA will be permanent and inherited by future generations of the damaged cell. The mutations will inactivate the cell surface proteins that block tumor formation; however, this does not relate to the speed of replication, making Choice *A* incorrect. Multiple mutations are common; however, since timing is the determinant of the inheritable cell defects, Choice *B* is incorrect. The mutations most often increase, rather than decrease, the rate of cellular proliferation, making Choice *D* incorrect.

145. D: Extravasation with vinca alkaloids, such as vincristine, respond better to the application of a warm compress to the injection site since it encourages the absorption of any extravasated medication into circulation. Choice *A* is incorrect because the arm is recommended to be elevated to prevent swelling of the extremity. Choice *B* is incorrect because application of a tourniquet above the insertion site is not indicated for extravasation. Choice *C* is incorrect because hyaluronidase would be the recommended antidote for vinca alkaloid extravasation. Sodium thiosulfate can be used to treat extravasation of medications such as cisplatin, cyclophosphamide, or dacarbazine.

146. D: In allogeneic transplants, the patient receives bone marrow, peripheral blood cells, or umbilical cells from a donor that closely matches their HLA. Since the cells are not coming from the patient, they do not need to undergo any collection, making Choice *A* incorrect. HLA testing is performed to ensure compatibility between the donor and recipient. Patients have a 1 in 4 chance of their sibling being a 10/10 antigen match; however, it is not guaranteed, making Choice *B* incorrect. Recipients of allogeneic transplant will need to be immunosuppressed afterward to prevent graft-versus-host disease, making Choice *C* incorrect.

147. B: Cancer patients are most likely to experience chronic DIC due to receiving regular rounds of treatment and the suppression of immunity caused by cancerous cells and aggressive treatments, which affect their body's natural healing abilities. Choices *A*, *C*, and *D* are not the most common type of DIC.

148. C: Melatonin, a supplement commonly used to assist with sleep, is the least likely to have an adverse impact on platelet count. In fact, some research suggests that melatonin could have a positive effect on platelet count for individuals experiencing thrombocytopenia. Choice *A* is incorrect since chamomile, a supplement used to calm and encourage sleep, has been shown to influence coagulation and can also reduce platelet activity, potentially increasing the risk of bleeding. Choice *B* is not the correct answer since American ginseng, an herbal supplement used to manage cancer-related fatigue, can reduce platelet aggregation and has resulted in rare cases of thrombocytopenia. Choice *D* is also incorrect since ginger may also reduce platelet aggregation and potentially increase the risk of bleeding.

149. C: Online support groups can be very beneficial for patients that live in small towns or do not have in-person support. Melvin can easily find support and camaraderie through an online group consisting of people who are going through his situation or have been there before; he does not have to continue to feel alone and distressed until treatment ends. Additionally, it is unlikely that an insurance company will pay for extended hospital stays that are not vital to survival, making Choice *A* incorrect. Rest may help Melvin's health, but it is not a substitute for a supportive community, which makes Choice *B* incorrect. Moving is not a realistic or easy solution to alleviate Melvin's distress, making Choice *D* incorrect.

150. D: Ben initially shows symptoms of sciatica, which can be a precursor to cauda equina syndrome. Loss of feeling and bladder control are telltale signs of cauda equina syndrome, a nerve issue that affects the lower half of the body and requires immediate medical attention. This condition may be caused by the presence of a tumor. Choices *A*, *B*, and *C* are not correct in Ben's case.

151. C: It is possible that cancerous cells had spread before the mass from Paula's cervix was removed. Therefore, she will need to be monitored to ensure cancerous cells are not found or growing larger in other parts of her body. Choices *A*, *B*, and *D* make assumptions that the case facts do not support.

152. D: Processed and red meats, in addition to other processed foods, are associated with the development of cancer; therefore, limiting or avoiding these foods is recommended as a primary prevention strategy. Aged cheese and red wine are not associated with the development of cancer, making Choices *A* and *B* incorrect. The oxalate in vegetables such as spinach binds to calcium and iron, making the calcium and iron biologically unavailable; however, there is no evidence that this reaction is associated with cancer prevention, making Choice *C* incorrect.

153. A: Cancer survivors are more likely to be in debt or bankruptcy than other demographics, often due to job loss, loss of insurance, disability, or other reasons that make earning income difficult. Choices *B*, *C*, and *D* are incorrect.

154. B: A male patient with stage III squamous cell carcinoma of the larynx would be the most likely candidate for prophylactic placement of a gastrectomy tube prior to treatment. Patients with head and neck cancers who undergo chemotherapy and radiation therapy tend to be at very high risk for malnutrition and dehydration, due to treatment-related toxicities such as severe mucositis. Choices *A*, *C*, and *D* are incorrect because prophylactic placement of a gastrostomy tube is not routinely recommended for patients with cancers of these anatomical locations.

155. D: Choice *D* is the most appropriate choice, as the listed aspects of the program are all evidence-based ways to increase emotional resilience, which is a major aspect of preventing staff burnout and compassion fatigue. Choices *A*, *B*, and *C* are not the correct answers because the program objectives are less directly related to patient satisfaction, error rates, or standards of practice. However, it is important to note that taking steps to increase staff resilience and prevent nursing burnout can have a positive impact on patient satisfaction, error rates, and the maintenance of standards of practice.

156. B: Lumbar puncture utilizes a syringe to draw fluid out of the spinal space. Examining the fluid can show whether there is excess fluid in the intracranial space, and removal can relieve some pressure. Choices *A*, *C*, and *D* are not used to decrease intracranial pressure.

157. A: The patient is describing anticipatory nausea and vomiting (ANV), which is a conditioned response that some patients experience prior to the administration of emetogenic chemotherapy treatment. This response is typically triggered by certain environmental stimuli, such as smells, being cared for by a specific staff member, or being treated in a specific location. This type of nausea responds best to benzodiazepine treatment and deconditioning. Choices *B*, *C*, and *D* are incorrect, as ANV does not respond well to traditional antiemetic treatment.

158. C: The patient's statement indicates that they are working through a potential spiritual dilemma. Choice *C* would be most appropriate, as chaplains specialize in questions, concerns, or crises of a spiritual nature. Choice *A* would not necessarily be indicated, as this patient is not mentioning a risk for harm or a medical need requiring physician notification. Choice *B* is not the best choice, as the patient's statement is realistic and does not indicate the presence of a psychiatric condition. Lastly, although palliative care (Choice *D*) may be appropriate for this patient based on his history, it is not the most appropriate option since the patient is only speaking about a spiritual dilemma.

159. A: Choice *A* is the most appropriate response because it addresses the patient's comments with concern and identifies that they should be addressed with a provider. The patient is voicing suicidal ideation, including a realistic plan, and would be a significant suicide risk. The nurse should remain with the patient to ensure safety and call for assistance, per facility policy. Choice *B* is incorrect, as it would not be safe for the nurse to leave the patient unattended to retrieve assistance. Choice *C* is incorrect because this statement can feel invalidating and does not address the patient's ideation or plan. While Choice *D* does provide empathy, it does not address the safety concern associated with the patient's comments.

160. A: The assessment section of a patient's medical care plan should include their current symptoms and pain level. Choices *B*, *C*, and *D* refer to responsibilities of the care team that would be found in other areas of the patient's medical care plan.

161. A: Palliative surgery refers to procedures that aim to improve the quality of life for patients who are not candidates to undergo cancer-fighting surgeries or treatments. Choice *B* refers to curative or primary surgery, which attempts to remove the entire tumor and surrounding tissue. Choice *C* refers to an endoscopy, while Choice *D* refers to more invasive forms of surgery and does not apply here.

162. A: Changes in chemotherapy dosing should never be received as a verbal order. The nurse should be familiar with facility policy on what orders, if any, are allowed to be received verbally. Choices *B*, *C*, and *D* are more likely to be permitted as verbal orders, since they include holding treatment, non-chemotherapy premedication orders, and orders for hydration.

163. B: One of the ways that malignant cells can sustain growth is by triggering the release of substances from adjacent tissues that inactivate the cells of the immune system. The action of antibodies would indicate normal immune functioning, making Choice *A* incorrect. The malignant cells are capable of initiating angiogenesis; however, this process most commonly begins when the tumor density reaches one million cells. The release of immune cell suppressants would be necessary to promote the early development of the tumor, making Choice *C* incorrect. As the tumor matures, cellular contact inhibition is lost, which allows the malignant cells to invade surrounding tissues. Cellular contact inhibition is therefore decreased, rather than increased, making Choice *D* incorrect.

164. D: Administration of bevacizumab for the purpose of controlling the growth of glioblastoma would be considered treatment of the condition; this would be generally discontinued upon transitioning to hospice care. Choices *A*, *B*, and *C* are examples of palliative treatments that address the patient's side effects and could possibly be continued upon transitioning to hospice care.

165. A: The number one cause for bladder cancer is the use of cigarettes. While obesity (Choice *B*), chronic urinary tract infections (Choice *C*), and exposure to environmental chemicals (Choice *D*) do present some risk for bladder cancer, they do not represent the most common cause.

Practice Test #2

1. A patient's wife calls to state that her husband is short of breath, increasingly tired, and has a dry, unproductive cough. Looking at his chart, the nurse sees that he was started on an immune checkpoint inhibitor six weeks ago for non-small cell lung cancer. The nurses recognizes that the patient is likely exhibiting symptoms of:

   a. Sepsis
   b. Pneumonia
   c. Advancing disease
   d. Pneumonitis

2. Which of the following causes of thrombocytopenia is considered an immunological cause?

   a. Folate deficiency
   b. Drug side effects
   c. Acute respiratory distress syndrome
   d. Viral infection

3. Malignant cells can exhibit all of the following qualities EXCEPT:

   a. The ability to grow blood supply
   b. The ability to invade into surrounding tissues
   c. Differentiation to carry out a specific function
   d. Failure to undergo apoptosis

4. What amount of blood loss is considered life-threatening and will throw a patient into hypovolemic shock?

   a. 1/8
   b. 1/7
   c. 1/5
   d. 1/10

5. Neoadjuvant therapy can be used before surgery but can result in prolonged wound healing. What does the nurse understand about this type of treatment?

   a. Neoadjuvant therapy eliminates cancer before restorative surgery can be performed.
   b. Neoadjuvant therapy is used to decrease the size or improve the margins of a tumor.
   c. Neoadjuvant therapy prepares the patient for chemotherapy and/or radiation.
   d. Surgery for cancer is always done after neoadjuvant therapy.

6. Myelosuppression is often an acute side effect of cytotoxic chemotherapy. What is the name of the time frame in which cytotoxic chemotherapy is at its greatest efficacy and causes the most myelosuppression?

   a. Pancytopenia
   b. Neutropenia
   c. Nadir
   d. Hematopoiesis

7. The nurse is reviewing morning labs during the patient report. Which patient should the nurse see first?
   a. ANC: 500 cells/mcL, temperature: 100.5°F, HR: 92
   b. K: 3.5 mEq/L, BP: 150/90 mmHg, HR: 120
   c. ANC: 1500 cells/mcL, temperature: 100.1°F, HR 60
   d. ANC: 500 cells/mcL, BP: 92/60 mmHg, HR: 72

8. Radiation safety principles should be followed by radiation providers. What are the three components of these safety principles?
   a. Shielding, personal alarm, and exposure limits
   b. Time, distance, and shielding
   c. Immobilization, positioning, and fractionation
   d. Positioning, shielding, and personal alarm

9. A nurse is seeing a patient for a surveillance visit who is eight years out from treatment of bladder cancer. The patient notes that the past year has been significant due to a diagnosis of congestive heart failure. The nurse understands this to be a long-term effect of which treatment?
   a. Bleomycin
   b. Methotrexate
   c. Doxorubicin
   d. Gemcitabine

10. A nurse is counseling a patient on their risk factors for colon cancer. Which of the following statements would the nurse identify as a risk factor?
   a. "I try to stay away from alcohol except for the occasional glass of red wine with my friends. This is usually a once-a-month experience."
   b. "My grandmother had breast cancer when she was 64 years old. Luckily, it was localized, and she was cured with surgery."
   c. "I try to eat several servings of fruits and vegetables, but I have to be cautious of what causes my Crohn's disease to flare."
   d. "I dislike exercise but still manage to walk at least 30 minutes a day."

11. The nurse is performing an assessment on a 27-year-old patient diagnosed with ovarian cancer. The patient becomes emotional and tells the nurse, "I'm not sure I want treatment. My opportunity of ever becoming a mom would be gone." Which of the following is the best response by the nurse?
   a. "It is too early for you to worry. You will be fine after your treatment."
   b. "You can still have a fulfilling life without becoming a mom."
   c. "I know this is difficult for you. Would you like me to call one of your support systems?"
   d. "I will make sure your provider discusses all of the treatment options with you."

12. The husband of a patient who recently died expresses confusion about the different terms he has been hearing in relation to the grief process. Which of the following statements indicates a need for further education?
   a. "Mourning is the outward expression of loss."
   b. "Bereavement is the process through which you accept loss."
   c. "When loss cannot be acknowledged, grief occurs."
   d. "Loss is the permanent absence of a person, relationship, or possession."

13. A patient has been receiving RCHOP (rituximab, cyclophosphamide, doxorubicin, vincristine, and prednisone) for diffuse large B-cell lymphoma. He presents for therapy and complains of intense abdominal pain and cramping. He states that he is unsure when his last bowel movement was. You suspect which of the following?
   a. Ileus related to vincristine infusion
   b. SVC syndrome related to disease progression
   c. Tumor lysis syndrome related to cyclophosphamide
   d. Hypersensitivity reaction related to rituxan

14. A nurse is floating to a different floor to administer chemotherapy due to a lack of qualified staff on the floor. As the patient is receiving the drug, the nurse notes symptoms of a hypersensitivity reaction. To provide effective emergency care to the patient, the nurse can expect to use what type of leadership style?
   a. Transactional
   b. Autocratic
   c. Democratic
   d. Strategic

15. There is a 3 percent loss of muscle mass within the thigh muscles within 7 days of bedrest, and contractures begin within 3 weeks. This is an example of which of the following?
   a. Immobility
   b. Decompression syndrome
   c. Deconditioning
   d. Debilitation

16. A nurse is discussing smoking cessation with a patient at an annual check-up. The nurse notes that smoking is linked to all of the following cancer types EXCEPT:
   a. Bladder
   b. Liver
   c. Pancreatic
   d. Lymphoma

17. A patient will be receiving a hematopoietic stem cell transplant. The patient understands that they will be receiving bone marrow from an unrelated donor. What is the name of this type of bone marrow donation?
   a. Autologous
   b. Allogeneic
   c. Volunteer
   d. Stem cell donor

18. A 75-year-old male who has completed treatment for colorectal cancer is meeting with the nurse for a surveillance visit. He notes that despite having completed treatment six months ago, he continues to feel moderately fatigued every day. What is an appropriate response from the nurse?

a. "The fatigue is likely due to your blood counts being low from chemotherapy. We may consider a transfusion to return your hemoglobin to normal."
b. "It is normal to feel fatigue for an extended time after treatment. To help mitigate the fatigue, you should get plenty of rest and utilize caffeine to stay awake."
c. "It is normal to feel fatigue for an extended time after treatment. To help mitigate the fatigue, you should participate in regular physical activity."
d. "It is unusual to have fatigue that is so impactful this long after treatment. We can discuss this with your provider because further testing will be needed to determine the cause."

19. The nurse listens to a patient as she tells him that she feels very dizzy when she stands up and has to do so very slowly. The nurse recognizes what type of low blood pressure may be occurring?

a. Hypovolemic
b. Postural
c. Neural
d. Postprandial

20. Mucositis can be incredibly painful and prevents patients from eating, drinking, and even speaking. What action can the patient take to help prevent mucositis?

a. Vigorously brush and floss with a hard toothbrush
b. Use an alcohol-based mouth rinse regularly
c. See a dentist before treatment and follow an oral hygiene regimen
d. Use a lidocaine mouth rinse before each meal

21. Which of the following ethical principles is MOST closely related to advocacy?

a. Distributive justice
b. Beneficence
c. Nonmaleficence
d. Fidelity

22. Which of the following is released into the bloodstream in the event of tumor lysis syndrome?

a. Potassium
b. Platelets
c. Calcium
d. Uric acid

23. A nurse is caring for a patient who will be discharged home and receiving hospice care. The patient has been asking questions about what to expect. Which of the following statements by the nurse is correct concerning hospice care?

a. "Hospice will not provide medical equipment and supplies, so it is important to have those ready at home."
b. "You may only spend six months in hospice care."
c. "Hospice is there to provide pain and symptom control while you undergo additional treatments."
d. "Hospice focuses on enhancement of quality of life for both patients and caregivers."

24. T. F. is a 52-year-old female preparing to undergo a core needle breast biopsy. The nurse understands that this procedure will involve which of the following?
   a. Removing the entirety of the tumor to clear margins
   b. Using a small needle to remove fluid for testing
   c. Using a large needle to aspirate bone marrow for testing
   d. Using a needle to remove tissue for testing

25. The Synergy Model views the practice of expert nurses as which of the following?
   a. Being able to anticipate the patient needs
   b. Being able to address change
   c. The point where clinical reasoning and clinical inquiry are inseparable
   d. Being able to incorporate research findings

26. A patient with non-small cell lung cancer (NSCLC) is experiencing acute dyspnea with associated anxiety. What should the nurse do as the priority intervention to reduce the patient's dyspnea?
   a. Raise the head of the bed and administer supplemental oxygen
   b. Administer prescribed inhalers
   c. Administer prescribed anxiolytic
   d. Set up a fan pointed at the patient

27. Which of the following is true of a germline mutation?
   a. DNA damage accumulates over time.
   b. It is associated with inherited cancers.
   c. The potential for malignancy is restricted to reproductive organs.
   d. It is associated with malignancy in people over 50 years old.

28. You are caring for a small cell lung cancer patient who received chemotherapy treatment that included cisplatin and etoposide one week ago. He complains of swelling and tenderness in his right arm for several days. You recognize that his condition is likely which of the following?
   a. Extravasation
   b. Venous thromboembolism
   c. Central line infection
   d. Hypersensitivity reaction to chemotherapy

29. Which of the following cancer types does NOT have an associated screening activity?
   a. Stomach
   b. Prostate
   c. Lung
   d. Cervical

30. The nurse is providing care to a patient with testicular cancer who is receiving chemotherapy. The patient tells the nurse, "I don't have any libido and I feel it's affecting my partner. I don't know what to do." Which of the following is the best response by the nurse?
   a. "This is an expected side effect of chemotherapy."
   b. "Are you thinking about stopping treatment?"
   c. "Have you spoken to your partner about your feelings?"
   d. "Your partner should be more supportive of your treatment."

31. In a patient with brain metastasis, what is the earliest indication of increased intracranial pressure (ICP)?
   a. Vomiting
   b. Vision changes
   c. Confusion and behavior changes
   d. Sluggish response of the pupils to light

32. After the removal of a breast tumor and surrounding lymph nodes, a patient begins to develop swelling and enlargement of her left arm. The nurse recognizes that this is likely lymphedema. What can the nurse and patient do to minimize the lymphedema?
   a. Use compression on the affected limb
   b. Use the left arm less so that it can rest
   c. Use hot compresses
   d. Use cold compresses

33. A nurse is caring for a patient with neutropenic fever on an overnight shift. The nurse documents in the note "BP 85/57, patient reports mild dizziness with position changes." The nurse notifies the provider and executes orders for fluid resuscitation, blood cultures, and continued monitoring. The nurse becomes busy during the shift and fails to document any additional information. What is the nurse at risk of legal action for?
   a. Negligence
   b. Defamation
   c. Slander
   d. Disclosure of information

34. Checkpoint inhibitors (CPIs) disrupt proteins used by tumors to disguise themselves from the immune system. These proteins are also used by healthy cells to avoid being targeted by the body's own immune system. In what way do checkpoint inhibitors reveal tumors to the immune system?
   a. Tumor cells have their phospholipid membrane disrupted by CPIs.
   b. CPIs return recognition of proteins on tumors to T-cells to encourage immune response.
   c. CPIs alter proteins on cancer cells to cause immune system recognition.
   d. Proteins used by cancer cells for cloaking are removed by CPIs.

35. The nurse is performing an assessment on a patient diagnosed with recurrent colon cancer. The patient tells the nurse, "It is so hard to talk to my family about my condition. They don't understand what I am going through." Which of the following is the best response by the nurse?
   a. "Do you have any friends who are willing to listen to you?"
   b. "You can't expect your family to know what you are going through."
   c. "There are community support groups for people who share your same experience."
   d. "Why do you think they don't understand your condition?"

36. A patient who is newly diagnosed with cancer can have difficulty dealing with such a life changing disease, which can result in significant depression and anxiety. Physicians may prescribe antidepressant medication for this problem. What is the most important side effect that the nurse should teach the patient to report immediately if it occurs?
   a. Suicidal ideation
   b. Fatigue
   c. Dizziness
   d. Weight gain

37. A nurse is caring for a patient with breast cancer who is receiving her last dose of radiation treatment. Which of the following statements made by the patient's partner indicates a need for further education?
   a. "She has been having more skin tenderness from the radiation. We'll hold off on strenuous activity for a bit longer."
   b. "We extended our leaves of absence from our employers for a few more weeks to deal with additional side effects."
   c. "I'm glad we won't be driving to the clinic every day, but it may take time before she's feeling back to normal."
   d. "It's great that this is the last treatment! She'll be able to go on a hike with me this weekend."

38. A nurse is caring for a 73-year-old patient who is admitted for management of cord compression. The nurse understands that this diagnosis will require collaboration with multiple specialties. Which of the following is NOT an example of the nurse providing collaborative care?
   a. Requesting a referral for physical therapy after the patient expresses concerns with ambulating stairs at home
   b. Encouraging early ambulation by the nurse upon admission
   c. Providing pain medication as prescribed an hour prior to radiation therapy
   d. Participating in daily rounds with updates on patient status from overnight reports

39. Proton therapy is more precise than traditional radiation, with selective cell destruction; however, proton therapy is also more expensive, and facilities that offer this treatment are harder to find. Which type of cancer is typically treated with proton therapy?
   a. Central nervous system, ocular, and skull-based cancers
   b. Esophageal, oral, and thyroid cancers
   c. Heart, sternal, and lung cancers
   d. Bladder, prostate, and rectal cancers

40. Palliative care contains many components, including decisions about goals of care, advanced directives, and maintaining quality of life. Which of the following is NOT part of palliative care?
   a. Pain and symptom management
   b. Determining the best lifesaving treatment
   c. Maintaining or improving quality of life
   d. Establishing values and priorities of the patient

41. Which of the following medications is most likely to cause hypersensitivity or anaphylaxis in oncology patients?
   a. Carboplatin
   b. Cyclophosphamide
   c. Daptomycin
   d. Vincristine

42. J. B. is a 47-year-old male currently undergoing treatment for Hodgkin lymphoma. He calls the triage line to report a nonproductive cough, shortness of breath, and sharp chest pain that worsens with breathing. The nurse reviews his chart and notes that he is a never smoker; he received doxorubicin, bleomycin, vinblastine, and dacarbazine; and he is undergoing radiation treatment to a mediastinal mass. The nurse recognizes which of the following as a risk factor for pulmonary toxicities?
   a. Chemotherapy regimen with radiation to lungs
   b. Smoking history
   c. 47 years of age
   d. Male gender

43. A nurse would expect to find a Gleason score for which patient?
   a. A 56-year-old female with colorectal cancer
   b. A 67-year-old male with prostate cancer
   c. An 82-year-old female with clear cell renal cancer
   d. A 26-year-old male with testicular cancer

44. Radiation can cause dermatitis to the skin. Acute radiation dermatitis can be painful, causing erythema, swelling, and itching. Which intervention can ease discomfort for the patient?
   a. Applying lotion that the patient brought from home
   b. Washing the area with antimicrobial soap and patting dry
   c. Applying mild corticosteroid cream as prescribed
   d. Taking oral antihistamines as prescribed

45. A nurse is taking a phone call from the wife of a patient undergoing treatment for colorectal cancer. The patient has had significant side effects with the current therapy, and the nurse is concerned that the caregiver will experience burnout. Which statement by the wife indicates the greatest risk for burnout?
   a. "It's been tough to manage his symptoms the past few days. Our son has come to live with us for a few weeks, but my husband doesn't want him to see how sick he is."
   b. "We have a great group of friends and family willing to help, but my husband doesn't want to burden them by asking for help."
   c. "Can we move his appointment to the afternoon instead? I've had to take time off work, and I'm falling behind on deadlines."
   d. "When his symptoms were worse, I wasn't getting much sleep. Hopefully we can get him feeling better, and I can catch up this week like I have in the past."

46. A patient is receiving chemotherapy and radiation for recently diagnosed breast cancer. The patient begins having blood in her urine and pain with urination. She recognizes that she needs to contact the doctor right away. Which chemotherapy drug is likely causing hemorrhagic cystitis in this patient?
   a. Carboplatin or cisplatin
   b. Bleomycin or mitomycin
   c. Cyclophosphamide or ifosfamide
   d. Doxorubicin or daunorubicin

47. Patients may consider trying complementary and alternative medicine (CAM) to treat their cancer or alleviate their symptoms. Meditation is one modality of CAM treatment that has been studied and shown to provide benefits to patients. Which of the following is NOT a benefit of meditation?
   a. Relief of muscle tension
   b. Decreased feelings of stress
   c. Boosted immune function
   d. Reduced cancer proliferation

48. A lung cancer patient with facial edema, jugular venous distention, and shortness of breath at rest likely has which of the following?
   a. Tumor lysis syndrome
   b. Cancer metastasis
   c. Superior vena cava syndrome
   d. Syndrome of inappropriate diuretic hormone

49. What serological marker indicates, with high specificity, that cardiac muscle tissue has been damaged and cell contents are being released into the bloodstream?
   a. Creatinine
   b. BUN
   c. Creatine kinase
   d. Troponin

50. Kidney dysfunction can occur during or after cancer treatment. This can occur due to medication or chemotherapy, such as cisplatin. What is the most important intervention to teach the patient and family to prevent kidney dysfunction or improve kidney function?
   a. Reduce fluid intake to rest the kidneys
   b. Drink plenty of fluids during and after administration of cisplatin
   c. Void frequently to keep the kidneys functioning
   d. Monitor for signs or symptoms of kidney dysfunction

51. Chimeric antigen receptor therapy (CAR-T) uses T-cells from a patient's peripheral blood. These T-cells are reprogrammed to add tumor antigen receptors which allow for the targeting of tumor cells. Large quantities of these cultured cells are then infused back into the patient. Which of the following processes programs the T-cells?
   a. DNA vector processes
   b. Antigen growth processes
   c. RNA vector processes
   d. T-cell manipulation processes

52. The nurse notices the site around the patient's peripheral IV has become puffy, cold, and tight. She suspects what has occurred?

a. Infection
b. IV infiltration
c. Allergic reaction
d. Nothing, this is a normal assessment of peripheral IV

53. A patient is participating in a clinical trial and has been randomized to treatment group A. Group A will receive one treatment, while group B is allocated to a different treatment. Which type of randomized trial design does this represent?

a. Parallel group trial design
b. Crossover design
c. Factorial design
d. Randomized withdrawal design

54. A nurse is preparing for a chemotherapy education session with a Spanish-speaking patient. Which of the following is a best practice to provide culturally congruent care?

a. Asking the patient about their preferred language in which to receive written education
b. Researching common cultural considerations when caring for Hispanic patients
c. Requesting that a family member serves as the interpreter to provide familiarity
d. Speaking loudly and slowly

55. Often, a patient who has been undergoing treatment for cancer will have low blood cell counts, including red cells, white cells, and platelets. What treatments can be prescribed by the provider to assist in recovery from low blood cell counts?

a. Anticoagulants
b. Myeloid growth factors
c. Antibiotics
d. Fresh frozen plasma, platelets, and red blood cell infusion

56. Intravenous access is important when administering chemotherapy or biotherapy. An implanted port is a good option for a patient who will be receiving these treatments. Which of the following is true regarding the initial access of a port for therapy?

a. It is accessed with a Luer lock syringe.
b. It is accessed with a butterfly needle.
c. It is accessed with a non-coring needle.
d. It is accessed with a peripheral intravenous catheter.

57. The nurse is performing a follow-up assessment on a patient who underwent a total pelvic exenteration two months ago. The patient tells the nurse, "I'm having doubts about the choice I made. I don't feel I will ever be able to have sex with a partner again." Which of the following is the best action by the nurse?

a. Encourage the patient to discuss future reconstructive surgery with their provider.
b. Assure the patient that sex with a partner can resume in a few months.
c. Redirect the patient to appreciate the medical benefit of treatment.
d. Prepare the patient for a pelvic exam by the provider.

58. Pain associated with cancer and cancer treatments can be treated both medically and with alternative treatments. Which of the following is NOT an effective alternative treatment?
   a. Physiatry
   b. Meditation
   c. Acupuncture
   d. Exercise

59. Small-molecule inhibitors are generally available orally and are molecularly smaller than monoclonal antibodies. In addition to these characteristics, which feature of small-molecule inhibitors differentiates them from monoclonal antibodies?
   a. Small-molecule inhibitors are used for extracellular targets.
   b. Small-molecule inhibitors are able to target intracellular molecules.
   c. The bioavailability of monoclonal antibodies is less than that of small-molecule inhibitors.
   d. Unlike monoclonal antibodies, small-molecule inhibitors are synthetic.

60. A nurse is caring for a 68-year-old black male with stage II esophageal cancer. His social history includes that he has worked as a dry cleaner for the past 15 years, has a history of GERD, and is a non-smoker. After completing chemotherapy and surgery, the patient learned that he has no evidence of disease. The nurse understands which of the following to be a favorable prognostic factor?
   a. The patient had complete resection of the tumor.
   b. The cancer was diagnosed at a late stage.
   c. The patient is a black male.
   d. The patient has significant environmental exposures working as a dry cleaner.

61. A patient undergoing cytotoxic chemotherapy is found to have a low platelet count of <75,000/mm^3. This puts the patient at serious risk of bleeding. What actions should the patient avoid in order to reduce the risk of bleeding?
   a. Using a soft toothbrush
   b. Implementing a bowel regimen
   c. Walking in bare feet or open toed shoes
   d. Using only electric shavers

62. Exposure to chemotherapy during administration is a major concern for nurses and an occupational hazard. What is the MOST significant result of accidental exposure?
   a. Contact dermatitis and rash
   b. Increased risk for malignancies or embryo-fetal toxicities
   c. Neurological changes
   d. Heart rhythm changes

63. Oncology patients can be at risk for infection while receiving cytotoxic chemotherapy and other therapies. This risk is often mitigated by using prophylactic antimicrobial medications. Which of the following actions should the patient take to reduce their risk of infection?
   a. Avoid leaving their house
   b. Wipe front to back after voiding or having a bowel movement
   c. Frequently visit the doctor's office to check for infection
   d. Cut their fingernails and toenails frequently to monitor skin integrity

64. A 47-year-old woman has been recommended to undergo hormone replacement therapy (HRT) to address symptoms of menopause. She asks the nurse if there are any cancer risks associated with starting this therapy. The nurse understands which statement to be true?

   a. HRT use can lower the risk for ovarian cancer.
   b. The risk of lung cancer increases with long term use of HRT.
   c. HRT can increase the risk for breast cancer.
   d. Estrogen may have a role in preventing pancreatic cancer.

65. The hospice nurse is performing an in-home assessment on a patient with end-stage liver cancer. The patient's caregiver states, "I love my partner very much, but it seems like I haven't slept in three months with everything I have to do." Which of the following is the best action by the nurse?

   a. Instruct the caregiver to prioritize which daily errands need to be completed first.
   b. Encourage the caregiver to take frequent naps.
   c. Help the caregiver make a list of daily tasks that can be delegated to family and friends.
   d. Emphasize the importance of taking care of the patient.

66. A patient is receiving doxorubicin for breast cancer and complains of burning pain during the infusion. Which of the following should be the first action by the nurse?

   a. Flush the site with 30 cc sodium bicarbonate.
   b. Stop the infusion and aspirate any remaining drug.
   c. Stop the infusion and apply a cold compress to the site.
   d. Decrease the rate of the infusion until the patient feels more comfortable.

67. A nurse is caring for a patient who is recovering from a prostatectomy earlier in the day. The nurse works with the patient to identify a goal to complete their first ambulation during the nurse's shift. This is an example of which step in the nursing process?

   a. Outcome identification
   b. Implementation
   c. Planning
   d. Assessment

68. Patients undergoing treatment for cancer can experience cognitive changes. They may take longer to complete tasks, not remember things as clearly, or not think as fast as they did before treatment. What strategy can patients use to improve their cognition during and after cancer treatment?

   a. Increase nutritional supplements
   b. Use stimulants such as methylphenidate
   c. Avoid exercise and ensure adequate rest
   d. Perform cognitive training

69. A patient is undergoing conditioning for a bone marrow transplant. The goal of preparation is to eliminate any remaining malignancy, suppress the immune system, and open space within the bone marrow. What is the name of this dose-intense conditioning?

   a. Marrow ablative
   b. Maintenance therapy
   c. Initial therapy
   d. Reduction therapy

70. Patients with cancer are commonly found to have a decrease in muscle mass or muscle wasting called sarcopenia. To slow the progression of sarcopenia, which intervention should the patient avoid?
   a. Resting, turning every two hours
   b. Resistance exercise
   c. Nutritional supplements
   d. Hormone replacement

71. A patient asks their nurse about the purpose of accreditation by The Joint Commission (TJC). The nurse correctly responds with which of the following statements?
   a. "Accreditation by TJC indicates an organization's commitment to nursing within an interdisciplinary team."
   b. "TJC accreditation indicates the organization's commitment to cancer research with rigorous standards for developing new and better approaches to prevention, diagnosis, and treatment."
   c. "TJC's objective is to evaluate processes in healthcare organizations to provide measures and assessments of safe, high-quality care for patients."
   d. "Accreditation by TJC shows high-quality care for outpatient hematology-oncology practices within the United States."

72. The nurse is orienting a new oncology nurse who is administering paclitaxel to a newly diagnosed ovarian cancer patient. The patient starts to complain that she feels warm, and her face appears flushed. She begins to cough and complain of tightness in her chest. Which of the following is the priority intervention?
   a. Reassure the patient that it is normal to be nervous during the first treatment.
   b. Decrease the rate of paclitaxel by 25 percent.
   c. Administer 25 mg of IV Benadryl and stop the infusion.
   d. Immediately stop the infusion and notify the provider.

73. A patient undergoing cancer treatment with Cytarabine (ara-C, cytosine arabinoside) begins to develop symptoms of dyspnea and hypoxia. The nurse can hear coarse crackles in both sides of the lungs. The patient has a chest X-ray that shows increasing pulmonary edema. Which of the following would be the priority in order to provide relief for the patient and reverse hypoxia?
   a. Obtaining a stat arterial blood gas
   b. Administering fluids as ordered
   c. Administering oxygen and furosemide
   d. Managing hypertension

74. Certain diagnostic tests must be completed to determine the appropriate biotherapy for a patient. Which is not a companion diagnostic that must be used to determine the correct biotherapy?
   a. Biological characteristics
   b. Molecular characteristics
   c. Genetic characteristics
   d. Chemical characteristics

75. Peripheral neuropathy caused by chemotherapy can be treated with medications prescribed by a physician. Which of the following medications is NOT used to treat peripheral neuropathy?

a. Anticonvulsants (gabapentin, pregabalin)
b. Antidepressants (tricyclic, SNRIs)
c. Opioids (oxycodone, hydrocodone)
d. Medication patches (lidocaine, capsaicin)

76. A nurse manager is creating a resilience program for the staff on an oncology unit. To incorporate evidence-based self-care practices, the manager should include all of the following recommendations EXCEPT which of the following?

a. Aromatherapy
b. Mindfulness
c. Art therapy
d. Pedicures

77. A patient develops a cardiovascular symptom of bilateral lower leg edema due to chemotherapy. What can the patient do to help reduce the amount of swelling?

a. Wear loose fitting clothing
b. Stand frequently
c. Follow a diabetic diet
d. Elevate legs above the level of the heart

78. An oncology nurse navigator is working with a 48-year-old female with newly diagnosed metastatic melanoma. Which would be the most appropriate next step for the nurse to discuss with the client based on her current stage within the care continuum?

a. Educate the patient on sun exposures to reduce risk.
b. Ensure orders for stage-appropriate testing.
c. Assess barriers and access to care.
d. Discuss surveillance recommendations.

79. Peritoneal catheters may be used for chemotherapy infusion. This type of catheter must be placed by interventional radiology or done in surgery. Which of the following is NOT a feature of peritoneal catheters?

a. Peritoneal catheters can be tunneled or can use a port for infusion access.
b. Peritoneal catheters are typically one lumen and have many fenestrations.
c. Peritoneal catheters are placed low and directed upward.
d. Peritoneal catheters may be temporary or permanent.

80. The clinic nurse is performing an intake assessment on a patient with recurrent breast cancer. The patient is visibly in distress and tells the nurse, “My pain is so excruciating that I plan on taking the full bottle of pills when I get home so I won’t feel anything anymore.” Which of the following actions does the nurse take first?

a. Review the patient’s medical record for information on next of kin
b. Request immediate counseling services for the patient
c. Ask the patient how long they have been feeling depressed
d. Document the patient’s statement in the medical record

81. Cachexia is unintended weight loss and often accompanies anorexia, resulting in cancer anorexia-cachexia syndrome (CACS). Which of the following is an intervention used for patients with this condition?

a. Encouraging the patient to eat three large meals each day
b. Administering megestrol (Megace)
c. Encouraging sugar-free vitamin drinks
d. Encouraging a high fat, high calorie diet

82. A nurse is providing education regarding the HPV (human papillomavirus) vaccine. The nurse notes that HPV is a risk factor for which cancers?

a. Liver cancer and non-Hodgkin lymphoma
b. Gastric cancer and gastric mucosa-associated lymphoma
c. Lung cancer and Kaposi sarcoma
d. Oropharyngeal cancer and cervical cancer

83. A patient has recently seen an oncologist after her mother was diagnosed with breast cancer. The oncologist revealed to her that she is BRCA1 positive. What will likely be her course of treatment?

a. Yearly MRI and mammogram screenings
b. Medications that reduce the risk of cancer
c. Double mastectomy
d. Healthy lifestyle changes

84. A patient had a radical colectomy to remove an adenocarcinoma from the descending colon. This resulted in the patient having a temporary colostomy placed on the lower left quadrant of his abdomen. To avoid skin breakdown around the ostomy, what is the most important teaching point for proper care of the ostomy site?

a. Prevent constipation
b. Eat a low residue diet
c. Change the bag every day
d. Appropriately size and apply the wafer of the ostomy device

85. A new nurse is taking care of a patient with diffuse large B-cell lymphoma (DLBCL) who is hospitalized for induction chemotherapy. The nurse reports several abnormalities in the patient's morning labs. Upon review, it is suspected that the patient is likely in tumor lysis syndrome based on which of the following lab results?

a. K: 3.7, Na: 140, Ca: 13
b. K: 6.4, Phos: 5.2, Ca: 4.0
c. K: 3.0, Hgb: 7.5, Mag: 1.4
d. K: 3.5, BUN: 15, Ca: 10

86. Which of the following is a type of growth factor that promotes the growth of blood vessels on a tumor?

a. TK
b. VEGF
c. EGFR
d. HER2

87. Cardiotoxicity can be an adverse reaction to biotherapy when using some monoclonal antibodies. What is one test that is done prior to starting biotherapy to help identify patients at risk of developing cardiotoxicity?
   a. Cardiac stress test
   b. Electrocardiogram
   c. Echocardiogram
   d. Computed tomography scan

88. A nurse is providing education on the side effects of androgen deprivation therapy (ADT) to a 71-year-old man with prostate cancer. Considering the side effect profile for this drug, how should the nurse best approach concerns related to sexuality?
   a. Information on this topic is not needed because the patient is too old to be sexually active.
   b. Allude to sexual side effects and instruct the patient to call the clinic for more information. The patient will feel more comfortable talking about this topic over the phone.
   c. Inform the patient of expected sexual side effects and provide him with information, resources, and referrals as needed.
   d. Ask the patient if he has any questions regarding sexual side effects and address the topic only if the patient asks about it. The patient will ask questions if they wish to know more.

89. Which response should the nurse make when a patient with advanced pancreatic cancer and a poor prognosis asks why she is receiving chemotherapy?
   a. "Your chance of remission is increased with chemotherapy."
   b. "There is always the chance that chemotherapy can cure your cancer."
   c. "Chemotherapy will keep your cancer from advancing further."
   d. "Chemotherapy is being used to help manage your pain."

90. The nurse is providing discharge instructions to the caregiver of a patient who will require daily transportation to radiation therapy for a malignant spinal tumor. The patient is paralyzed and requires total care. What should the nurse include in the discharge packet to provide the caregiver with support?
   a. A list of discounted transportation companies
   b. A pamphlet with information about medical insurance options
   c. A copy of the patient's in-network home health agencies
   d. A folder with a caregiver resource guide

91. Patients undergoing cancer treatment with chemotherapy often lose weight. One cause of this is due to changes in their taste. What can patients safely do to make food more palatable?
   a. Eat spicy foods to increase taste
   b. Increase meats to hide unpleasant flavors
   c. Use spices and flavorings to improve flavors
   d. Use more dry foods

92. Some cancer patients are treated by accessing their cerebral spinal fluid. Rather than repeatedly accessing the cerebral spinal fluid through lumbar puncture, an intraventricular port or reservoir may be placed. This allows for repeated and direct access to cerebral spinal fluid more safely. What is this type of access called?

a. Ommaya reservoir
b. Epidural port
c. Tunneled access catheter
d. Implanted power port

93. A nurse is providing end-of-life care and notices that the patient, who has been minimally responsive to stimuli, is appearing increasingly agitated, grimacing, and experiencing increased work of breathing. After reviewing the orders, the nurse prepares to administer which medication?

a. PO acetaminophen
b. Sublingual ondansetron
c. IV dexamethasone
d. IV morphine

94. A new nurse who is caring for a patient with multiple myeloma states that the patient seems increasingly confused and weaker overnight while continuing to complain of thirst. Morning labs show Hgb: 7.9, K: 3.6, Ca: 15, Mag: 2.1, and glucose: 135. You recognize that this patient is likely showing signs of which of the following?

a. Brain metastasis
b. Hypercalcemia
c. Anemia
d. Diabetes insipidus

95. A nurse is caring for a patient with stage IV pancreatic cancer who is currently full code. The patient notes that they do not wish to have CPR and would like to die a natural death. The nurse best advocates for the patient by doing which of the following?

a. Recommending that the patient discuss this with their doctor during the next rounds
b. Facilitating a discussion with the doctor regarding change in code status and providing patient information about advanced directives
c. Providing education about CPR statistics and recommending that the patient think about it further before deciding
d. Calling the patient's next of kin to discuss the decision

96. TNM classification is used in which of the following cancer types?

a. Liver
b. Leukemia
c. Brain
d. Ovarian

97. Peripheral neuropathy is a symptom that can develop after a patient receives certain types of chemotherapy. What can the patient do to reduce the uncomfortable sensations caused by neuropathy?

a. Massage affected areas regularly
b. Wear tight clothing on the affected areas
c. Use ice and heat to reduce discomfort
d. Protect hands and feet from extreme temperatures

98. Hematopoietic stem cells (HSCs) are infused into a patient after they have been prepped with marrow ablative treatment and the bone marrow transplant has been prepared. In what setting are the HSCs delivered?
   a. Outpatient infusion clinic
   b. Surgical suite
   c. Inpatient hospital room
   d. Oncology office

99. A nurse is assessing a new patient for familial history and genetic risk factors. Which finding would prompt the recommendation for genetic testing?
   a. A maternal aunt died of colorectal cancer at 56 years of age.
   b. A paternal grandfather was diagnosed with localized, hormone-sensitive prostate cancer at 70 years of age.
   c. A paternal cousin was diagnosed with HER2 positive breast cancer at 55 years of age.
   d. A mother of Ashkenazi Jewish ancestry was diagnosed with breast cancer at 47 years of age.

100. The nurse is caring for a patient with small cell lung cancer who reports nausea, tiredness, and confusion. Her urine output remains less than 30 ml/hr despite an aggressive IV fluid bolus of normal saline. The nurse recognizes that this patient may be experiencing which of the following?
   a. The patient may be experiencing Syndrome of Inappropriate Antidiuretic Hormone Secretion (SIADH), so low sodium levels are anticipated.
   b. The patient may be experiencing increased fluid retention related to the saline solution, so an increase in BNP is anticipated.
   c. The patient may be experiencing kidney metastases, so an increase in creatine levels is anticipated.
   d. The patient may be experiencing dehydration, so an increase in potassium is anticipated.

101. A nurse is counseling a patient who continues to have diarrhea three weeks after the completion of radiation. The nurse understands that chronic diarrhea puts the patient at risk for all of the following EXCEPT which outcome?
   a. Skin breakdown
   b. Increased absorption of medications
   c. Social isolation
   d. Impaired immune function

102. A patient has been recently diagnosed with early-stage adenocarcinoma of the colon. What is the first line of treatment in this patient's case?
   a. Small bowel resection
   b. Chemotherapy
   c. Chemotherapy and radiation concurrently
   d. Colon resection surgery

103. Apnea and loss of normal oxygenation during a spontaneous breathing trial are signs that what should occur?
   a. Sedation should be increased.
   b. The breathing trial should continue for a few more minutes.
   c. An antidote for respiratory distress should be administered.
   d. Mechanical ventilation should continue.

104. The nurse is preparing to discharge a patient with instructions for outpatient chemotherapy. The patient tells the nurse, "I am not sure I will have enough money for transportation to my appointments." Which of the following actions does the nurse immediately take?

a. Call the provider to delay the outpatient therapy appointments
b. Arrange for the case manager to meet with the patient prior to discharge
c. Document the patient's statement in the medical record
d. Ask the patient to sign the discharge paperwork

105. Patients undergoing treatment for cancer often feel weak, which may lead to a patient staying in one position too long. This can lead to the development of pressure injuries. What is the most important thing to teach families of those who have a pressure injury?

a. To put extra blankets under pressure areas
b. To massage pressure areas thoroughly
c. To wear shoes to bed to protect heels from pressure
d. To ensure that the patient is repositioned every two hours

106. Biotherapies are made from living beings or derived in a laboratory. They include a very broad range of cancer treatments. What is the goal of biotherapy in cancer treatment?

a. To increase the incidence of cell death
b. To regulate the use of proteins by cells
c. To prevent nausea and vomiting
d. To prevent cell growth or cell proliferation

107. Brain metastases are most common in which cancer?

a. Melanoma
b. Prostate
c. Bladder
d. Stomach

108. Radiation therapy includes extensive treatment planning. The process of simulation is part of this planning. Which of the following is NOT part of that process?

a. Complete CT scan
b. CT and virtual planning
c. Immobilization of patient
d. Complete PET scan

109. Patients with bone metastasis can develop pathological fractures of the bone. This can be due to tumor proliferation, treatment side effects, or metabolic changes from cancer. To prevent further damage, what is the most important action to take for a patient who has pathological fractures?

a. Taking calcium supplements
b. Maintaining a safe environment
c. Controlling pain with medications as ordered
d. Performing weight-bearing exercise

110. A patient who has been receiving chest radiation for lung cancer presents with a BP of 75/40, jugular distention, and muffled heart sounds. You recognize that this patient likely has which of the following conditions?

a. SVC syndrome
b. Pneumonitis
c. Cardiac tamponade
d. SIADH

111. A patient who is undergoing cancer treatment is experiencing generalized pain. The patient's physician prescribed acetaminophen and cyclobenzaprine, an adjuvant medication. Two weeks later, the patient visits the doctor again, this time complaining of 7/10 pain. According to the next step of the World Health Organization's (WHO) pain ladder, which of the following would the provider prescribe next for pain management?

a. Opioid for severe pain, acetaminophen, and cyclobenzaprine
b. Opioid for mild pain, acetaminophen, and cyclobenzaprine
c. Ibuprofen, acetaminophen, and cyclobenzaprine
d. Opioid for severe pain, cyclobenzaprine, and lorazepam

112. Peripherally inserted central catheters (PICCs) can be used to deliver medications, including chemotherapy and biotherapy, for an extended period. Which of the following is NOT an advantage to using a PICC line?

a. PICC lines can be used for up to one year.
b. PICC lines are less likely to become infected than implanted ports.
c. PICC lines can be sterilely inserted by nurses.
d. Blood can be drawn for labs from PICCs.

113. An oncology nurse navigator is counseling a 35-year-old man who recently completed treatment for testicular cancer. The patient has been referred to cancer rehabilitation, which the nurse correctly explains as which of the following?

a. A service to wean patients off of narcotic pain medication
b. A supportive care program to minimize disability and improve quality of life
c. A service that will replace the patient's oncologist moving forward
d. A short-term physical therapy service

114. The nurse is assessing a patient with a recent history of bowel carcinoma and poor prognosis. During the interview, the patient tells the nurse, "I frequently experience heart palpitations and shortness of breath, but all tests come back normal. The symptoms go away when I relax and stop thinking about when I'm going to die." Which is the best response by the nurse?

a. "What kind of help are you receiving for your anxiety?"
b. "How long have you been feeling depressed?"
c. "What kind of tests are ordered when this happens?"
d. "Why do you think you are going to die?"

115. Urinary incontinence is a very disruptive symptom that can occur with cancer and cancer treatments. This symptom can be particularly difficult for formerly continent patients. What can help reduce the incidence of incontinence for patients?

a. Bladder training
b. Wearing incontinence briefs or pads
c. Drinking caffeinated drinks only in the morning
d. Using a straight catheter to fully empty the bladder

116. Alkylating agents, such as ifosfamide, can be used to treat testicular cancer. How does this class of drug affect cells?

a. Alkylating agents insert themselves into DNA, inhibiting DNA repair.
b. Alkylating agents bind with DNA, inhibiting DNA and RNA synthesis.
c. Alkylating agents interfere with DNA replication.
d. Alkylating agents block DNA production and prevent cell division.

117. A nurse is counseling a 25-year-old female Hodgkin lymphoma survivor. The nurse notes that the patient received significant radiation to the chest. Which of the following recommendations would the nurse make?

a. Complete breast imaging annually starting at age 25.
b. Have a skin evaluation completed every five years.
c. Complete a lung cancer screening CT every five years.
d. Have a screening colonoscopy every five years starting at age 35.

118. All EXCEPT which of the following are components of Virchow's triad?

a. Heart disease
b. Hypercoagulability
c. Endothelial injury/dysfunction
d. Hemodynamic changes such as stasis or turbulence

119. Checkpoint inhibitors (CPIs) can result in adverse reactions, such as rash, fatigue, pneumonitis, hepatic toxicity, and gastrointestinal toxicity. What is the cause of these adverse events?

a. Overactive immune system stimulated by CPIs
b. CPIs are toxic to the body
c. CPIs cause dysregulation of the immune system
d. Attack of healthy cells by CPI activated T-cells

120. A nurse is caring for a patient experiencing chemotherapy-induced nausea and vomiting. Which of the following actions best represents evidence-based practice?

a. The nurse asks the charge nurse for their experience in treating nausea.
b. The nurse reassures the patient that nausea and vomiting are signs that the chemotherapy is working.
c. The nurse researches the emetogenic potential of the patient's regimen and provides antiemetics at strategic timepoints.
d. The nurse recommends ginger tea to treat nausea.

121. A patient who is undergoing treatment with 5-fluorouracil (5FU) for adenocarcinoma of the large intestine develops severe diarrhea. The patient reports having eight to ten liquid stools every day. What patient teaching is important to reduce the incidence and severity of diarrhea?

a. The importance of using loperamide as prescribed
b. Going to the emergency department when diarrhea occurs
c. Using wipes instead of paper to reduce skin irritation
d. Increasing consumption of fatty food and fruit juices

122. A nurse is caring for a patient in hospice at home and is providing education to the family on non-pharmacologic comfort measures. When discussing management of secretions, the nurse should include which information?

a. Secretions may result in an audible rattle. This is normal and not distressing to the patient.
b. Position the patient flat on their back to manage secretions.
c. Secretions can be thinned by giving fluids to the patient.
d. A fan blowing on the patient's face can be helpful for drying out excess secretions.

123. For vinca alkaloid extravasations, once the infusion has been stopped and the drug has been aspirated, what should the nurse do next?

a. Remove the IV line and apply a compression bandage.
b. Administer hyaluronidase and apply heat for twenty minutes four times daily.
c. Administer DMSO and apply cold for twenty minutes four times daily.
d. Administer dexrazoxane.

124. Patients undergoing cancer treatment who spend extended time in the hospital are at risk for developing delirium. What can patients and/or nurses do to reduce the risk of delirium in the hospital?

a. Maintain a schedule, use available glasses or hearing aids, and maintain adequate sleep
b. Restrain patients to prevent delirium
c. Provide adequate stimulation, such as television or radio
d. Maintain ample lighting and reassure the patient every two hours

125. Which of the following is NOT true about people with cancer under the Americans with Disabilities Act (ADA)?

a. When interviewing applicants for a job, employers may request to know what specific treatment the potential employee is undergoing.
b. The ADA allows people with cancer to work during and after treatment if they can perform the functions of their job.
c. Cancer is covered under the ADA due to the physical or mental changes caused by the disease or treatments.
d. Although it applies to private employers with fifteen or more employees, the ADA does not apply to US federal government executive branch employees.

126. When administering chemotherapy, a nurse ensures proper PPE by donning which of the following?

a. One pair of sterile gloves
b. An N-95 mask
c. Surgical booties
d. A polyethylene-coated gown

127. Occasionally, surgery is performed for a patient to reduce tumor size. This can create symptom relief for the patient and help them maintain function. What is this type of surgery called?

a. Palliative surgery
b. Oncoplastic surgery
c. Curative surgery
d. Preventative surgery

128. A cancer patient notices swelling in their left calf. The nurse assesses the leg and finds redness, heat, and a positive Homan's sign. After an ultrasound, a deep vein thrombosis (DVT) is identified. What intervention is likely to treat this problem and prevent new thrombi from forming?

a. Sequential compression devices applied to bilateral lower extremities
b. Anticoagulant medication, such as a low-molecular-weight heparin
c. Placement of an inferior vena cava filter (IVC filter)
d. Frequent walking and exercise

129. A patient who is being treated for stage IV lung cancer tells the nurse that his legs have been weaker and his back aches all the time. Which action should the nurse take first?

a. Give the patient the prescribed PRN opioid.
b. Teach the patient strengthening and stretching exercises.
c. Assess for sensation and strength in his legs.
d. Notify the doctor about the patient's symptoms.

130. Both targeted therapy and chemotherapy have a goal of limiting or stopping the spread of cancer. However, they also have distinct differences. Which of the following does NOT describe the function of targeted therapy?

a. Cytotoxic
b. Specific
c. Targets molecules
d. Cytostatic

131. After receiving chemotherapy to treat testicular cancer, with which secondary malignancy is the patient at a higher risk of being diagnosed?

a. Melanoma
b. Leukemia
c. Prostate cancer
d. Rectal cancer

132. The nurse is admitting a patient status post-fall after receiving chemotherapy. The patient states, "I wanted to shower by myself even though I felt weak. I don't like depending on my caregiver." Which of the following is the best action by the nurse?

a. Provide the patient with a list of assistive devices to help with activities of daily living.
b. Urge the patient to find another caregiver to help with activities of daily living.
c. Re-educate the patient on the risks of performing activities of daily living by themselves.
d. Encourage the patient to highlight activities of daily living that they are able to perform independently.

133. A nurse is educating the family of a patient in hospice care about things to expect as the patient progresses towards death. The patient's wife voices concern that her husband has not been drinking enough or eating full meals in the past week. Which of the following is an appropriate response by the nurse?

a. "It is a normal part of the dying process for people to lose appetite and thirst. It is ok if he is not eating and drinking as normal, and these actions should not be forced."
b. "We want to see him staying hydrated. If he is not drinking at least 32 ounces of liquids, we should start him on IV fluids."
c. "It's likely that he has had taste changes. You should make his favorite foods and encourage him to eat."
d. "We can discuss placement of a feeding tube with the doctor. It is important that he maintain an appropriate caloric intake."

134. An oncology nurse is training a new nurse to the unit. Which statement surrounding hypersensitivity reactions indicates a need for further education?

a. "My patient is receiving cycle 8 of carboplatin. I will be on the lookout for signs of a hypersensitivity reaction."
b. "I will watch for symptoms of a hypersensitivity reaction within the first 5 to 30 minutes of the infusion."
c. "I will give the pre-medications to the patient a few minutes before starting the chemotherapy."
d. "If the patient shows signs of a reaction, I will first stop the infusion."

135. Biotherapy improves or boosts the body's immune system to reduce or eliminate cancer. Which of the following is NOT a benefit of using biotherapy over chemotherapy?

a. It targets cancer cells only.
b. It is used for any type of cancer.
c. It has fewer or lessened side effects.
d. It causes cancer cells to act like healthy cells.

136. A nurse is caring for a patient who is being evaluated for a small-bowel obstruction. Which of the following assessment findings is consistent with this condition?

a. pH 7.32, PCO_2 38, HCO_3 20
b. Serum osmolality 285 mOsm/kg
c. Serum sodium 128 mmol/L
d. Lower abdominal distention

137. Complementary and alternative medicine (CAM) can be used by patients to alleviate the discomforts of cancer or cancer treatment. Why is it important to educate the patient to report the use of CAM therapy?

a. Dance therapy can cause fatigue.
b. Acupuncture can interfere with lymphatic drainage.
c. Herbal therapy can interfere with cancer treatment.
d. Massage can cause damage when neuropathy is present.

138. The nurse is admitting a patient with suspected early sepsis. Which nursing intervention should be the first priority?

a. Blood cultures
b. Antibiotics
c. IV fluids
d. Vasopressors

139. A clinic nurse is educating a patient about molecular tumor profiling. The patient asks about the purpose of the test. The nurse correctly explains with which of the following responses?

a. "Molecular testing is performed to determine your likely response to different chemotherapies."
b. "Molecular testing is primarily completed to determine if you definitively carry an inheritable mutation that you may pass to your children."
c. "Molecular testing is performed to see if there is a specific biomarker that we have an effective targeted therapy for."
d. "Molecular therapy is run to profile your likely side effects of immunotherapy."

140. A nurse is educating a patient who is preparing to undergo a colonoscopy. The patient asks about the qualities that make a screening test effective. Which of the following responses is the BEST reply from the nurse?

a. "Screening tests should be sensitive enough to detect no disease in a negative result."
b. "Screening tests should be directed toward a serious health problem with minimal treatment options."
c. "Screening tests are often expensive and difficult to find but are worth it to identify problems at early stages."
d. "Screening tests should be safe, sensitive, specific, reliable, and have benefits that outweigh the risks."

141. The nurse is educating a patient post-complete bladder resection with a urostomy creation for stage 3 bladder cancer. The patient becomes tearful and tells the nurse, "I don't think I can ever go out in public again and be judged with this bag hanging from my body." Which is the BEST response by the nurse?

a. "Tell me about what you think the public's perception of you will be."
b. "You don't have to worry. The urostomy is only temporary."
c. "I understand how you feel; I had a family member who went through this."
d. "It's completely safe for you to be out in public with your urostomy."

142. Taxol and other taxanes are commonly used for breast cancer. These drugs end in -taxel and are in the class of antimicrotubule agents used to slow down the growth of cancer cells. How does this class of drug affect cells?

a. Taxanes inhibit mitosis and therefore prevent cell division.
b. DNA and RNA synthesis are inhibited with taxanes.
c. Taxanes inhibit protein synthesis.
d. DNA repair is inhibited.

143. A patient who is experiencing a fever of 101°F, chills, and malaise is admitted to the hospital for neutropenic fever. What is the priority intervention to treat this patient's neutropenic fever and chills?

a. Place wet washcloths on the patient and point a fan at them.
b. Apply ice packs to the patient's groin, axilla, and neck.
c. Increase fluid intake to prevent dehydration.
d. Administer acetaminophen.

144. When providing chemotherapy education, the nurse recognizes which of the following techniques to be effective?

a. Primarily asking closed-ended questions
b. Using written education and instructions only
c. Presenting data from clinical trials to all patients
d. Utilizing frequent teach-back methods

145. The oncology nurse is caring for a patient with chronic kidney disease. Which of the following should the nurse consider when caring for a patient receiving hemodialysis?

a. Monitoring the patient's respiratory status
b. Providing the patient with high potassium, sodium, and phosphoric-containing foods
c. Monitoring the patient's blood pressure
d. Encouraging the patient to consider a kidney transplant

146. A patient diagnosed with lung cancer is scheduled for radiation. The patient understands that they are scheduled every day for thirty days because of what type of dosing?

a. Total dose
b. Dosimetry
c. Absorbed dose
d. Fractionation

147. Palliative care is intended to improve quality of life for patients. Which of the following is NOT considered palliative treatment?

a. Surgery
b. Chemotherapy
c. Radiation treatment
d. Curative treatment

148. A 35-year-old patient with metastatic breast cancer reports numbness in her feet and new urinary incontinence. The nurse suspects which of the following?

a. Spinal cord compression
b. Bladder infection
c. Peripheral neuropathy
d. Bone metastasis

149. A patient undergoing treatment for cancer has an absolute neutrophil count (ANC) of <1000 per microliter. What is the most important intervention for the patient to perform to prevent infection?

a. Proper hand washing technique
b. Wearing a mask at all times
c. Limiting all visitors
d. Bathing at least twice a day

150. A patient is preparing for bone marrow transplantation and understands that they will remain in the hospital for a period of time after the transplant. The patient knows that this time is for what purpose?

a. To harvest autologous bone marrow for future use
b. For infusion of chemotherapy and symptom management
c. To prohibit visitors and prevent exposure to infection
d. To support the patient during marrow aplasia

151. The nurse is counseling a patient who recently lost their child to leukemia. During the interview, the patient states, "I can't focus at work and haven't been sleeping well. It seems like the walls are caving in on me." Which is the best response by the nurse?

a. "I will ask the provider to prescribe you something for sleep."
b. "What coping skills are you using to process your grief?"
c. "Everyone goes through loss at some point in their life."
d. "Are you concerned about losing your job?"

152. Monoclonal antibodies are named using specific nomenclature to describe their mechanism, target, derivation, and components. Where is the target of the monoclonal antibody trastuzumab?

a. The circulatory system
b. The pulmonary system
c. The immune system
d. On the tumor

153. A nurse is caring for a patient undergoing a phase I trial. The nurse understands the goal of therapy to be which of the following?

a. Comparing an experimental drug with the standard of care
b. Evaluating safety during the post-marketing period
c. Determining whether a treatment provides benefit
d. Finding the best dose with the fewest side effects

154. A patient is receiving cyclophosphamide for lymphoma treatment. The nurse recognizes that this patient should also have an order for which of the following?

a. Fluid restriction
b. Mesna
c. EKG prior to administration
d. Ondansetron

155. A nurse is caring for a female patient receiving chemotherapy. When the patient develops a low neutrophil level, which of the following instructions is a priority for the nurse to give the patient?

a. Use a safety razor
b. Take iron supplements
c. Avoid crowds
d. Drink plenty of fluids

156. While performing an assessment, the nurse observes a non-raised, purple rash on the patient's chest and upper back. The nurse suspects that the patient may be experiencing disseminated intravascular coagulation (DIC) and anticipates orders for which laboratory studies?

a. PT, PTT, CBC, Fibrinogen
b. BNP, Lipase, Amylase
c. CBC, Ferritin, Hgb
d. BMP, CBC, Type and Screen

157. A nurse is discussing a POLST form with a patient who is transitioning to hospice care. Which of the following statements by the client indicates a need for further education?

a. "It is important for me to participate in advanced planning and communicate my wishes since I am seriously ill."
b. "This is a legal document relaying my wishes if I am unable to make decisions."
c. "This form is 'portable' and can communicate my wishes regardless of the care setting."
d. "This will help translate my wishes for CPR, intubation, and artificial nutrition if I am unable to communicate for myself."

158. A nurse is working in an outpatient oncology clinic that prides itself on having a culture of safety. The nurse understands that this includes which of the following?

a. Investigations of errors to understand who should take the blame
b. Hiring employees with strong skills to reduce the need for training opportunities
c. Slow response time to safety concerns to understand if a pattern is in place
d. Implementation of policies and procedures that support safe care

159. A nurse is counseling a patient who has completed radiation for tonsillar cancer about long-term effects of treatment. The nurse should include which of the following?

a. "Since the radiation was directed at your tonsils, you are not at higher risk for osteoradionecrosis."
b. "Long-term side effects can include dry mouth and gum disease, so regular dental check-ups are important."
c. "The radiation treatment may impact your eyesight, so it is important to have regular check-ups with an eye doctor."
d. "It is important to use regular mouth rinses of salt and water even after treatment ends."

160. The clinic nurse is performing an intake assessment on a transgender patient recently diagnosed with prostate cancer. The patient tells the nurse, "I am afraid that no one will be able to lead me in the right direction when I start chemotherapy. As a transgender person, I already struggle with finding unbiased medical care as it is." Which is the best follow-up intervention by the nurse?

a. Provide the patient with a list of community support groups.
b. Request a consult for a patient navigator.
c. Inform the provider that the patient is undecided about receiving treatment.
d. Explain treatment options to the patient.

161. A nurse receives a phone call from the family of a patient in hospice. The family reports that the patient has been restless today and has suffered from ongoing nausea. The nurse recommends that the family administer which previously prescribed medication?

a. Acetaminophen
b. Atropine
c. Morphine
d. Lorazepam

162. Immunotherapy uses the body's own defenses to target cancer cells. Which of the following is NOT one of the pathways that is used in immunotherapy?

a. Antivirals
b. T-cells and B-cells
c. Lymph nodes
d. Cytokines

163. A nurse navigator is preparing educational information for a community health fair. Which statement about modifiable risk factors should be included?

a. Tobacco use increases the risk of several cancers, including liver, bladder, and pancreas.
b. Consuming three or more servings of vegetables daily is associated with a lower risk of breast cancer.
c. Occupational exposure for steel workers increases the risk for prostate cancer.
d. Increased alcohol consumption is linked to kidney cancer.

164. Which of the following is true regarding sarcoma metastasis?

a. Sarcoma has a good prognosis when metastases are present.
b. Brain metastases are very common with sarcoma.
c. The axial skeleton is a common site for early metastasis.
d. Distant metastases are associated with less aggressive disease.

165. The nurse is taking care of a patient with newly diagnosed stage 3 lung cancer who is head of the household. The patient tells the nurse, "My doctor told me I can't work while receiving treatment, but I have to provide for my spouse and two children. I am feeling very stressed." Which is the best intervention by the nurse?

a. Encourage the patient to clarify the instructions from their doctor.
b. Educate the patient on the risks of refusing treatment.
c. Provide the patient with a list of local service organizations.
d. Call the patient's spouse to discuss the concerns.

Answer Explanations #2

1. D: Immunotherapy medications work by stimulating the body's immune system to attack cancer cells; however, sometimes the immune system will attack healthy tissue of the lungs, resulting in pneumonitis. Pneumonitis is swelling and irritation of the lungs that can affect patients after treatment has ended. Symptoms include a dry, unproductive cough, shortness of breath, and chest pain when taking a breath. Choices *A*, *B*, and *C* are incorrect.

2. D: There are two categories of causes for thrombocytopenia: immunologic and nonimmunologic. A viral infection is considered an immunologic cause as the immune system is weakened by the viral infection and thrombocyte levels drop as a result. Nonimmunological causes arise from a source outside of the immune system, such as sepsis and acute respiratory distress syndrome. Folate deficiency is unrelated to thrombocytopenia but rather a cause for anemia.

3. C: Differentiation is the process of maturing to carry out a particular function. Cancer cells grow and divide too rapidly to fully mature; therefore, they do not differentiate. Cancer cells can influence growth of vasculature toward tumors, do not stop growing when they encounter other cells, and ignore signals to stop growing or dividing (apoptosis or cell death). Therefore, Choices *A*, *B,* and *D* are incorrect.

4. C: Losing 1/5 or 20% percent of one's blood volume will throw a person into hypovolemic shock and is considered life-threatening. Organ failure with profound hypotension will likely follow; fluid resuscitation and blood transfusions will be needed as soon as possible.

5. B: Neoadjuvant therapy consists of chemotherapy or radiation that is administered before surgery to improve the margins of or reduce the size of a tumor. This can lead to better success in surgery. Choice *A* is incorrect because neoadjuvant therapy is not done before restorative surgery. Choice *C* is incorrect because neoadjuvant therapy itself involves chemotherapy and/or radiation, not a preparation for them. Choice *D* is incorrect because neoadjuvant therapy is not always part of a treatment plan that includes surgery.

6. C: The nadir is the time frame in which blood cell counts are lowest after cytotoxic chemotherapy. The nadir can vary but generally occurs seven to ten days after administration of cytotoxic chemotherapy. Choice *A* is incorrect since pancytopenia refers to the actual low counts of white cells, red cells, and platelets in the blood, not what the specific time frame is called. Choice *B* is also incorrect since neutropenia describes a low white blood cell level which may be a result of cytotoxic chemotherapy, but it is not the name of the time frame in which it happens. Choice *D*, hematopoiesis, refers to the process of blood cell production.

7. A: A patient with an ANC of 500 cells/mcL is severely neutropenic and at high risk of infection. Since neutropenic patients' immune systems are unable to defend against infection, a temperature of 100.4°F or higher may be a sign of infection. This patient takes priority over the patients listed in Choices *B*, *C*, and *D*.

8. B: Time, distance, and shielding are principles that guide radiation safety. It is most important to reduce the time of exposure, increase distance from the radiation source, and have effective shielding. Choices *A*, *C*, and *D* are incorrect since they do not correctly list the radiation safety principles for providers.

9. C: Anthracyclines, such as doxorubicin, carry a risk of cardiotoxicities after completion of therapy, sometimes up to twenty-five years later. The risk of developing anthracycline-associated cardiotoxicity increases with the total cumulative dose. Other drugs that increase the risk of late-effect cardiotoxicities include trastuzumab, high-dose cyclophosphamide, mitomycin, and platinum agents. Choices *A, B,* and *D* do not carry high risk for cardiotoxicities.

10. C: Personal history of inflammatory bowel disease, including Crohn's disease, increases the risk of colon cancer. This is due to prolonged inflammation of the colon over time. Therefore, patients with IBD should start screening earlier. Choice *A* is incorrect since limiting the intake of alcohol to no more than one drink per day for women or two drinks per day for men does not increase the risk for colon cancer. Choice *B* exhibits no familial history of colon cancer, and a breast cancer diagnosis over the age of 50 is not alarming for hereditary conditions. Choice *D* shows regular physical activity, which reduces the risk of colon cancer.

11. D: Choice *D* is the best response by the nurse because the statement encourages patient advocacy and ensures that all treatment options are discussed with the patient. Choice *A* is not the best response by the nurse because the statement ignores the patient's concern and provides false reassurance. Choice *B* is not the best response by the nurse because the statement disregards other treatment options and negatively validates the patient's fear. Choice *C* is not the best response because the patient's immediate concerns about her illness and treatment options cannot be addressed by her support systems.

12. B: Bereavement is the state of experiencing loss of a person, relationship, or possession. It can entail loss, grief, and the associated processes. Grief, not bereavement, is commonly thought of as the process through which a person responds to loss. The nurse can provide education regarding the terminology to assist the patient's husband in processing the loss. Choices *A, C,* and *D* are all accurate statements.

13. A: When a patient is receiving vincristine, they should be prescribed a prophylactic stool softener to prevent gastrointestinal motility disorders and ileus. A patient who is receiving RCHOP without a stool softener regime is likely to develop a paralytic ileus, which may present with abdominal pain, constipation, and abdominal distress. Choices *B, C,* and *D* are not represented by the scenario.

14. B: In an emergency situation, an autocratic style of leadership, where there is a clear leader who has control of the situation, is often the most effective. In this case, there is a limited number of nurses on the floor who have experience with chemotherapy, so it would be best for the floating nurse to take control of the situation. While they may be effective leadership styles in other cases, Choices *A, C,* and *D* are not the most appropriate choices for this scenario.

15. C: Deconditioning is the term for muscle wasting and debilitation caused by bedrest. Immobility is the limited ability to move freely, which may lead to deconditioning. Decompression syndrome is a physiological condition caused by a rapid decrease in surrounding pressure and is unrelated to these symptoms. Debilitation describes a loss of strength, not necessarily muscle wasting, and thus is not the best choice to explain the described changes.

16. D: Tobacco use is linked to over fifteen types of cancers. However, it has not been linked to lymphoma. The risk for bladder, liver, pancreatic, leukemia, and many other solid tumor cancers are directly linked to tobacco use. It is important to recommend and support smoking cessation to patients at every point of the care continuum.

17. B: Allogeneic is correct, as this comes from a healthy related or unrelated donor. Choice *A* is incorrect because the patient themselves would be the donor in an autologous donation. Choices *C* and *D* are not names of hematopoietic stem cell sources.

18. C: Fatigue is a common side effect of many treatments; while some patients see improvement after the completion of treatment, many patients experience fatigue that lingers for months or years after. Physical activity (specifically at least 150 minutes of moderate activity or 75 minutes of vigorous activity per week) can help to lessen the fatigue. Fatigue may persist despite normalization of lab values, making Choice *A* incorrect. Choice *B* is incorrect because patients should be counseled to return to normal activity as soon as possible, rest appropriately, and avoid caffeine. Choice *D* is incorrect because fatigue after treatment is normal, and there are limited tests to determine causes of fatigue.

19. B: Low blood pressure that occurs when a patient changes position from sitting to standing is called postural hypotension and may be caused by cardiac or neurological disease. Postprandial hypotension results after one eats. Neural hypotension arises from neurological deficits and is not positional. Hypovolemic hypotension is a type of low blood pressure that is caused by low circulating blood volume.

20. C: The patient should be instructed to have a dental exam before starting treatment and develop an effective and consistent oral hygiene regimen. Choice *A* is incorrect since using a hard toothbrush can break down the oral mucosa and cause irritation. Choice *B* is incorrect since alcohol-based mouth rinses can be painful and do not prevent mucositis. Choice *D* is incorrect since lidocaine mouth rinses also cannot prevent mucositis.

21. A: Distributive justice refers to the allocation of scarce resources, and advocacy is support for policies that protect at-risk populations. The nurse understands that scarce resource allocation may be sub-standard in certain populations. In nursing, nonmaleficence refers to the act of inflicting the least amount of harm possible in order to reach a favorable result. Fidelity refers to faithfulness but does not specifically address resources or the patient population.

22. D: Tumor lysis syndrome is characterized by an increase in uric acid levels triggered by acute cell lysis from cancer treatment. Patients are treated with rasburicase or allopurinol and aggressive hydration. Choices *A*, *B*, and *C* are incorrect.

23. D: Hospice care is based on the understanding that death is a natural part of the life cycle, and quality of life should be promoted for the patient and their caregivers during this time. This is accomplished through care for physical, psychosocial, and spiritual symptoms. Choice *A* is incorrect because hospice will provide medical equipment and supplies, including a hospital bed. There is no limit to the amount of time a person can spend in hospice, but they do need to have regular reassessments to meet eligibility criteria, making Choice *B* incorrect. Hospice care does focus on pain and symptom control; however, patients may not be simultaneously undergoing treatment. Therefore, Choice *C* is incorrect.

24. D: A core needle biopsy entails using a needle to extract a small piece of tissue for examination by a pathologist to determine diagnosis. Choice *A* refers to an excisional biopsy, in which the goal is complete removal of the tumor for pathology. Choice *B* refers to a fine needle aspiration, while Choice *C* describes a bone marrow biopsy.

25. C: Expert nurses are those who reach the point in their clinical practice where clinical reasoning and inquiry are intertwined, allowing the nurse to make clinical judgements quickly and appropriately, according to best practice standards.

26. A: Oxygen administration can help reduce dyspnea, and raising the head of the bed can reduce the work of breathing by better allowing the chest to expand. Choices *B* and *C* are incorrect since administering prescribed medication, including inhalers and anxiolytics, is important but should not be the first intervention. Choice *D* can increase the comfort of the patient but is not a priority intervention for dyspnea.

27. B: Germline mutations are mutations found in the DNA of egg or sperm cells and are present at conception. These mutations are passed to future generations. Choice *A* is incorrect, as it is somatic cell mutations that accumulate over an extended time. Germline mutations are incorporated into every type of tissue, resulting in the potential for malignancy in multiple tissue types, making Choice *C* incorrect. Choice *D* is incorrect, as germline mutations are commonly associated with malignancies in those under 50 years of age.

28. B: Individuals with certain malignancies (especially brain, breast, pancreatic, and lung) are at higher-than-average risk for deep vein thrombosis and venous thromboembolism. Chemotherapy and the presence of venous access devices can increase that risk further. Unilateral edema of a limb with possible associated warmth, erythema, and tenderness indicates a likely DVT in the affected extremity.

29. A: Stomach cancer does not have a routine screening activity associated with diagnosis. For men between 55 and 69 years of age, PSA testing is used to screen for prostate cancer. A low-dose CT is used to screen for lung cancer in men and women with significant smoking history. HPV tests and Pap smears are used to screen for cervical cancer between 21 and 65 years of age. Therefore, Choices *B, C,* and *D* are incorrect.

30. C: Choice *C* is the best response by the nurse because the question encourages the patient to talk openly about their feelings and promotes therapeutic communication. Choice *A* is not the best response by the nurse because stating a fact of therapy does not address the patient's concern. Choice *B* is not the best response by the nurse because the question encourages the patient to think about ending necessary medical treatment before other interventions are explored. Choice *D* is not the best response by the nurse because the statement speaks negatively about the patient's partner.

31. C: Early signs of increasing intracranial pressure include confusion, behavior changes, and headache. Vomiting and pupillary or vision changes are considered late indications of intracranial pressure, making Choices *A*, *B*, and *D* incorrect.

32. A: Using compression can move fluids toward the trunk of the body where they can be removed and processed. Choices *B*, *C*, and *D* are incorrect, as these interventions would only further increase the lymphedema.

33. A: Negligence is an unintended deviation from a professional standard of care. By not documenting communication, plan, intervention, or resolution of symptomatic hypotension, the nurse has no proof that attention was provided to this patient in the presence of abnormal findings. Choice *B* refers to making false statements to harm the reputation of another and is incorrect. Choice *C* is a defamatory statement made verbally and is incorrect. Choice *D* refers to the right that patients have to privacy and the expectation of confidentiality. The nurse did not violate privacy, so Choice *D* is incorrect.

34. C: CPIs restore the ability of T-cells to recognize the tumor by disrupting proteins and eliminating its ability to cloak itself. Choices *A*, *B*, and *D* are incorrect, as these answers do not depict how CPIs work with the body's immune system.

35. C: Choice *C* is the best response by the nurse because speaking with other people who share the same experience and understand the condition can bring comfort and support to the patient. Choice *A* is not the best response by the nurse because asking if there is someone else who is willing to listen deflects from the patient's concern. Choice *B* is not the best response by the nurse because the statement places blame on the patient and does not promote therapeutic communication. Choice *D* is not the best response by the nurse because asking the patient to explain a lack of understanding by others does not address the main concern.

36. A: Suicidal ideation, Choice *A*, is critical to report to the patient's provider. Suicidal ideation is an infrequent side effect of antidepressants but can result in the patient's death. It is important to stop a medication that is causing this side effect. Choices *B*, *C*, and *D* are all possible side effects that warrant discussion with the provider; however, they are not the most important side effects to report.

37. D: Even though patients are no longer receiving active treatment, it can take time for the body to heal and recover. Many patients and family members are unprepared for the extended recovery time. It is important for them to understand the timeframe to lessen worry, frustration, and disappointment. Choices *A*, *B*, and *C* all indicate understanding of the time that will likely be required to heal.

38. B: Patients hospitalized for management of spinal cord compression are often on bed rest with log-rolling techniques and use of neutral spine alignments to protect the spinal cord. Nurses should collaborate with the team, including physicians and physical therapists, before ambulating patients. Choice *A*, *C*, and *D* are all examples of collaborative care of patients with spinal cord compression.

39. A: Proton therapy is usually reserved for central nervous system, ocular, and skull-based cancers because it is the most precise. Choices *B*, *C*, and *D* are not typically treated with proton therapy.

40. B: Palliative care is used to maintain or improve quality of life for patients with a life threatening or terminal disease. The treatments included in palliative care are not curative. Choices *A*, *B*, and *C* are all incorrect. Pain and symptom management are used in palliative care to increase quality of life. Establishing the values and priorities of a patient is crucial when engaged in palliative care. The patient determines the goals and what they consider to be quality of life.

41. A: Platinum-based chemotherapies, such as carboplatin, are frequently associated with hypersensitivity reactions. These drugs are associated with a high risk of hypersensitivity (10%–27%) that almost always occurs after several courses of treatment. Choices *B*, *C*, and *D* have less frequent hypersensitivity reactions.

42. A: Bleomycin, doxorubicin, and vinblastine are chemotherapies that predispose a patient to pulmonary toxicities. When combined with radiation to the lungs, the risk of toxicities increases. Choice *B* is incorrect because the patient is a never smoker, which lessens the risk for pulmonary toxicities. Female patients who are over seventy years of age are at higher risk for pulmonary toxicities, making Choices *C* and *D* incorrect.

43. B: The Gleason score is a grading system used in prostate cancer to predict the aggressiveness of the tumor. The lower the score, the less aggressive the cancer is thought to be. The Gleason score is not used for colorectal, renal cell, or testicular cancers, making Choices *A, C,* and *D* incorrect.

44. C: Applying mild corticosteroid cream is the first line treatment for radiation dermatitis. Choice *A* is incorrect since lotions with any fragrances or harsh chemicals should be avoided. Choice *B* is incorrect since antimicrobial soap should not be used, as it is typically harsher on skin. Soap that has a pH of 5 can be used safely on radiation dermatitis. Choice *D* is incorrect because oral antihistamines have not been shown to have any symptom relief or benefit for radiation dermatitis.

45. C: Financial stress and employment obligations are risk factors for burnout in caregivers. In addition to the financial strains of treatment and travel to treatment centers, many caregivers are not able to maintain productivity and need to reduce work hours to manage. Choices *A* and *B* indicate that there is support available for the wife, lessening the concern for burnout. Choice *D* alludes to sleep disturbances; however, the wife indicates that she has experienced this before and has the means to cope with it, lessening the concern for burnout.

46. C: Cyclophosphamide and ifosfamide both have toxicity that can result in hemorrhagic cystitis. Choice *A* is incorrect since carboplatin and cisplatin can cause renal toxicity. Choice *B* is incorrect, as bleomycin and mitomycin are associated with pulmonary toxicity and injury. Choice *D* is also incorrect; doxorubicin and daunorubicin are well known for their cardiotoxicity.

47. D: Studies have not shown that CAM therapies reduce cancer proliferation. However, Choices *A*, *B*, and *C* have all been proven to be benefits of meditation for cancer patients.

48. C: Superior vena cava syndrome occurs due to compression of the superior vena cava where it enters the right atrium, resulting in edema and retrograde blood flow. The compression and obstruction of blood flow causes collateral veins to form in the neck, the axillary vessels to dilate, and the jugular vein to distend. Facial swelling is the most common symptom of SVC syndrome. Patients may also present with symptoms such as cough, dyspnea at rest, hoarseness, chest and shoulder pain, and swelling or discoloration of the neck and upper extremities. Choices *A, B*, and *D* are not represented by the scenario.

49. D: Troponin is a muscle cell protein that is released when cardiac tissue is broken down during an ischemic event. Elevated levels of troponin in the bloodstream indicate cardiac muscle damage. Creatinine and BUN are waste products of the body, and higher levels of these in the bloodstream indicate kidney failure or damage, not heart damage. Creatine kinase is an enzyme found in muscle tissue. One form of the enzyme, CK-MB, is a cardiac enzyme, but its structure is similar to creatine kinase found in skeletal muscle. Therefore, it's a less specific indicator of cardiac muscle damage.

50. B: The patient should be instructed to drink plenty of fluids to help flush the kidneys. Choice *A* is incorrect; low intake of fluids can cause toxins to build up in the kidneys, causing further damage. Choice *C* is incorrect, as the patient should void as needed. It is not necessary to void more often than needed. Choice *D* is also incorrect. While monitoring for signs and symptoms of kidney dysfunction is important, it is not the most important intervention for the patient to learn.

51. A: DNA vector processes are used to program T-cells with tumor antigen receptors. Choices *B, C,* and *D* are incorrect and are not used in CAR-T treatment.

52. B: The nurse suspects that the IV has infiltrated, meaning the catheter tip has become dislodged and IV medication and/or fluids are leaking into the surrounding tissues. The nurse should stop the infusion, remove the IV, and dress the site. An allergic reaction or infection would be warm, not cold, due to the inflammatory response present in such conditions. This is not a normal assessment of a peripheral IV.

53. A: Parallel group designs have participants randomized to one of several treatment groups, and each group is administered a different intervention. This is opposed to crossover design (Choice *B*), where participants receive more than one treatment, but the order is randomized. Factorial design (Choice *C*) allows multiple factors to be studied simultaneously. Randomized withdrawal design (Choice *D*) allows all participants to receive an experimental treatment during the first phase. In the second phase, non-responders are dropped, and the remaining participants are randomized to receive either the intervention or a placebo.

54. A: Asking questions regarding patient preference rather than making assumptions is important in providing culturally congruent care. Choice *B* is incorrect because the nurse should ask the patient about their preference instead of researching. Choice *C* is incorrect because, whenever possible, family members should not be interpreting information to the patient. It is unnecessary to speak in a different manner than the nurse would for an English-speaking patient, so Choice *D* is incorrect.

55. B: Myeloid growth factors are medications that stimulate myeloid cells to produce more red cells and white cells. This can help reduce or alleviate myelosuppression. Choice *A* is incorrect, as anticoagulants are contraindicated in patients with low platelet counts. Choice *C* is incorrect; while antibiotics may be used prophylactically to prevent infection, they will not stimulate an increase in blood cells. Choice *D* is also incorrect; while these blood products can increase blood cells to safe levels, they do not stimulate the production of white cells, red cells, or platelets by the patient's body.

56. C: A non-coring needle is used to puncture through the skin and into the self-sealing septum of the implanted port. Choice *A* is incorrect, as this cannot access an implanted port by itself. Choice *B* is incorrect, as a butterfly needle should not be used to access the port. Choice *D* is also incorrect since peripheral intravenous catheters will cause damage to the self-sealing septum of the port.

57. A: Choice *A* is the best action by the nurse because encouraging the patient to discuss future reconstructive surgery with their physician will provide options for sexual activity. A total pelvic exenteration removes all organs within the pelvic cavity, including the vagina. Choice *B* is not the best action by the nurse because the nurse cannot predict the patient's recovery or promote false reassurance. Choice *C* is not the best intervention by the nurse because the action does not address the patient's concerns regarding intimacy. Choice *D* is not the best action by the nurse because the intervention ignores the patient's main concern regarding intimacy.

58. A: Physiatry is a recognized medical specialty that aids in the treatment of pain; therefore, it is not an alternative therapy. Choices *B*, *C*, and *D* are all effective alternative treatments for pain management.

59. B: Small-molecule inhibitors are able to penetrate cell membranes and target intracellular molecules due to their molecular size. Choice *A* is incorrect because small-molecule inhibitors target smaller intracellular molecules. Choice *C* is incorrect; bioavailability is lessened in small-molecule inhibitors because of the typical oral route of administration. Choice *D* is incorrect; while some monoclonal antibodies are derived from living sources, others are made in labs.

60. A: Favorable prognostic factors for esophageal cancer include early-stage disease and complete resection. Stage II is still considered early stage, making Choice *B* incorrect. Choice *C* is associated with higher mortality rates; therefore, it is not a positive prognostic indicator. Choice *D* refers to risk factors for development of esophageal cancer, not prognosis; thus, it is incorrect.

61. C: Patients with thrombocytopenia should always wear shoes to avoid injury to the feet. Choices *A*, *B*, and *D* are all incorrect. Bleeding precautions include using a soft toothbrush, implementing a bowel regimen to avoid constipation, only using electric razors, preparing the environment to reduce fall risk, and avoiding activity that can result in bleeding.

62. B: Accidental chemotherapy exposure increases the risk for malignancies in nursing staff and can result in embryo-fetal toxicities in pregnant nurses. Choice *A* is incorrect; while accidental exposure can result in contact dermatitis, it is not the most significant problem with exposure. Choices *C* and *D* are incorrect because neurological changes and heart rhythm changes are not significant complications associated with accidental chemotherapy exposure.

63. B: The patient should follow hygienic techniques to assist in eliminating sources of infection, including wiping front to back after using the restroom. Choice *A* is incorrect because the patient does not need to always stay inside their house. However, they may choose to wear a mask around others who may be sick or when around crowds. Choice *C* is incorrect, as this would expose the patient to more possible sources of infection. Choice *D* is incorrect because it is not important to cut fingernails or toenails to monitor skin integrity. In fact, if the skin was nicked by clippers, the wound could provide an opportunity for infection.

64. C: HRT has been linked to an increased risk of breast cancer in post-menopausal women, who are also more likely to be diagnosed with advanced disease. HRT has been linked to a slightly higher risk of ovarian cancer, making Choice *A* incorrect. Choice *B* is incorrect because long-term use of HRT has not been shown to increase the risk of lung cancer. Choice *D* is incorrect because estrogen may have a role in preventing colorectal cancer, but it has not been shown to have an impact on pancreatic cancer.

65. C: Choice *C* is the best action for the nurse to take because the caregiver's statement suggests burnout. Delegating tasks to family and friends will assist the caregiver with completing their daily routine. Choice *A* is not the best action by the nurse because prioritizing daily errands does not correct the issue of caregiver burnout. Choice *B* is not the best action by the nurse because this statement advocates for the caregiver's needs only. Choice *D* is not the best action by the nurse because the caregiver's statement does not suggest a lack of understanding about the importance of taking care of their loved one.

66. B: Pain, burning, stinging, and erythema are common with extravasation. Early recognition and intervention at the site can minimize damage. The infusion should immediately be stopped and the line aspirated to remove as much drug from the site as possible and limit tissue exposure.

67. A: The creation of goals happens in the outcome identification phase. The nurse recognizes that early ambulation is an expected outcome for a post-operative patient. The planning phase involves prescribing strategies to attain the goals, which have not yet been identified in this scenario; therefore, Choice *C* is incorrect. After the planning phase is completed, the nurse moves into the implementation phase, and the plan is carried out, which makes Choice *B* incorrect. Assessment is the first step in the nursing process, in which the nurse gathers necessary data and information. In this scenario, the assessment phase is not the active phase in place, making Choice *D* incorrect.

68. D: Performing cognitive training can contribute to improved cognition. Choices *A* and *B* are incorrect because increasing nutritional supplements and using stimulants have not been shown to improve cognition in cancer patients. Choice *C* is also incorrect. Avoiding exercise will not help improve cognition; in fact, regular exercise may help with cognition.

69. A: Marrow ablative conditioning is used to prepare a patient for bone marrow transplantation. Choices *B, C,* and *D* are incorrect because these are not associated with bone marrow transplants.

70. A: Resting and turning every two hours should be avoided and replaced with resistance exercise. Choices *B, C,* and *D* are all incorrect and should not be avoided by the patient. Studies show that resistance training with nutritional support and the use of hormone therapy allows the patient to improve muscle mass.

71. C: The Joint Commission provides accreditation for healthcare organizations to ensure the delivery of safe, high-quality patient care. They conduct unannounced surveys where surveyors may pull patient records and trace their care through the clinic, often asking questions of doctors, nurses, and other staff who have interacted with the patients. Choice *A* most closely aligns with Magnet Recognition, which is focused on an organization's commitment to nursing care and scope of practice. Choice *B* refers to National Cancer Institute (NCI) accreditation, which focuses on research standards in cancer care. Choice *D* refers to the Quality Oncology Practice Initiative (QOPI), which focuses on outpatient hematology-oncology practices in the United States by comparing practice performance against quality measures and standards established by experts in oncology.

72. D: Paclitaxel is a chemotherapy drug that is known to cause infusion reactions, resulting in flushing, chills, back pain, difficulty breathing, hypotension, and a scratchy feeling in the throat. The reactions can quickly progress to anaphylaxis, represented by tightness in the chest, bronchospasm, and shortness of breath. The priority intervention is to stop the drug and notify the provider immediately for further orders. Choice *A* is incorrect, as these symptoms are more likely to indicate an infusion reaction than an anxiety reaction. Choice *B* is incorrect, as the infusion should be stopped rather than slowed. Choice *C* is incorrect, as the provider should be contacted before administering additional medications.

73. C: Hypoxia should be treated with supplemental oxygen, and pulmonary edema should be treated with intravenous furosemide, a diuretic. Choice *A*, obtaining an arterial blood gas, is not the priority intervention to reduce dyspnea or improve oxygen saturation. Choice *B* is incorrect since fluids should be stopped and the doctor consulted if pulmonary edema occurs. Choice *D*, managing hypertension, is also incorrect. While hypertension may occur with pulmonary edema, it is not the priority intervention to reduce dyspnea or increase oxygen saturation.

74. A: Choice *A*, biological characteristics, is not used as a diagnostic to determine the appropriate biotherapy for a patient. Choices *B, C,* and *D* are not correct because they are all included in labeling instructions from the FDA for biotherapy and corresponding diagnostic tests.

75. C: Opioids do not provide relief for neuropathic pain and are higher risk medications. Choices *A, B,* and *D* are all incorrect choices since they are used in the treatment of peripheral neuropathy and neuropathic pain.

76. D: Effective self-care activities require the nurse to have the skills and knowledge to manage their stress. While many nurses still view self-care as getting pedicures and massages, other interventions such as aromatherapy, mindfulness practices, and art therapy have been shown to improve nursing resilience and act as effective tools for healthy coping. Therefore, Choice *D* is not an evidence-based self-care practice.

77. D: To reduce swelling, the patient should elevate the extremities above the level of the heart. This uses gravity to help return the fluid into the circulation. Choice *A* is incorrect, as loose-fitting clothing will not affect swelling. Instead, using compression stockings or TED hose will assist in reducing swelling. Choice *B* is incorrect, as standing will cause more fluid to collect in the lower legs. Choice C is also incorrect, as following a diabetic diet will not help to reduce swelling. Instead, a heart healthy, low sodium diet is recommended for these patients.

78. C: Since the client is newly diagnosed, assessing barriers to care is the most sensible next step. Choice *A* is incorrect because education on prevention is currently not the most appropriate step. Choice *B* refers to the diagnosis phase—which the client has already gone through—making this an incorrect choice. Choice *D* is an appropriate step for a client who has completed treatment and is entering the surveillance phase. It is not the best discussion for someone who is newly diagnosed.

79. C: Peritoneal catheters are placed at the level of the umbilicus and directed downward to allow for more distribution within the peritoneal cavity. Choices *A*, *B*, and *D* are all characteristics of peritoneal catheters.

80. B: Choice *B* should be the first action by the nurse because the patient has expressed suicidal ideation with a plan. Immediate counseling services are needed to assess the patient's mental and emotional state. Choice *A* is not the correct immediate action by the nurse because the next of kin should be contacted after ensuring the patient's safety and only if consent for contact is obtained from the patient. Choice *C* is not the correct immediate action by the nurse because the patient is voicing suicidal ideation with a plan. Asking about the length of their symptoms does not immediately assist in crisis management. Choice *D* is not the correct immediate action because documentation of the patient's statement should occur after the patient's safety is secured and all other interventions have been performed.

81. B: Administration of megestrol can increase a patient's appetite, which would be helpful to improve the patient's condition. Choice *A* is incorrect. The patient should be encouraged to consume five to six small meals each day; however, their appetite may prevent this amount of consumption. Choices *C* and *D* are incorrect. Sugar-free vitamin drinks will not provide enough nutrition, and a high-fat diet will not provide enough variation in nutrition. The patient should be encouraged to consume nutritional supplement drinks and snacks that are high in protein and calories.

82. D: HPV has been linked to multiple cancers, including anal, bladder, cervical, head and neck, penile, vaginal, and vulvar cancers. Choice *A* refers to cancers linked to the hepatitis virus. Choice *B* refers to cancers linked to *Helicobacter pylori* infections. Choice *C* refers to cancers associated with human immunodeficiency virus (HIV) infections.

83. C: Double mastectomy in BRCA1 or BRCA2 positive patients is the most effective option for preventing breast cancer. Choice *A* is incorrect because MRI and mammograms may catch this type of cancer too late and are not the best option. Choice *B* is incorrect; although there are medications that can reduce the risk in this population, they are not as effective. Healthy lifestyle changes are good but cannot prevent breast cancer; therefore, Choice *D* is incorrect.

84. D: It is crucial to size and cut the wafer to the appropriate size, which prevents stool from having contact with the skin and causing skin breakdown. While Choices *A* and *B* are important for stool management with an ostomy, they are not the most important part of preventing skin breakdown around the ostomy site. Choice *C* is incorrect since the bag should be changed every five to seven days. More frequent changes can cause skin breakdown of the ostomy site.

85. B: Tumor lysis syndrome is a rare but life-threatening complication of chemotherapy and typically occurs when cancer cells are killed rapidly, leading to the release of metabolic byproducts and intracellular ions within 12 to 72 hours of initial therapy. The release of tumor intracellular contents leads to rapidly induced electrolyte imbalances, including hyperkalemia, hyperphosphatemia, hypocalcemia, and hyperuricemia. The nurse would expect to treat the patient with aggressive IV hydration to protect kidney function, administer allopurinol or rasburicase to reduce uric acid, and treat the electrolyte abnormalities. Choice *B* correctly represents hyperkalemia, hyperphosphatemia, and hypocalcemia. Choices *A*, *C*, and *D* do not represent the lab values associated with tumor lysis syndrome.

86. B: Vascular endothelial growth factor (VEGF) is a growth factor that is upregulated in cancer cells, allowing for the growth of blood vessels to the tumor. Choices *A*, *C*, and *D* are types of receptors found on the cell that allow for increased cell division but are not specific to angiogenesis.

87. C: An echocardiogram can determine how well the heart is functioning at baseline, including ejection fraction, and would be used prior to starting biotherapy. Choices *A* and *B* are incorrect because these tests would not identify existing heart failure. Choice *D* is also incorrect because this test would not provide imaging about the function of the heart.

88. C: Discussions about sexuality related to cancer and cancer treatments should be factual and normalized. Sexuality is not limited to intercourse; it also includes sexual response, sexual self-concept, and sexual/intimate relationships. It is also not defined by a particular age range; therefore, Choice *A* is incorrect. Nurses should bring up the information directly and address the patient's questions. Asking patients to call later is not therapeutic, making Choice *B* incorrect. Many patients are hesitant to ask questions about sexual function for many reasons, including embarrassment, lack of education, and belief that it is the clinician's role to bring up the topic. Nurses should bring up the topic and provide space for open communication, making Choice *D* incorrect.

89. D: In advanced stages of cancer, even when the prognosis is poor, chemotherapy may be able to manage pain and suffering. Choices *A*, *B*, and *C* are not correct, because the chance of remission, cure, or halting the advance of cancer in advanced stages with a poor prognosis is low, and the nurse should not give the patient false hope.

90. D: Choice *D* is the best action because the patient's physical status and medical treatment is complex. The nurse recognizes that there is a high likelihood of caregiver stress, and providing a resource guide will offer support to the caregiver. Choice *A* is not the best action because there is no indication that the caregiver needs financial assistance with transportation. Choice *B* is not the best action because there is no indication that the patient is uninsured. Choice *C* is not the best action because home health services require a provider order and provide specialized services. The caregiver will be responsible to provide care to the patient around the clock.

91. C: Patients should experiment with spices and flavoring to see what is appealing. Choice *A* is incorrect, as spicy food may be harmful to the oral mucosa. Choice *B* is also incorrect, as meat can also be unappetizing and alternative sources of protein should be explored. Choice *D* is also incorrect because the patient should eat moist food, including soups and gravies.

92. A: An Ommaya reservoir allows for long-term access to cerebral spinal fluid. Choices *B*, *C*, and *D* are not ways to access the cerebral spinal fluid.

93. D: Agitation and grimacing are often signs of patient discomfort, and patients can experience air hunger at the end of life. Morphine is used to address both symptoms, so it would be a reasonable choice of medication. Choice *A* is incorrect because an oral medication is not appropriate for a minimally responsive patient. Choice *B* is incorrect because the patient is not experiencing nausea. Although sometimes used to address pain, dexamethasone would not help with agitation and can often worsen it; therefore, Choice *C* is incorrect.

94. B: Hypercalcemia, presenting with a serum calcium level of more than 10.5 mg/dL, occurs in roughly a quarter of patients with cancer. It is often associated with multiple myeloma, and symptoms include progressive decline in mental function, weakness, anorexia, thirst, constipation, and nausea. Choices *A*, *C*, and *D* are not represented by the scenario and lab values.

95. B: As patient advocates, it is important for nurses to listen to and respect patients' wishes. By providing further education and requesting that the doctor come speak to the patient about changing code status, the nurse is giving the patient the tools and support to make the decision that is best for them. In Choices *A, C,* and *D,* the nurse is not respecting the patient's autonomy and decision making, thus exemplifying poor examples of advocacy.

96. A: Liver cancer uses TNM classification. TNM is a system used to describe the amount and spread of cancer in the body using largest tumor size, extent of lymph node involvement, and presence of distant metastasis. Brain and spinal cord, leukemia, and gynecological cancer use alternative classification systems. Therefore, Choices *B*, *C*, and *D* are incorrect.

97. D: It is important to protect hands and feet of patients with neuropathy from extreme temperatures. Not only can the sensations be uncomfortable, they can also result in injuries, including burns. Choice *A* is incorrect, as massaging or stimulating the areas affected by neuropathy will cause discomfort. Choice *B* is incorrect, as wearing tight clothes will cause more stimulation and therefore more discomfort. Choice *C* is incorrect since extreme temperatures should be avoided.

98. C: The patient would need marrow ablative therapy before infusion, and the hospital is where the patient will be during that process as well as during the period of marrow aplasia. Choices *A*, *B*, and *D* are not appropriate settings for a marrow transplant.

99. D: A diagnosis of prostate or breast cancer in an individual with Ashkenazi Jewish heritage indicates a need for genetic testing due to the risk of BRCA gene mutation. Colorectal cancer is associated with a genetic link when diagnosed in people under 50 years old, meaning Choice *A* is not an indication for genetic testing. Prostate cancer is associated with a genetic link when diagnosed in men younger than 65 years old or when a patient is metastatic at diagnosis, making Choice *B* incorrect. For familial traits, cousins are considered third-degree relatives and are at a lower risk for a hereditary cancer. Additionally, triple negative breast cancers are associated with genetic mutations; therefore, a HER2 positive breast cancer would be of average risk, making Choice *C* incorrect.

100. A: Syndrome of Inappropriate Antidiuretic Hormone Secretion (SIADH) occurs when the body is unable to regulate the amount of antidiuretic hormone, causing water excretion to be impaired. If fluid intake exceeds the amount excreted, the patient would experience hyponatremia. SIADH can be found in 10 to 15% of small cell lung cancer patients. Low sodium concentration can lead to symptoms such as nausea, fatigue, and confusion. Choices *B*, *C*, and *D* are not represented by this scenario.

101. B: Chronic diarrhea can cause a decrease in absorption of oral medications, as motility of the gut is increased, and medications have a lower chance of moving through the lining of the GI tract. Choices *A, C,* and *D* are all risks associated with chronic diarrhea and should be addressed by the nurse during their evaluation.

102. D: Choice *D* is correct because the most common first-line treatment for early-stage colon cancer is colon resection surgery to remove the tumor. This is sometimes followed by chemotherapy. Choice *A* is incorrect because a small bowel resection is not a treatment for colon cancer. Choices *B* and *C* are not correct, as these are not first-line treatments in early-stage colon cancer.

103. D: If a patient becomes apneic and oxygenation drops off during a spontaneous breathing trial, it is a sign that the patient should be placed back on mechanical ventilation, as they are not ready to breathe on their own. Increasing the sedation will worsen the patient's breathing function. Continuing the breathing trial will lead to organ damage due to lack of oxygenation and perfusion. An antidote is not appropriate in this scenario.

104. B: Choice *B* is the best action by the nurse because all of the patient's concerns should be addressed before discharge, especially if outpatient treatments may be delayed due to financial concerns. The patient's case manager can assist with transportation arrangements or community resources. Choice *A* is not the best action because calling the provider to delay the appointments will hinder the patient's treatment. Choice *C* is not the best action because documenting the patient's statement in the medical record should occur after all interventions are performed and all of the patient's concerns are addressed. Choice *D* is not the best action because the patient should be asked to sign the discharge paperwork after all of the patient's concerns are addressed and all instructions are understood by the patient.

105. D: The patient should be repositioned frequently to avoid or aid in healing pressure injuries. Choice *A* is incorrect; putting extra blankets under the patient can create new pressure areas. It is better to use pillows under the patient, alternating right and left every two hours. Choice *B* is incorrect, as pressure areas and pressure injuries should not be massaged since this can increase the incidence of pressure injuries. Choice *C* is also incorrect, as shoes can create new pressure areas and do not protect the feet from pressure injuries.

106. D: The purpose of biotherapies is to prevent or slow the growth and proliferation of cancer cells. Choice *A* is incorrect because this is typical of chemotherapy and cytotoxic treatment. Choices *B* and *C* are incorrect because these items are not the goal of biotherapy treatment.

107. A: Metastatic melanoma is commonly associated with brain metastasis. The brain is a less common metastatic location in prostate, bladder, and stomach cancers, making Choices *B, C,* and *D* incorrect.

108. D: A PET scan is not involved in the planning of radiation. Choices *A*, *B*, and *C* are all part of treatment planning and simulation.

109. B: The patient's priority should be to maintain a safe environment to avoid falls and accidents that could result in further bone damage. Choice *A* is incorrect, as the patient should not take any supplements without first discussing it with their physician. Choice *C* is incorrect, as pain control will not prevent further pathological fractures. Choice *D* is also incorrect, as weight-bearing exercise can help to build muscle but will not prevent pathological fractures.

110. C: This patient is presenting with Beck's Triad: hypotension, jugular vein distension, and muffled heart sounds. Beck's Triad is a classic physical finding in cardiac tamponade. Choices *A*, *B*, and *D* are incorrect.

111. B: Using the WHO pain ladder, the second step includes a mild opioid, with or without a non-opioid and with or without an adjuvant medication. The medications listed in Choice *B* follow step two in the WHO ladder appropriately. Choice *A* is incorrect, as opioids for severe pain are the third step in WHO's pain ladder. Choice *C* is incorrect, as two non-opioids and an adjuvant medication does not correctly move up the ladder to treat the patient's continued pain. Choice *D* is also incorrect because it skips the second step on the WHO ladder and contains two adjuvant medications.

112. B: Choice *B* is correct because PICCs are more likely to develop infections than implanted ports. Choices *A*, *C*, and *D* are incorrect, as they are all advantages of a PICC line.

113. B: Cancer rehabilitation services are used to identify impairments caused by cancer history or treatment and to develop a plan that promotes health and reduces the severity of actual or potential impairments. Their services can include pain control; however, the main purpose is not to wean patients off of narcotics, making Choice *A* incorrect. Cancer rehabilitation works in tandem with the patient's primary oncology team, especially during the active surveillance period, making Choice *C* incorrect. While the rehabilitation plan often utilizes physical therapy, it is not solely a physical therapy service, making Choice *D* incorrect.

114. A: Choice *A* is the best response by the nurse because the patient's statement is indicative of anxiety related to their diagnosis. The question encourages open dialogue and therapeutic communication. Choice *B* is not the best response by the nurse because the patient's symptoms describe anxiety, not depression. Choice *C* is not the best response by the nurse because the question does not address the patient's underlying concern. Choice *D* is not the best response by the nurse because the question negatively supports the patient's concern with death.

115. A: Bladder training helps reduce incontinence and includes routine voiding, practicing suppression of the urge to urinate, Kegel exercises, and decreasing fluid intake in the evening. Choice *B* is incorrect; wearing briefs or pads assists in preventing accidents or leaks but does not reduce the frequency of incontinence. Choice *C* is incorrect, as the patient should be advised to avoid caffeine and other bladder irritants. Choice *D* is also incorrect. Using a straight catheter should not be a routine practice for incontinence because it can lead to infection.

116. C: Alkylating agents disrupt the DNA strand, causing them to be unable to replicate. Choice *A* is incorrect; antimetabolites incorporate into the DNA chain and inhibit repair. Choice *B* is incorrect; inhibiting DNA and RNA synthesis is true of antitumor antibiotics. Choice *D* is incorrect; plant alkaloids (vinca alkaloids) block DNA replication and prevent cell division.

117. A: Radiation to the chest as a child, adolescent, or young adult (before 30 years of age) increases the risk of a subsequent breast cancer diagnosis. The patient should receive annual breast imaging beginning at 25 years of age. Annual skin examinations should be completed to assess for skin cancers, making Choice *B* incorrect. Childhood radiation does not necessitate regular lung cancer screening, so Choice *C* is incorrect. This patient had radiation to the chest; therefore, they would be at normal risk for colorectal cancer and should follow normal screening practices, making Choice *D* incorrect.

118. A: Virchow's triad identifies factors that contribute to the thrombotic process associated with deep venous thrombosis (DVT) and pulmonary embolism (PE). The triad consists of hypercoagulability, endothelial injury/dysfunction, and hemodynamic changes such as stasis and turbulence. Heart disease is a risk factor for DVT and PE, but it is not part of Virchow's triad.

119. D: CPIs can cause T-cells to attack healthy cells as well as cancer cells. The targeted proteins that cancer cells use to avoid immune response are also used by healthy cells. Choices *A* and *C* are incorrect because CPIs do not cause an overactive immune system or a dysregulated immune system. Choice *B* is incorrect because CPIs themselves are not toxic.

120. C: Evidence-based practice relies on up-to-date research and knowledge rather than traditional methods, advice from colleagues, and personal beliefs to provide holistic, high-quality care. Choice *C* utilizes pharmacologic data to administer antiemetics on a schedule where they will be most effective. Choice *A* utilizes advice from colleagues rather than evidence. Choice *B* perpetuates a common myth surrounding chemotherapy-induced nausea and vomiting. While ginger has often been used to treat nausea and vomiting, the effectiveness has not been proven and should be used in a complementary fashion per patient preference, making Choice *D* incorrect.

121. A: Diarrhea after 5FU is due to mucositis of the gastrointestinal tract (GIM). Loperamide can reduce the number of occurrences or eliminate diarrhea, so the patient should be instructed about its use. It is important to stop the diarrhea to prevent further complications, such as dehydration. Choice *B* is incorrect. The patient should notify the oncologist, not go to the emergency department, if loperamide is not effective after twenty-four hours of use (maximum dose 16 mg per day). Choice *C* is incorrect. The priority is to reduce or eliminate the diarrhea to prevent further complications, not just to treat the resulting symptoms of diarrhea, including skin breakdown. Choice *D* is also incorrect. The patient should be educated on avoiding fatty foods and fruit juices, which can increase the incidence of diarrhea.

122. A: At the end of life, secretions often build up in the airway as the patient becomes too weak to clear them. This creates an audible noise often referred to as a "death rattle." This is not thought to be concerning to the patient, although it can cause distress to those caring for the patient. Choice *B* is incorrect because positioning a patient on their side can assist in mobilizing the secretions from the airway. IV fluids and enteral feedings should be stopped to decrease secretions; therefore, Choice *C* is incorrect. A fan blowing across the face can be helpful for breathing; however, movement of air is unlikely to have an impact on the secretions as they are typically deeper in the airway, making Choice *D* incorrect.

123: B: The nurse should administer hyaluronidase and apply local heat for twenty minutes four times daily for one or two days. Although the IV should be removed, this should occur after administration of hyaluronidase, making Choice *A* incorrect. Cold should not be used in cases of extravasation of vinca alkaloids because it can cause further tissue damage, making Choice *C* incorrect. Dexrazoxane is not the correct medication to administer, making Choice D incorrect.

124. A: Maintaining a routine, reducing sensory deficits, and having adequate sleep can help prevent delirium. Choice *B* is incorrect, as putting patients in restraints can worsen delirium. Choice *C* is also incorrect since stimulation should be kept to a minimum. Choice *D* is incorrect. Adequate lighting should be provided during the daytime; however, the patient should have the lights out and be allowed to sleep. Reassuring the patient every two hours will not allow the patient to have adequate sleep.

125. A: Employers cannot ask if an applicant is disabled, the type or severity of the disability, if they have ever had cancer or a past illness, or what type of medicines they take when applying for a job. They *can* ask about the ability to perform a job or task. Choices *B, C,* and *D* are correct statements about the ADA.

126. D: A disposable gown made of a low-permeability fabric, such as polyethylene-coated material, should be worn to prevent transfer of chemotherapy agents onto clothes and skin. Two pairs of disposable gloves that have been tested for use with hazardous drugs should be used for administration, making Choice *A* incorrect. A NIOSH-approved respirator is not necessary for administration but should be used in scenarios where inhalation is possible, such as a spill, making Choice *B* incorrect. Surgical booties are not necessary for administration, making Choice *C* incorrect.

127. A: Palliative surgery improves comfort when cancer is not curable. Palliative surgery can include debulking, decompression, or diversion around tumors. Choice *B* is restorative plastic surgery that improves the appearance of a defect caused by cancer or other surgeries for cancer. Choice *C* is done only when curative measures are possible. Choice *D* is incorrect because preventative surgery is performed in cases when patients have genetic causes of cancer, such as BRCA genes.

128. B: After a deep vein thrombosis is identified, the patient will begin receiving low molecular weight heparin subcutaneously. Unfractionated heparin may also be used in addition to aspirin or other anticoagulants. Choice *A* is incorrect; placing sequential compression devices on a leg with a DVT results in a risk of dislodging the clot, which can then travel through the body and cause a pulmonary embolism (PE). Choice *C* is incorrect. An IVC filter is placed for hypercoagulable patients in order to prevent a DVT from traveling to the lungs and causing a PE; it will not prevent new DVTs from forming. Choice *D* is incorrect. While walking and exercise are good interventions to prevent DVTs from forming, walking and frequent exercise can dislodge an existing DVT and could result in a PE.

129. C: Spinal cord compression is an oncological emergency in which the tumor invades or puts pressure on the epidural space. The nurse must first assess for decreased sensation and strength, then notify the doctor of the new symptoms and administer pain medication, making Choices *A* and *D* incorrect. Teaching the patient about stretching and strengthening exercises is not the correct next step in this scenario, making Choice *B* incorrect.

130. A: Unlike targeted therapy, chemotherapy is cytotoxic because it causes cell death and damages different types of cells. Choices *B, C,* and *D* are incorrect because they are all ways in which targeted therapy functions. Targeted therapy is cytostatic (does not kill cells), specific to certain cells, and works on molecular targets.

131. B: Chemotherapy treatment for testicular cancer typically includes cisplatin and etoposide, which are linked to leukemia. The risk increases if the patient is also treated with radiation. Melanoma is an uncommon secondary malignancy in this scenario, making Choice *A* incorrect. Prostate and rectal cancers are linked to radiation treatment, not chemotherapy, making Choices *C* and *D* incorrect.

132. D: Choice *D* is the best response by the nurse because the action encourages the patient to speak about activities that make them feel independent and promotes personal control. Choice *A* is not the best action by the nurse because providing a list of assistive devices further discourages the patient from feeling independent with their activities. Choice *B* is not the best action by the nurse because there is no indication that the patient is not content or safe with their current caregiver. Choice *C* is not the best action by the nurse because there is no indication that the patient needs re-education on the topic. The patient's main concern is loss of independence.

133. A: It is normal for people to have decreased appetite and thirst as they progress through the dying process. Food is a sensitive topic, and it is often distressing for the family to see their loved one not eating or drinking. While providing their favorite meals may encourage them to eat, it is often emotionally distressing for the patient if they cannot meet their loved ones' expectations and physically distressing if they are not digesting normally. For these reasons, Choice *C* is incorrect. Interventions such as feeding tubes and IV hydration can lead to complications that increase physical suffering without prolonging life. Choices *B* and *D* are incorrect for this reason. It is important for nurses to educate family members on the dying process and its effect on nutritional status.

134. C: Pre-medications should be given with enough time to take effect prior to the chemotherapy infusion to prevent hypersensitivity reactions. This is typically at least 30 minutes prior, and it is important that new staff being certified in chemotherapy administration understand the role of pre-medications. Choices *A, B,* and *D* are correct statements about hypersensitivity reactions.

135. B: Biotherapy is not always appropriate for all types of cancer, and the benefits can vary from patient to patient, depending upon their cancer's characteristics. Choices *A, C,* and *D* are all benefits of using biotherapy over chemotherapy.

136. C: Small-bowel obstruction is associated with severe fluid and electrolyte losses. The normal serum sodium level is 135 to 145 mEq/L; therefore, Choice *C* is indicative of deficient serum sodium and severe alterations in fluid balance. Small-bowel obstruction is manifested by metabolic alkalosis due to the loss of acids with vomiting. Choice *A* is consistent with metabolic acidosis, not alkalosis, and is therefore incorrect. As noted, small-bowel obstruction is associated with fluid volume deficits; however, the reported serum osmolality of 285 mOsm/kg is within the normal range for serum osmolality (275–295 mOsm/kg); therefore, Choice *B* is incorrect. Abdominal distention in large-bowel obstruction most commonly occurs in the lower abdomen, while abdominal distention in the small bowel most commonly occurs in the epigastric or upper abdominal area; therefore, Choice *D* is incorrect.

137. C: Some herbal supplements can interfere with chemotherapy or biotherapy. It is important for patients to discuss their use of these products so any interactions can be prevented. Choice *A* is incorrect. Although dance therapy does take energy, it also lifts the spirits of those who enjoy it. Choice *B* is also incorrect, as acupuncture has been shown to aid in lymphatic drainage. Choice *D* is incorrect, as massage is not a risk for cancer patients with neuropathy.

138. A: The first priority for a patient who may have sepsis is to collect blood cultures followed by antibiotic administration. While IV fluids and vasopressors may be appropriate, blood cultures should be the primary intervention to determine the cause of the infection and which targeted antibiotics might be necessary. Therefore, Choices *B, C,* and *D* are incorrect first steps.

139. C: Molecular tumor profiling is used to evaluate whether the tumor is expressing biomarkers for which there are known effective targeted therapies. It is not useful for determining response to chemotherapies, as chemotherapy acts on cells at various stages of division, making Choice *A* incorrect. Choice *B* is incorrect, as molecular testing is not used to test exclusively for germline (hereditary) variants. Some variants are both germline (hereditary) and somatic (acquired). When these are present, further testing may be required to determine the source of the variant. Choice *D* is incorrect since molecular testing cannot predict side effects of treatments.

140. D: Sensitivity in screening tests is necessary and indicates the ability of a test to detect disease—in other words, the test should be able to provide a true positive result. However, Choice *A* indicates specificity, making it incorrect. Choice *B* is incorrect because screening should be conducted to identify important health problems, especially those with treatments that are more effective at early stages. Choice *C* is incorrect because testing should be readily available and inexpensive.

141. A: Choice *A* is the best response by the nurse because the statement encourages the patient to speak openly about their feelings and supports therapeutic communication. Choice *B* is not the best response by the nurse because the statement provides false reassurance to the patient. Urostomies are permanent after a complete bladder resection. Choice *C* is not the best response by the nurse because the statement focuses on the nurse's experience, not the patient's concern. Choice *D* is not the best response by the nurse because the statement ignores the patient's main concern regarding their body image.

142. A: Taxol and other taxanes interfere with microtubules, inhibiting mitosis and cell division. Choice *B* is incorrect, as this describes antitumor antibiotics. Choice *C* is not a result of taxanes. Choice *D* is also incorrect, as this is not a result of taxanes but of antimetabolites.

143. D: It is important to administer the medication to reduce the fever for the patient's comfort. Choices *A* and *B* are incorrect, as this can cause rapid cooling resulting in increased chills. The chills could cause the body to warm, and fever could recur. Choice *C* is also incorrect. While this intervention is important after a fever, it will not help to reduce the fever.

144. D: The teach-back method is the evidence-based standard tool used to assess patient comprehension when providing patient education. Closed-ended questions limit responses to single-word answers. While closed-ended questions have their place in conversations, asking open-ended questions can lead to a better understanding of a patient's thoughts and comprehension, thereby making Choice *A* incorrect. It is best to assess a patient's needs and offer the media modality that best matches those needs. While this may often be written information, it can also include videos, demonstrations, or explanations, making Choice *B* incorrect. While referring to data may be helpful in some instances, it is often too technical for patients to understand, and health literacy should be assessed first. Therefore, Choice *C* is not a correct technique.

145. C: Hemodialysis is used for patients with chronic kidney disease that may not be able to receive a kidney transplant. The kidneys of these patients are unable to filter waste through their kidneys. In hemodialysis, blood is removed from the patient, filtered through what is called a dialysis membrane, and returned to the patient. Due to the large amount of blood that is out of the body at one time, it is important to make sure that blood pressures are assessed throughout the dialysis process to ensure that the patient does not experience hypotension or disequilibrium syndrome. Although monitoring respiratory status may be important in other areas of nursing, it is not a priority in dialysis care, making Choice *A* incorrect. Patients who are undergoing dialysis should avoid foods with high potassium, sodium, and phosphor levels because dialysis alters the electrolyte levels within the blood. High levels of these electrolytes can potentially become dangerous, making Choice *B* incorrect. Choice *D* is also incorrect because kidney transplants may not be an option for many patients—the nurse should not discuss this with the patient at this time.

146. D: Fractionation refers to the total dose given over a certain time frame and determines the frequency of the patient's visits. Choice *A* is incorrect, as that is the sum of the fractionation. Choice *B* is incorrect because dosimetry refers to all measurements involving the total dose. Choice *C* is incorrect, as this does not explain the frequency of visits.

147. D: Curative treatment is not included in palliative care. Palliative care can begin when a life-threatening or life-limiting illness, such as cancer, is diagnosed. Choice *A* is incorrect because surgery can be used to reduce symptoms and increase quality of life. Choices *B* and *C* are also incorrect, as chemotherapy and radiation can be used to reduce tumor burden to increase quality of life.

148. A: Spinal cord compression symptoms include changes in urinary function, weakness, and changes in sensation of the lower extremities. Choices *B*, *C*, and *D* are not represented by the scenario.

149. A: The most important intervention for the patient to use is effective hand washing techniques to prevent infection. Choice *B* is incorrect, as the patient does not need to wear a mask at all times; however, they should avoid crowds and wear a mask if they will be around potentially ill people. Choice *C* is incorrect. The patient does not need to limit all visitors, but they should limit visitation of anyone who is sick, especially children. Choice *D* is also incorrect. Neutropenic patients do not need to bathe twice a day; instead, they should bathe at least once a day and follow good personal hygiene practices.

150. D: Supporting the patient during marrow aplasia can last from ten to thirty days. This time is used to lessen complications that may arise, such as graft-versus-host disease or sinusoidal obstructive disease. Choices *A* and *B* are incorrect because these procedures would happen prior to the bone marrow transplant. Choice *C* is incorrect; while avoiding infection is important, the patient is not kept to prevent visitors. Visitors will be required to follow isolation precautions.

151. B: Choice *B* is the best response by the nurse because the patient is experiencing symptoms of grief after the loss of their child. It is important for the nurse to explore the patient's coping skills to assess the need for further interventions. Choice *A* is not the best response by the nurse because the patient's coping mechanisms should be assessed prior to suggesting medical treatment. Choice *C* is not the best response by the nurse because the statement is insensitive to the patient's individual experience. Choice *D* is not the best response by the nurse because asking about loss of employment ignores the main concern of processing grief.

152. D: Choice *D* is correct because the nomenclature of naming monoclonal antibodies is as follows: prefix + substem 1 target location + substem 2 monoclonal antibody derivation + stem. The substem "tu" within trastuzumab indicates that the target is located on the tumor. Choice *A* is incorrect because the substem "ci" indicates a circulatory target. Choice *B* is incorrect because the pulmonary system is not included as a target in the nomenclature. Choice *C* is also incorrect; the substem "li" indicates a target located on the immune system.

153. D: Phase I trials are first in human therapies and are used to determine optimal dosing for safety and tolerance. Choice *A* refers to phase 3 trials. Choice *B* best describes phase 4 trials. Choice *C* refers to phase 2 trials.

154. B: Mesna is administered before high doses of cyclophosphamide and for multiple doses after to inhibit the hemorrhagic cystitis caused by cyclophosphamide. Adequate hydration during treatment and for twenty-four hours post-treatment is important to ensure sufficient dilatation of the drug in the urinary system to prevent toxicity, making Choice *A* incorrect. An EKG is not required for treatment with cyclophosphamide, making Choice *C* incorrect. While nausea may be a side effect of cyclophosphamide for which ondansetron can be helpful, administration of Mesna is the priority order. Therefore, Choice *D* is incorrect.

155. C: Since chemotherapy may affect the bone marrow, the patient receiving chemotherapy may have low red blood cell, white blood cell, and platelet counts. This patient has a low neutrophil count, which means the patient does not have enough white blood cells in her body. Since white blood cells help the body fight infection, the patient is at risk for infection and should avoid being in crowds, especially during influenza season. Choice *A* is not correct; using a safety razor reduces the risk of bleeding due to a low platelet count. Choice *B* is not correct; iron supplements help in the production of red blood cells, not white blood cells. Although the patient may benefit from drinking fluids, this instruction will not reduce the risk of infection.

156. A: Petechiae are pinpoint red or purple hemorrhagic spots on the skin that indicate microvascular bleeding. This indicates to the nurse that the patient may be experiencing disseminated intravascular coagulation (DIC), a systemic syndrome characterized by excessive clotting and bleeding. The clotting cascade of DIC is characterized by low platelet (thus the order for the CBC) and fibrinogen levels as well as prolonged PT, PTT, and thrombin times. Therefore, Choices *B*, *C*, and *D* do not represent the correct laboratory orders.

157. B: POLST forms are medical orders that specify preferences for CPR and medical interventions, such as intubation, ventilation, artificial nutrition, and hospitalization. They are portable, making them valid in settings across the care continuum, including inpatient, outpatient, residential care facilities, and at home. Unlike advance directives or living wills, a POLST is not a legal document; rather, it is a complement to a will that should be used when patients are seriously ill. Choices *A, C,* and *D* are accurate statements.

158. D: A culture of safety indicates that safety is an explicit organizational goal; as a result, processes that build trust and accountability through all levels of professional collaboration have been established. Key factors include confidential and nonpunitive investigations into errors, frequent training and reassessment of processes, evaluating errors and near misses in a timely manner, and clear policies and procedures to support safe care. Therefore, Choices *A, B,* and *C* are incorrect.

159. B: Since radiation to the head and neck impacts the jawbone, salivary glands, and teeth, it is important to have good dental hygiene and regular dental check-ups before, during, and continuously after radiation treatment. Radiation to the tonsils can impact surrounding tissues, including the jawbone, but radiation is unlikely to impact eyesight; therefore, Choices *A* and *C* incorrect. While continuing oral hygiene after treatment is important, the use of saltwater rinses is recommended for treatment of mucositis and is unnecessary to continue after treatment has ended.

160. B: Choice *B* is the best intervention by the nurse because patient navigators help patients navigate through the health system and provide unbiased guidance for obtaining the care they need. Choice *A* is not the best intervention by the nurse; while community groups help the patient feel supported, these groups are not the best option to help guide the patient medically. Choice *C* is not the best intervention by the nurse because the patient has not voiced being undecided about receiving treatment. Choice *D* is not the best intervention by the nurse because the statement does not address the patient's concern, and explaining treatment options is not within the scope of the nurse's job.

161. D: Lorazepam is effective for treating agitation and can also treat nausea. The nurse should counsel the family that it may cause drowsiness. Choice *A* would be used for pain and fevers. Choice *B* would be used to help manage secretions and noisy breathing. Choice *C* can be used for pain and air hunger.

162. A: Antivirals are not part of the immune system that are used in immunotherapy. Choices *B, C,* and *D* are all used in direct immune-mediated targeting of tumors.

163. A: Tobacco use is the single most preventable cause of disease and death within the United States and is linked with an increased risk of many cancers, such as lung, larynx, esophagus, stomach, liver, pancreas, bladder, and kidney. Choice *B* is incorrect because there is no correlation between vegetables and breast cancer, although consumption of vegetables decreases the risks of other cancers. Choice *C* is incorrect because steel workers are at a higher risk for lung cancers, not prostate cancers. Choice *D* is incorrect because alcohol has not been linked to kidney cancer but to mouth, pharynx, larynx, esophagus, liver, colorectum, pancreas, stomach, and breast cancers.

164. C: The axial skeleton (spine, ribs, pelvis) is a common site of early metastasis. As with most cancers, sarcoma has a poor prognosis if there are metastases. If the metastatic site is distant from the primary site, this is an aggressive tumor, as it has quickly spread to other sites. The brain is not considered to be a common metastatic site for sarcoma. Therefore, Choices *A, B,* and *D* are incorrect.

165. C: Choice *C* is the best intervention by the nurse because local service organizations can provide the patient with options for financial assistance, such as grants, aids, or fundraisers. Choice *A* is not the best intervention by the nurse because the patient did not voice a misunderstanding of the provider's instructions. Choice *B* is not the best intervention by the nurse because the patient's statements do not suggest that they are refusing treatment. Choice *D* is not the best intervention by the nurse because calling the patient's spouse violates the patient's privacy and does not promote patient advocacy.

OCN Practice Tests #3 - #25

To keep the size of this book manageable, save paper, and provide a digital test-taking experience, the 3rd – 25th practice tests can be found online. Scan the QR code or go to this link to access it:

testprepbooks.com/online387/ocn

SCAN ME

The first time you access the tests, you will need to register as a "new user" and verify your email address.

If you have any issues, please email support@testprepbooks.com.

Dear OCN Test Taker,

Thank you for purchasing this study guide for your OCN exam. We hope that we exceeded your expectations.

Our goal in creating this study guide was to cover all of the topics that you will see on the test. We also strove to make our practice questions as similar as possible to what you will encounter on test day. With that being said, if you found something that you feel was not up to your standards, please send us an email and let us know.

We would also like to let you know about other books in our catalog that may interest you.

Medical Surgical Nurse

This can be found on Amazon: amazon.com/dp/1637754647

CEN

amazon.com/dp/1637757891

CNOR

amazon.com/dp/1637753004

We have study guides in a wide variety of fields. If the one you are looking for isn't listed above, then try searching for it on Amazon or send us an email.

Thanks Again and Happy Testing!
Product Development Team
support@testprepbooks.com

Online Resources

Included with your purchase are multiple online resources. This includes the practice tests in an interactive format and a convenient study timer to help you manage your time.

Scan the QR code or go to this link to access this content:

testprepbooks.com/online387/ocn

SCAN ME

The first time you access the page, you will need to register as a "new user" and verify your email address.

you have any issues, please email support@testprepbooks.com.

nk you for letting us be a part of your studying journey!

Printed in Dunstable, United Kingdom

91220105R00125